Youth Drinking Cultures in a Digital World

Social media has helped boost the culture of intoxication, a central aspect of young people's social lives in many Western countries. Initial research suggests that these technologies enable highly nuanced, targeted marketing and innovations – creating new virtual spaces that alter the dynamics and consequences of drinking cultures in significant ways.

Youth Drinking Cultures in a Digital World focuses on how pervasive social networking technologies contribute to drinking cultures. It brings together international contributions from leading researchers in this emerging field to explore how new technologies are reconfiguring the key themes, traditional interests, practices and concerns of alcohol-related research with young people. It is particularly concerned with three important areas, namely:

*   identities, social relations and power
*   alcohol marketing and commercialisation
*   public health and regulating alcohol promotion.

This innovative book includes original research and commentary and is a must-read for academics and researchers in the areas of public health, psychology, sociology, media studies, youth studies and alcohol studies.

Antonia C. Lyons is Professor of Psychology at Massey University, New Zealand.

Tim McCreanor is an Associate Professor and senior researcher at Social and Health Outcomes Research and Evaluation (SHORE) and Whāriki Research Centre, College of Health, Massey University, New Zealand.

Ian Goodwin is a Senior Lecturer in the School of English and Media Studies at Massey University, New Zealand.

Helen Moewaka Barnes (Te Kapotai, Ngaphui-nui-tonu) is a Professor, the Director of Whāriki and Co-director of the Social and Health Outcomes Research and Evaluation (SHORE) and Whāriki Research Centre, at the College of Health, Massey University, New Zealand.

Routledge Studies in Public Health

Youth Drinking Cultures in a Digital World

Alcohol, social media and cultures of intoxication

Edited by Antonia C. Lyons, Tim McCreanor, Ian Goodwin and Helen Moewaka Barnes

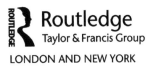

Routledge
Taylor & Francis Group
LONDON AND NEW YORK

First published 2017
by Routledge

2 Park Square, Milton Park, Abingdon, Oxfordshire OX14 4RN
52 Vanderbilt Avenue, New York, NY 10017

Routledge is an imprint of the Taylor & Francis Group, an informa business

First issued in paperback 2019

British Library Cataloguing-in-Publication Data
A catalogue record for this book is available from the British Library

Library of Congress Cataloging in Publication Data
Names: Lyons, Antonia C., author. | McCreanor, Tim, author. | Goodwin,
Ian, author. | Moewaka Barnes, Helen, author.
Title: Youth drinking cultures in a digital world : alcohol, social media and
cultures of intoxication / Antonia Lyons, Tim McCreanor, Ian Goodwin,
Helen Moewaka Barnes.
Other titles: Routledge studies in public health.
Description: Abingdon, Oxon ; New York, NY : Routledge, 2017. | Series:
Routledge studies in public health | Includes bibliographical references and
index.
Identifiers: LCCN 2016035268| ISBN 9781138959040 (hardback) | ISBN
9781315660844 (ebook)
Subjects: | MESH: Alcohol Drinking--psychology | Alcohol Drinking--
prevention & control | Adolescent | Social Marketing--ethics | Social
Media--ethics | Social Media--legislation & jurisprudence
Classification: LCC HV5135 | NLM WM 274 | DDC 362.292--dc23
LC record available at https://lccn.loc.gov/2016035268

ISBN: 978-1-138-95904-0 (hbk)
ISBN: 978-0-367-22410-3 (pbk)

Typeset in Times New Roman
by Saxon Graphics Ltd, Derby

Contents

Contributors

Lin Bailey is a Senior Lecturer in Psychology at Southampton Solent University in the UK. Her research interests include new forms of gendered and classed social inequalities, consumption and subjectivities with a particular interest in young people's drinking cultures. In conjunction with the local authority in Southampton and with the involvement of local charities for young people and colleges, she is currently supervising a PhD exploring drinking cultures of young people aged 16 to 18 years old from a diverse range of social locations.

Nicholas Carah is a Senior Lecturer in Media and Communication at the School of Communication and Arts, University of Queensland. His work examines media technologies, alcohol consumption and promotion, and everyday culture.

Hélène Cherrier is currently Associate Professor at RMIT, Australia. Her research interests focus on bringing about a more sustainable and just society and involve changes in consumption lifestyles, social and environmental activism, practices of re-use and re-purposing, and issues at the nexus of marketing and sustainability, social justice and well-being. She has published her work in high-quality refereed academic journals including the *Journal of Business Research*, the *European Journal of Marketing* and the *Journal of Public Policy and Marketing*.

Ian Goodwin is a Senior Lecturer in the School of English and Media Studies, Massey University Wellington. With a background in cultural studies Ian's research is wide ranging and often inter-disciplinary, yet centres on understanding the societal changes associated with the rise of 'new' media technologies. He is interested in exploring intersections between contemporary media forms, identity politics, popular culture, activism, citizenship, media policy, consumption, health and well-being, and space/place.

Brendan Gough is a Critical Social Psychologist and Qualitative Researcher interested in men and masculinities. Now based at Leeds Beckett University, he has published many papers on gender identities and relations, mostly in the context of health, lifestyles and well-being. He is co-founder and co-editor of the journal *Qualitative Research in Psychology*; he edits the Critical Psychology section of the journal *Social & Personality Psychology Compass*, and is associate editor for the journal *Psychology of Men and Masculinity*. He has co-authored/edited three books in the areas of critical social psychology (with McFadden, McDonald), reflexivity in qualitative research (with Finlay), and men's health (with Robertson).

Christine Griffin (PhD University of Birmingham, UK) is Professor of Social Psychology at the University of Bath. She is a member of the UK Centre for Tobacco and Alcohol Studies funded by the UK Clinical Research Collaboration. She has a long-standing interest in young people's experiences, as shaped by gender, class, race and sexuality, and the relationship between identity and consumer culture. She was a founding member of the editorial group that launched the international journal *Feminism and Psychology* in 1991. She is currently investigating alcohol marketing to young people via social media funded by Alcohol Research UK.

Derek Heim is a Professor of Psychology at Edge Hill University. Utilising quantitative and qualitative research methods, his work focuses on social, cultural and contextual influences on substance use, health and well-being. He is editor-in-chief of *Addiction Research and Theory*, the leading outlet for research and theoretical contributions that view addictive behaviour as arising from psychological processes within the individual and the social context in which the behaviour takes place as much as from the biological effects of the psychoactive substance or activity involved.

Jo Lindsay is Associate Professor of Sociology in the School of Social Sciences at Monash University. She specialises in the sociology of families, consumption and the environment. Over-consumption is a central theme of her research and she has conducted several studies on the social dynamics of youth drinking. Books include *Consuming families: Buying, making, producing family life in the 21st century* with JaneMaree Maher and *Families, relationships and intimate life* with Deb Dempsey.

Antonia Lyons is Professor of Psychology at Massey University, Wellington, New Zealand. Her research focuses on the social and cultural contexts of behaviours related to health and their implications for gendered identities and embodied subjectivities. Antonia is a co-editor of the journal *Qualitative Research in Psychology* and an associate editor of *Health Psychology Review* and *Psychology and Health*.

Sarah Mart is a public health advocate, researcher, writer, and director. She has directed research and policy analysis, programs, and publications on topics including pinkwashed alcohol products, industry domination of alcohol regulator groups, "drink responsibly" messaging, and alcohol promotion in social media. Her peer-reviewed journal publications include articles in *Addiction, Substance Use* and the *Journal for Global Drug Policy and Practice*. She also presents and facilitates around public health, policy and social justice for international, national, state and community audiences.

Tim McCreanor is an Associate Professor and senior researcher at SHORE and Whāriki Research Centre, College of Health, Massey University. His broad public health orientation and interest in the social determinants of health and well-being provide a platform for social science projects that support and stimulate social change. Discourse analysis and action research methods have been a key approach to studies of racial discrimination, youth well-being, alcohol marketing, media representations and social cohesion.

Carla Meurk is a postdoctoral research fellow at the University of Queensland where she co-leads the Policy and Research Translation Group at the Queensland Centre for Mental Health Research. Her research spans mental health and addiction and is focused on the prospective evaluation of innovations and new technologies; consumer research and co-design; implementation planning; policy analysis; and the development of research methods to understand and improve health policy.

Nina Michaelidou is a Reader in Marketing at Loughborough University, UK. Her research interests lie in the area of consumer behaviour and include personality traits, perceptions and attitudes, image and emotions. She is the Chair of the Academy of Marketing Special Interest Group on Consumer Psychology and Cross-Cultural Research and has published papers in various journals including *European Journal of Marketing*, *Journal of Business Research* and the *International Marketing Review*.

Helen Moewaka Barnes (Te Kapotai, Ngaphui-nui-tonu) is a Professor, the Director of Whāriki and Co-director of the SHORE and Whāriki Research Centre, College of Health, Massey University. Her research areas include natural environments and health, life-course approaches to health and well-being, health promotion, health services research, identity culture and nationhood, sexuality, parent and child health, growing Māori and Pacific research capacity and research use; developing methods and methodologies within Māori paradigms and evaluation research.

Rebecca Monk works as a Senior Lecturer in Psychology at Edge Hill University in the UK. Her main research interests relate to social health psychology and her work investigates the various ways in which social and environmental contexts shape people's alcohol-related cognitions and behaviours. In addition to using traditional survey and experimental research designs, her methodological repertoire encompasses context aware experience sampling methods hosted on Smartphone applications.

Marjatta Montonen is a Researcher at the National Institute for Health and Welfare in Finland who has a long track record of research around alcohol on television and in the mass media and in particular the portrayal of alcohol on Finnish television. She is currently a senior specialist on the EU-funded multi-country project Joint Action on Reducing Alcohol Related Harm.

Patricia Niland is currently employed as a clinical knowledge translator in the biomedical field, and part-time academic at Massey University, NZ. Her doctoral research was a social constructionist Foucauldian analysis of young adults' friendships in relation to their Facebook and drinking practices. This research provided new knowledge of the complexities and work involved for young adults to do friendship within a technologically mediated social world, and within an entrenched societal drinking culture.

Richard Purves is a Research Fellow in the Institute for Social Marketing at the University of Stirling. He was previously a Research Associate at the Centre for Research in Education, Inclusion and Diversity at Moray House School of Education in Edinburgh. Since joining ISM in 2010 he has worked extensively in the area of alcohol marketing and policy and the impact of commercial marketing on addictive behaviours such as smoking, gambling and online gaming.

Andy Ruddock is a Senior Lecturer in Communications and Media Studies at Monash University in Melbourne. Author of *Youth and Media*, *Investigating Audiences* and *Understanding Audiences*, Andy has published in various anthologies and journals on topics such as school shootings, gaming, pornography, youth and moral panics, media sport, news and media violence, celebrity and political communication.

Lina Samu is a doctoral candidate within SHORE & Whariki Research Group in Auckland. She was born and educated in Aotearoa New Zealand and is a tulafale/alii matai with the title Tuiloma, an orator chief for her village, Sapunaoa in Samoa. Her research works with young adult Pasifika participants and seeks to understand how social media and online tools are being used. She is interested in how social media play out in their social lives, including influences on the ways in which alcohol may be used, as well as the effects on identity formation, family and community life.

Acushla Deanne Sciascia is a Māori academic and researcher with a keen interest in Kaupapa Māori research and studies of cultural impacts on online social communities of Indigenous peoples. Her doctoral research focused on Māori community engagement and interactions in online social media spaces and the impacts on culture, identity and protocols. Acushla plans to extend this research to understand online citizenship and how socially mediated spaces facilitate notions of membership, citizenship and community of Indigenous peoples.

Sian Supski is a Research Fellow in Sociology at Monash University. Her current research includes the sociology of domestic cultures, including domestic water practices, kitchens/food/writing and alcohol in Australia. She has written two books, *A Proper Foundation: A History of the Lotteries Commission of Western Australia* (Black Swan 2009) and *It Was Another Skin: The Kitchen in 1950s Western Australia* (Peter Lang 2007). She is a commissioning editor of the journal *Thesis Eleven: Critical Theory and Historical Sociology*. In 2015 Sian was a Visiting Scholar at the Stellenbosch Institute for Advanced Study, Stellenbosch, South Africa.

Ismo Tuominen is a Ministerial Counsellor and legal affairs expert at the Ministry of Social Affairs and Health in Helsinki, Finland where he is Director of Alcohol Policy.

Acknowledgements

The idea of attempting an edited volume in this domain arose from a seminar among interested researchers invited by Dr James Nicholl to Alcohol Research UK in London, August 2014. The meeting was made up of Scottish and English researchers, all of whom inspired and impressed Tim McCreanor and Ian Goodwin who were visiting from New Zealand on research leave. They were based at the University of Bath with Professor Christine Griffin. James guided and facilitated the meeting in such a manner that by the end of the proceedings we were happy to endorse the notion of a joint project and found ourselves offering to lead it! We offer special thanks therefore to James, for he certainly catalysed and supported the book as it developed.

We wish to thank all the chapter authors for their willingness to work collaboratively, and for their excellent contributions to this volume. The submitted chapters were of exceptional quality and revisions were attended to with despatch so that our editorial roles felt highly constructive and positive. We are very grateful to them for this experience.

We would also like to acknowledge the generous help and assistance provided by Lisa Morice (information specialist) and Jan Sheeran (office manager) at SHORE & Whariki Research Centre, Massey University. Lisa checked and managed referencing issues and Jan assisted with formatting of the text.

Thanks and acknowledgements also go to the School of Psychology and the School of English and Media Studies, Massey University, for their support of Antonia Lyons and Ian Goodwin (respectively) in undertaking this project. Antonia and Ian would also like to say a big thanks to Callum and Esme for their love, patience and distraction as we worked on this book.

We are also indebted to the Marsden Fund of the Royal Society of New Zealand for funding a three-year study in the area of young people, social media and drinking cultures (grant no. MAU0911). This provided for collaboration between the editors, Professor Christine Griffin, Dr Fiona Hutton, and Dr Kerryellen Vroman, as well as for funding three PhD students and research expenses. We would like to acknowledge all the members of this research team for their contributions, hard work and ongoing support.

Antonia, Tim, Ian and Helen

Introduction to youth drinking cultures in a digital world

Antonia C. Lyons, Tim McCreanor, Ian Goodwin and Helen Moewaka Barnes

In many Western countries, drinking cultures are central to young people's social lives. Since the mid-1990s an increasingly globalised, pervasive culture of intoxication has emerged amongst young people driven by deregulation of sale and supply, decreasing prices, wider ranges of products, decreased age of purchase, and increasingly sophisticated marketing of alcohol. These changes have seen increasing levels of consumption among young people across many Western nations, with important variations by gender, class and culture. Simultaneously, personalised, virtual, social media systems have developed and been taken up enthusiastically by young people in particular. These commercial platforms (e.g. Facebook, YouTube) have profoundly changed communications and relationships. But how do the pervasive social networking technologies contribute to contemporary drinking cultures? Do the new virtual spaces (with their associated targeted marketing and commercial innovations) alter the dynamics and consequences of drinking cultures in significant ways? The aim of this book is to bring together contributions from leading researchers in this emerging field, and explore how the new technologies are reconfiguring the key themes, traditional interests, practices and concerns of alcohol-related research with young people. In this introductory chapter we briefly outline the key concepts that form the focus of this edited volume, and consider the range and reach of research exploring this developing area. Different perspectives bring different emphases and sometimes fresh and new lenses through which to view the issues involved. We then describe three important areas that are involved in youth drinking cultures in a digital world, namely 1) identities, social relations and power; 2) alcohol marketing and commercialisation; and 3) public health and regulating alcohol promotion. These form the structure of this edited collection.

Social media are digital technologies that allow people to interact, share and consume online content. They include social networking sites such as Facebook, Twitter, YouTube and Instagram. Facebook is the most commonly used social media site in Western societies, reaching over a billion users in 2014 (Sedghi, 2014). It is a commercial platform that makes vast profits, with its net income in the first quarter of 2016 tripling to US$1.51 billion (Wong and Thielman, 2016). A *Guardian* newspaper article highlighted the value of advertising revenue to Facebook, stating that compared to the same period last year, as of the end of March 2016:

Ad revenue was up by more than half, from $3.3bn to $5.2bn. The company is at the forefront of trends toward greater mobile use and more significant video advertising revenue; monthly active users and daily active users were up in excess of 20% on mobile devices.

(Wong and Thielman, 2016)

The article goes on to note that just under one billion people (989m) check their Facebook site on their smartphones at least once a day (Wong and Thielman, 2016), demonstrating the ongoing shift to using social media on mobile devices.

Social networking is highly popular and almost ubiquitous among teenagers and young adults in Western societies. As social media are increasingly accessed on mobile devices (such as smartphones) they become more fully integrated into young people's everyday lives. Within social media, alcohol content is quite common and most of this content portrays alcohol and drinking in positive ways (see Westgate and Holliday, 2016 for a review). Students at college or university have been found to have particularly high alcohol-related content depicted on their Facebook pages (Ridout, 2016). There are also hundreds of publicly available alcohol-related smartphone apps, most of which promote alcohol use (Moreno and Whitehill, 2016), and a strong pro-alcohol presence has also been found on Twitter (Cavazos-Rehg et al., 2015). Taken together these findings illustrate the high level of alcohol-related content on social media, which contributes to the normalisation of drinking for young adults (Nicholls, 2012).

Westgate and Holliday's (2016) review highlights that research shows inconsistent findings regarding the relationship between *general* social media use and levels of alcohol consumption, but consistent positive associations between *engaging with alcohol content* on social media and alcohol consumption. Posting alcohol-related content on Facebook has also consistently been related to 'alcohol consumption, alcohol-related problems, cravings, and clinical measures of risk for alcoholism' (p. 28). Longitudinal studies show relationships between exposure to drinking content on Facebook and subsequent drinking behaviours. Westgate and Holliday (2016) suggest that these relationships may be due to creating individual and group identities, perceived social norms and direct digital marketing and alcohol promotion on social media sites. Additionally, Alhabash and colleagues (2016) showed that the mere exposure to alcohol messages on social media can affect people's intentions to consume alcohol and engage in alcohol-related behaviours, such experiences priming people to think about alcohol. This is consistent with Ridout's (2016) review of social media and alcohol use among college students, where he concluded that 'it is the sheer quantity of social networking sites' alcohol content (i.e. descriptive norms) that has the most significant effect on a student's own alcohol use' (p. 84). As we discuss below, the reach and volume of digital alcohol marketing messages on social media are of particular concern.

Before turning to the three main sections in the book, we briefly consider research conceptualisations of drinking culture and different disciplinary perspectives on this field. 'Drinking culture' is a major concept in alcohol research, although it is rarely defined. Around the world many policy documents discuss the need to 'change the drinking culture' to reduce the harms associated with alcohol, and the term has also been used increasingly in academic research since the early 2000s (Savic et al., 2016). Savic and colleagues' (2016) recent review of this concept concludes that research on drinking culture tends to focus on the national level, with much less attention paid to cultural groups below this level. They 'encourage a nuanced and multidimensional understanding of drinking cultures' (Savic et al., 2016: 2) and argue that the macro and micro levels of focus are best seen as complementary perspectives. They also note that increasingly we might be seeing a more globalised (and homogenising) drinking culture that is linked to those seen in national contexts. Simultaneously, multicultural societies are diverse and local drinking micro-cultures may vary in patterns of drinking, as well as in the meanings and values attached to drinking practices. These authors argue for the need to examine local situations and 'the meanings and practices associated with alcohol use that are culturally significant' (Savic et al., 2016: 7).

Savic and colleagues (2016) also critically analyse the use of the concept of 'drinking culture' in social research. This provides useful insights into the range of ways in which culture, alcohol and drinking practices have been studied, and the kinds of tensions that exist across different disciplinary perspectives and approaches. They note that fields such as sociology and anthropology have long investigated the role of culture in alcohol consumption. More recently, public health-oriented approaches have turned their attention to cultural aspects of drinking, in an effort to more fully understand consumption in order to better prevent and alleviate health and social problems that stem from alcohol (Savic et al., 2016). As a discipline, public health is concerned with prevention of health problems at the population level by attending to the upstream conditions, the 'causes of causes' (CSDH, 2008). With respect to alcohol policy, this social catchment is complex and contested, reflecting the diverse interests, values, norms, policies and practices that influence consumption. Public health organisations and institutions with responsibility for the health and well-being of the public are involved in efforts to manage consumption, which is most effectively achieved through regulation of the alcohol industry (Babor et al., 2010).

Public health research approaches have been critiqued for a number of reasons. Although their concern has been on upstream factors beyond the level of the individual, their traditional focus on environmental and structural factors 'has been relegated to the background in favour of a focus on the individual (and individual responsibility), behaviour change and unhealthy lifestyles, of which alcohol consumption is seen as a part (Hunt and Barker, 2001)' (Savic et al., 2016: 1). In addition, again arising primarily from their population focus, these approaches have been accused of discounting the pleasures of consumption (Hunt and Barker, 2001; Savic et al., 2016). Public health researchers, however, would argue that there are key reasons for discounting a focus on pleasure in the research, the most obvious of which is that the alcohol industry is deeply involved in promoting the premium enjoyment and excitement of consumption. For the industry, such research may validate their promotion of alcohol and lead to increased population harms; research of this nature has been appropriated to strengthen and advance alcohol sales. Preventable population level harms driven by commercial industries dealing in risky commodities (such as alcohol, tobacco and fast foods) are central to a public health agenda. Problem-focused dimensions of drinking culture are a key focus of public health and public policy, as are ways to identify interventions to minimise harm (Savic et al., 2016) or reduce drinking levels by altering the environments in which alcohol is consumed.

Researchers in other disciplines such as anthropology, sociology and cultural studies have argued for the importance of attending to the meanings, pleasures and contexts of alcohol use, and being aware of the pathologising accounts of intoxication (as risky and harmful) and scientific discourses (Race and Brown, 2016, forthcoming). They also are committed to examining the relation between social and cultural practices around drinking and social structure (Race and Brown, 2016, forthcoming). Tensions arise because, while drinking practices have very real health outcomes, focusing solely on health risks or prevalence misses key aspects of meanings of drinking, and can function to pathologise certain groups in society (Race and Brown, 2016, forthcoming). Such tensions inevitably lead to debates around the appropriate level of analysis and relevant points of focus. For example, by pathologising particular (often marginalised) subgroups in society, such as youth, attention gets turned on them as the 'problem' and these groups are 'othered' and made abject (while the structural contexts of their lives remain under-explored). This type of critical analysis is apparent across some of the chapters in this book, but sits rather uneasily with other chapters where the public health perspective of problematising alcohol consumption to reduce harms is viewed as crucially important. New and alternative perspectives highlight the complexities inherent in the field, the tensions that exist around practical utility and critical dissent and how policy developments are never simple or straightforward (Race and Brown, 2016, forthcoming). It is only with a range of perspectives that we will be able to explore the importance of the multidimensional nature of drinking culture and its meanings at both macro and micro levels (Savic et al., 2016).

Structure of this book

With this broader critical context in mind, the book has three main sections: 1) identities, social relations and power; 2) alcohol marketing and commercialisation; and 3) public health and regulating alcohol promotion. Within this structure, specific chapters consider the ways in which digital cultures and social networking sites are playing a role within micro (local), meso (national) and macro (global) drinking cultures. Contributors draw on social theories and empirical research to explore the ways that social networking systems, with multimodal affordances that incorporate both user-generated digital photos, video, audio and narrative text, as well as similar materials from other (often commercial) sources, have become increasingly central to online drinking cultures. The significance of evolving mobile technologies increasing people's access to virtual spaces (such as smartphones with mobile data platforms and geo-location features) is also considered, alongside their consequences for drinking norms and practices as well as identities, identity performances, and social relationships.

Part I: Identities, social relations and power

Young people are avid users of social media and these play a crucial role in identity construction (Zhao et al., 2008). In our New Zealand-based research, Facebook was central to young adults' social lives and their participation in local drinking cultures. Participants posted photos of drinking events, engaged in online communication and photo-sharing while they were pre-loading (drinking before they went out into commercial premises) and while they were consuming alcohol in bars and clubs. Afterwards they continued to share and comment on the night out and the photos posted for days and sometimes weeks (Lyons et al., 2014; McCreanor et al., 2015; Moewaka Barnes et al., 2016). These activities were crucial for friendships and bonding (Niland et al., 2014) as well as identities. The ways in which participants engaged with the online worlds of cultures of intoxication varied for people across structural and social locations (e.g. see Goodwin et al., 2016; Hutton et al., 2016; Lyons et al., 2016). The five chapters in Part I therefore explore how identities play out across drinking cultures and social media and how this is intimately linked to social relations and power.

In Chapter 1, Ian Goodwin and Christine Griffin question the extent to which the concept of neoliberalism is useful for interrogating the inter-relationships between identity, youth drinking practices and digital media. While there have been critiques of neoliberalism as an analytical term, here they demonstrate how it can provide a broader critical context to make sense of the developments taking place in this field. In Chapter 2, neoliberal theories of class that construct young workers as flawed consumers, in ways that link to their drinking cultures and social media practices, are critiqued by Lin Bailey and Christine Griffin. They deconstruct online and offline depictions of women as a focus of concern around respectable femininities, and of men as reckless drinkers and explore how such identities play out in particular working-class drinking contexts. Jo Lindsay and Sian Supski draw together recent scholarship in the area of pleasure, identity, consumption and femininities in Chapter 3. Social media are depicted as an extension of public drinking space where contradictory pressures from personal, societal and commercial networks are inflected in practices of drinking, identity and gender relations across online and offline environments. Chapter 4 turns the focus on men and masculinities. Here Antonia Lyons and Brendan Gough examine the links between masculinities, drinking and social networking, and consider how distinctive markers of traditional masculine identities may play out at the confluence of youth drinking cultures and social media use. The section ends with a chapter on culture/ethnicity by Helen Moewaka Barnes, Patricia Niland, Lina Samu, Acushla Dee Sciascia and Tim McCreanor. These contributors highlight the importance of ethnicity in drinking practices and their representation on social networking sites through analyses of focus group data with young Māori, Pasifika and Pākehā New Zealanders. Societal power relations within and across the three groups are seen as central to their drinking practices and their social media use.

Part II: Alcohol marketing and commercialisation

In 2015, *Adweek*, the US advertising trade publication, ran a story entitled 'With better targeting, alcohol brands bet big on digital' (Johnson, 2015). The article outlined the ways alcohol brands are 'stepping up their digital marketing', increasing proportions of their budgets to digital platforms; for example, Pernod Ricard 'increased its digital budget by more than 50% every year for the past few years'. Twenty-five percent of Heineken's marketing spend is digital, and they are working in partnership with different social media platforms including Facebook and Twitter 'to build mini profiles of users to target its ads against'. The piece also outlines how brands are 'zeroing in on location targeting too' through using geo-location technology in mobile phones, and creating geo-targeted ads. A recent article in the *Journal of Interactive Advertising* noted that 'the 14 leading alcohol brands [in the USA] spent in excess of $3.5 billion in marketing expenditures, with approximately eight investing heavily in digital media, which is a fourfold increase during the past few years (Federal Trade Commission, 2014)' (Alhabash et al., 2016: 44).

McClure and colleagues (2016) comment that, as alcohol companies shift their emphasis and budgets into the digital environment, there is greater engagement with consumers and much greater promotion of interactive relationships. This fundamentally alters the landscape of alcohol marketing, such that young people are no longer passive recipients but active in engaging with, co-creating and disseminating marketing messages (Dunlop et al., 2016). There is also greater exposure of such marketing to underage youth. As De Bruijn and colleagues (2016) point out, Heineken and Google's global partnership to increase Heineken's YouTube activity 'very likely means that at least 103 million minors around the world are being exposed to the harmful effects of alcohol marketing on a monthly basis (EUCAM, 2011)' (p. 6).

A burgeoning area of research aims to examine the impacts of digital alcohol marketing, highlighting consistent associations between exposure to online alcohol marketing and drinking behaviour in teenagers and young people (Moreno and Whitehill, 2014). A study examining this relationship among over 9,000 adolescents across four European countries (Germany, Italy, The Netherlands and Poland) demonstrated that these young people were frequently exposed to online alcohol marketing, and this was significantly related to starting to drink and binge drinking in the previous 30 days (De Bruijn et al., 2016). Perhaps unsurprisingly, active engagement with this type of marketing was more strongly linked to drinking outcomes. Similar findings were obtained in a sample of Australian young people (Jones et al., 2015) and a recent UK study demonstrated that digital alcohol marketing was able to reach young people more effectively than traditional alcohol marketing, and was strongly associated with the frequency of high levels of episodic drinking (Critchlow et al., 2016). In New Zealand, researchers found that 13 and 14 year olds who engaged with digital alcohol marketing had increased odds of being a drinker by 98%, while having an online allegiance to a particular brand was related to greater frequency of alcohol consumption and drinking larger quantities, and increased the odds of being a drinker by 356% (Lin et al., 2012). McClure and colleagues (2016) are the first to show a prospective relationship between engagement with digital alcohol marketing and drinking outcomes one year later.

Alcohol companies embed their brands into the everyday lives of young people through their activities on social media (Brodmerkel and Carah, 2013). In Part II of this book, the four chapters by leading researchers in this rapidly developing field explore how alcohol interests increasingly employ social media systems to create sophisticated marketing strategies, and the ways in which young people actively and passively engage with corporate content online. In Chapter 6, at the start of this section, Nina Michealidou provides an overview of the multiple issues involved in big alcohol use of social media. She then theorises the associations between social media and alcohol consumption that highlights their potentials for health and harm and the long-term implications of embedding social media practices into young people's drinking cultures. In Chapter 7, Nicholas Carah focuses in on specific activities of alcohol brands on social media to illustrate participatory, data-driven characteristics that appropriate the creativity of users for industry purposes. Drawing on industry and public good research and analysis, this chapter deftly scrutinises claims about commercial impact, the increasing invisibility of customised marketing and the challenges these dynamics present to public health research and policy. Chapter 8 turns to the evolution of social media within mobile platforms. Here Rebecca Monk and Derek Heim consider the ways alcohol marketing makes use of new mobile technologies and the affordances they offer. They review published public good research to explore the opportunities and threats of these mobile marketing developments, considering what impacts they might have for public health and related policy development. In the final chapter of this section – Chapter 9 – Richard Purves focuses on user-generated promotion and viral phenomena common on social media. He points out how difficult it can be to identify what influence commercial marketing is having in these spaces. He explores alcohol marketers' use of social media as part of their repertoire of marketing activities to create and reinforce powerful brands and how they work with users to co-create and distribute marketing messages.

Part III: Public health and regulating alcohol promotion

Most countries around the world do not regulate digital alcohol marketing by law, but rely on self-regulation by the alcohol industry (Finland is a notable exception, as discussed below). However, the research demonstrates that this does not protect young people from high exposure to online alcohol marketing, or from the impact of this exposure on their consumption (De Bruijn et al., 2016). Through social media, alcohol companies are able to reach underage and young people at vulnerable ages (De Bruijn et al., 2016; Moreno and Whitehill, 2014). Any effort to try to reduce young people's exposure to digital alcohol marketing will require targeting multiple areas (McClure et al., 2016), and Casswell (2012) has called for a global response to this issue. Given that teenagers and young adults are high users of social media, these platforms provide many opportunities for health promotion agencies and activities (Dunlop et al., 2016). As Dunlop et al. (2016) note, however, 'health promoters lag far behind commercial marketers in the extent and sophistication of their use of social media to communicate with young people about alcohol' (p. 8). Researchers also struggle to keep up with alcohol marketing on rapidly changing social media technologies, with time lags between technological changes and research analyses and dissemination of findings (Westgate and Holliday, 2016). There are also challenges in accurately measuring digital marketing exposure, engagement and interaction (Dunlop et al., 2016).

In this section of the book contributors to the five chapters consider the new challenges and possibilities that social media and digital technologies afford for health promotion, public health and health policy. Regulation and legislation is discussed in terms of the ineffective industry voluntary codes for the digital environment and the innovative regulation that Finland adopted from 2016 to control online alcohol marketing. Methodological and ethical issues that arise from undertaking research within this emerging arena are also considered. The section begins with Chapter 10 by Hélène Cherrier, Nicholas Carah and Carla Meurk, who outline some of the health communication efforts that have employed social media to intervene in problematic alcohol use. They describe the successful 'Hello Sunday Morning' project in Australia, an online website and intervention programme that encourages people to join and commit to a period of alcohol abstinence, while communicating, blogging and sharing their experiences. This programme is effective in providing support and enabling users to reflect on their own drinking, not drinking and alcohol more broadly. In Chapter 11, Andy Ruddock explores the complications social media bring to understanding the relationship between commercial messages and high levels of alcohol consumption. He draws on Gerbner's cultural indicators project to make sense of intoxicating cultures, and argues this approach is highly relevant for questions around youth, social media and alcohol within broader political aspects of media systems. He describes an empirical study to show how complaints about alcohol marketing provide us with insights into issues of access and participation in media culture.

Implications for public health are considered in Chapter 12. Here Marjatta Montonen and Ismo Tuominen provide an account of the introduction of a policy based ban on the use of alcohol marketing on social media in Finland. They describe the country's regulation of alcohol marketing, the rationale that was given to extend this to social media and the mechanism and limitations of the ban. They then provide some comments on the projected outcome of this policy. In Chapter 13, Sarah Mart, a pioneer in the study of alcohol marketing in social media in the USA, reviews developments since her 2009 landmark paper on this topic. She includes developments that have occurred among alcohol companies, social media corporations and policy makers. She offers a palette of possible solutions built around legislation, monitoring, enforcement and accountability that resonate with evidence offered by many of the chapters in this book. Chapter 14 is the final chapter of the section and the book, and is written by the editors. It presents an overview of issues concerning research methodologies and ethics that are apparent across the chapters presented in this volume, and more widely evident in the field. We explore the imbalance between industry and public good research as a way of highlighting the assets and possibilities that the latter brings to providing quality empirical foundations for new policy to manage the challenges of online alcohol marketing.

We end this chapter by acknowledging two important issues. First, this collection is focused on young people's drinking practices and social media use. This focus on young people is reflected in the research literature and is driven by their high levels of engagement with alcohol and social media and by the relative vulnerability of young people as they are recruited into alcohol use. Commercial sellers of alcohol have a strong interest in recruiting new generations of drinkers and are therefore constantly seeking new means of promotion. Currently we know little about different age groups, social media use and alcohol consumption (Westgate and Holliday, 2016), but it is likely that many of the possibilities, problems and challenges identified in this volume apply across other age bands. In this rapidly expanding field, researchers work across many disciplines, including media studies, psychology, sociology, public health, geography, education, criminology, cultural studies and so on. This raises tensions around the focus of research, research approaches, and meanings of key concepts and terms. These tensions are taken up in different ways, and/or with different emphases, by researchers working in diverse fields with their own disciplinary viewpoints. From our own standpoints, this is one of the positive aspects of working in this field, as we see the beneficial cross-fertilisation of ideas and development of theories and constructs across disciplinary boundaries, creating debates that help to create relevant and important knowledge and understandings.

References

Alhabash, S., McAlister, A., Kim, W., Lou, C., Cunningham, C., Quilliam, E., and Richards, J. (2016). Saw it on Facebook, drank it at the bar! Effects of exposure to Facebook alcohol ads on alcohol-related behaviors. *Journal of Interactive Advertising*, *16*(1), 44–58.

Babor, T., Caetano, R., Casswell, S., Edwards, G., Giesbrecht, N., Graham, K., Grube, J., Hill, L., Holder, H., Homel, R., Livingston, M., Osterberg, E., Rehm, J., Room, R., and Rossow, I. (2010). *Alcohol: No Ordinary Commodity Research and Public Policy* (2nd edn). Oxford: Oxford University Press.

Brodmerkel, S., and Carah, N. (2013). Alcohol brands on Facebook: The challenges of regulating brands on social media. *Journal of Public Affairs*, *13*(3), 272–281.

Casswell, S. (2012). Current status of alcohol marketing policy – an urgent challenge for global governance. *Addiction*, *107*, 478–485.

Cavazos-Rehg, P., Krauss, M., Sowles, S., and Bierut, L. (2015). 'Hey everyone, I'm drunk.' An evaluation of drinking-related Twitter chatter. *Journal of Studies on Alcohol and Drugs*, *76*(4), 635–643.

Critchlow, N., Moodie, C., Bauld, L., Bonner, A., and Hastings, G. (2016). Awareness of, and participation with, digital alcohol marketing, and the association with frequency of high episodic drinking among young adults. *Drugs: Education, Prevention and Policy, Published online 26 January*, DOI: 10.3109/09687637.09682015.01119247.

CSDH. (2008). *Closing the Gap in a Generation: Health Equity through Action on the Social Determinants of Health. Final Report of the Commission on Social Determinants of Health*. Geneva: World Health Organization.

De Bruijn, A., Engels, R., Anderson, P., Bujalski, M., Gosselt, J., Schreckenberg, D., Wohtge, J., and De Leeuw, R. (2016). Exposure to online alcohol marketing and adolescents' drinking: A cross-sectional study in four European countries. *Alcohol and Alcoholism*, first published online: 5 May, http://dx.doi.org/10.1093/alcalc/agw1020.

Dunlop, S., Freeman, B., and Jones, S. (2016). Marketing to youth in the digital age: The promotion of unhealthy products and health promoting behaviours on social media. *Media and Communication, 4*(3), 35–49.

Federal Trade Commission. (2014). *Self-Regulation in the Alcohol Industry: Report of the Federal Trade Commission*. Washington, DC. www.ftc.gov/system/files/documents/reports/self-regulation-alcohol-industry-report-federal-trade-commission/140320 alcoholreport.pdf.

Goodwin, I., Griffin, C., Lyons, A., McCreanor, T., and Moewaka Barnes, H. (2016). Precarious popularity: Facebook drinking photos, the attention economy, and the regime of the branded self. *Social Media + Society, 2*(1), doi: 10.1177/2056305116628889.

Hunt, G., and Barker, J. (2001). Socio-cultural anthropology and alcohol and drug research: Towards a unified theory. *Social Science and Medicine, 53*(2), 165–188.

Hutton, F., Griffin, C., Lyons, A., Niland, P., and McCreanor, T. (2016). 'Tragic girls' and 'crack whores': Alcohol, femininity and Facebook. *Feminism and Psychology, 26*(1), 73–93.

Johnson, L. (2015, 16 June). With better targeting, alcohol brands bet big on digital: Annual budgets increase as much as 50 percent. *Adweek*. Retrieved 15 April 2016, from www.adweek.com/news/technology/better-targeting-alcohol-brands-bet-big-digital-165357

Jones, S., Robinson, L., Barrie, L., Francis, K., and Lee, J. (2015). Association between young Australian's drinking behaviours and their interactions with alcohol brands on Facebook: Results of an online survey. *Alcohol and Alcoholism*, first published online: 19 October, doi: http://dx.doi.org/10.1093/alcalc/agv1113.

Lin, E.-Y., Casswell, S., You, R. Q., and Huckle, T. (2012). Engagement with alcohol marketing and early brand allegiance in relation to early years of drinking. *Addiction Research and Theory, 20*(4), 329–338.

Lyons, A., Goodwin, I., Griffin, C., McCreanor, T., and Moewaka Barnes, H. (2016). Facebook and the fun of drinking photos: Reproducing gendered regimes of power. *Social Media and Society, 1–13*. DOI: 10.1177/2056305116672888.

Lyons, A., McCreanor, T., Goodwin, I., Griffin, C., Hutton, F., Moewaka Barnes, H., O'Carroll, D., Samu, L., Niland, P., and Vroman, K.-E. (2014). Youth drinking cultures in Aotearoa New Zealand. *Sites: New Series, 11*(2), 78–102.

McClure, A., Tanski, S., Li, Z., Jackson, K., Morgenstern, M., Li, Z., and Sargent, J. (2016). Internet alcohol marketing and underage alcohol use. *Pediatrics, 137*(2).

McCreanor, T., Lyons, A., Moewaka Barnes, H., Hutton, F., Goodwin, I., and Griffin, C. (2015). 'Drink a twelve box before you go'*: Pre-loading among young people in Aotearoa New Zealand. *Kotuitui*, published online: 9 Jun 2015.

Moewaka Barnes, H., McCreanor, T., Goodwin, I., Lyons, A., Griffin, C., and Hutton, F. (2016). Alcohol and social media: Drinking and drunkenness while online. *Critical Public Health*, *26*(1), 62–76.

Moreno, M., and Whitehill, J. (2014). Influence of social media on alcohol use in adolescents and young adults. *Alcohol Research: Current Reviews*, *36*(1), 91.

Moreno, M., and Whitehill, J. (2016). # Wasted: the intersection of substance use behaviors and social media in adolescents and young adults. *Current Opinion in Psychology*, *9*, 72–76.

Nicholls, J. (2012). Everyday, everywhere: Alcohol marketing and social media—current trends. *Alcohol and Alcoholism*, *47*(4), 486–493.

Niland, P., Lyons, A., Goodwin, I., and Hutton, F. (2014). 'See it doesn't look pretty does it?' Young adults' airbrushed drinking practices on Facebook. *Psychology and Health*, *29*(8), 877–895.

Race, K., and Brown, R. (2016, forthcoming). Cultural studies perspectives [on Drugs and Alcohol]. In T. Kolind, B. Thom and G. Hunt (Eds.), *The Sage Handbook of Drug and Alcohol Studies* (Volume 1: Social Science Approaches).

Ridout, B. (2016). Facebook, social media and its application to problem drinking among college students. *Current Opinion in Psychology*, *9*, 83–87.

Savic, M., Room, R., Mugavin, J., Pennay, A., and Livingston, M. (2016). Defining 'drinking culture': A critical review of its meaning and connotation in social research on alcohol problems. *Drugs: Education, Prevention and Policy*, published online: 15 April, doi: 10.3109/09687637.09682016.01153602.

Sedghi, A. (2014, 4 February). Facebook: 10 years of social networking, in numbers. *The Guardian*. Retrieved 20 June 2016, from www.theguardian.com/news/datablog/2014/feb/04/facebook-in-numbers-statistics.

Westgate, E., and Holliday, J. (2016). Identity, influence, and intervention: The roles of social media in alcohol use. *Current Opinion in Psychology*, *9*, 27–32.

Wong, J., and Thielman, S. (2016, 27 April). Facebook's net income triples in first quarter of 2016. *The Guardian*. Retrieved 15 June 2016, from www.theguardian.com/technology/2016/apr/27/facebook-revenue-first-quarter-2016.

Zhao, S., Grasmuck, S., and Martin, J. (2008). Identity construction on Facebook: Digital empowerment in anchored relationships. *Computers in Human Behavior*, *24*(5), 1816–1836.

Part I

Identities, social relations and power

1   Neoliberalism, alcohol and identity

A symptomatic reading of young people's drinking cultures in a digital world

Ian Goodwin and Christine Griffin

A broad range of research has established the importance of youth drinking as an essentially social act with important implications for young people's identities. There is long-standing evidence that peer groups form an important part of young people's social lives generally (Kehily, 2007), and peer networks and friendship groups are central to youth drinking as a specific form of leisure practice which helps mark out identity and status, as well as a shared sense of communality (Douglas, 1987; Lyons and Willott, 2008; MacLean, 2016; Sheehan and Ridge, 2001). Such socially orientated practices are often enhanced by the embodied pleasures young people experience while being drunk (Griffin et al., 2009a; Szmigin et al., 2011). Moreover, 'after the fact', stories about drinking and drunken behaviour are often told and re-told amongst peer networks, playing a crucial additional role in the development and maintenance of friendships (Griffin et al., 2009b; Sheehan and Ridge, 2001) and ongoing forms of identity work (Lyons and Willott, 2008; McCreanor et al., 2005). As the other chapters in part one of this volume will go on to outline in detail, these processes are always overlaid with power relations which produce important differentiations in experience across genders, socio-economic groups, ethnicities and sexualities. Conceptions of identity, identity work and differentiated power relations that work through categories of identity are all central to understanding the complexity of young people's socially orientated drinking practices.

Over the past few decades the marketing campaigns launched by alcohol corporations have become increasingly aimed at aligning their branded messages with the meanings young people themselves form in their cultural practices and socialising. Young people have become increasingly familiar and comfortable with alcohol brands as a result, and take up and use brands in identity work across both personal and social settings (McCreanor et al., 2005; McCreanor et al., 2008). The concept of identity is also increasingly important to the way that alcohol, and in particular 'problematic' and 'risky' drinking by young people, is regulated and controlled. Alcohol consumption within the night-time economy, 'as well as being something experienced by participants', increasingly forms a key site of 'spectacle with gendered and classed dynamics', whereby certain forms of drinking and specific drinkers become identified by the state and subjected to a concerted regulatory gaze with direct policy implications (Haydock,

2015a: 1). Young people, and in particular young women, are often 'othered' and pathologised through such processes (Brown and Gregg, 2012). Equally, health policy interventions seeking to minimise alcohol-related harms experienced by young people are increasingly taking account of the importance of drinking for young people's sense of identity, and indeed it is argued that they must recognise the importance of peer-orientated socialising and associated processes of identity formation if they are to be effective (see Niland et al., 2013).

In sum, identity is well established in the literature as a key nexus, or lens, through which to analyse youth drinking cultures, both at the micro level of youth cultural practices and more broadly in terms of economics, marketing, regulation and policy. The growing centrality of digital media technologies to youth drinking practices has acted to enhance this broad relevance of identity as an analytical category. Many of the relevant online developments have been analysed in detail elsewhere in this volume, but the major issues related to identity are worth briefly recapping here. Social media have been appropriated by young people as a key site of online self-display where the pleasures, identity work, and socialising associated with their drinking cultures become extended and developed (Goodwin et al., 2016; Hebden et al., 2015; Niland et al., 2014). Analyses of self-displays and friendship in online drinking cultures have also found young people's online practices to be bound up in structural constraints and power relations around class, gender and ethnicity in a fashion that mirrors earlier research of offline drinking cultures (Goodwin et al., 2016; Hutton et al., 2016). Alcohol corporations have been quick to follow young people to social media, utilising sites like Facebook as a key space to engage with young people in order to enhance their sales and aid their marketing campaigns. Young people's everyday online activities now often seamlessly mesh with commercially driven alcohol promotion, blurring stark distinctions between user-generated and commercial content such that branded alcohol promotion is often a taken for granted, integral part of identity work and social life online (Carah et al., 2014; Nicholls, 2012). In opposition to these developments, social media are increasingly being considered as potentially important settings for engaging young people in forms of health promotion (Loss et al., 2014). Supplementing these shifts, new forms of more user-driven health campaign 'movements', like Hello Sunday Morning, 'ask participants to stop drinking for a period of time, to set a personal goal, and to record their reflections and progress on blogs and social networks' (Carah et al., 2015: 214). Meanwhile, a range of smartphone 'apps', such as 'Let's Get Wasted', intensify and extend the importance of alcohol consumption to young people's identities and social lives, both online and offline (Weaver et al., 2013).

Against this critical context, this chapter poses a key question: to what extent is the concept of neoliberalism useful for interrogating these broad inter-relationships between identity, youth drinking practices and digital media? We argue that setting alcohol-related identity issues in youth drinking cultures against the broader critical context suggested by the literature on neoliberalism is potentially highly useful. This is not least because neoliberalism as an analytical category highlights a series of productive *interconnections* between the contemporary (social, economic, political, policy) issues we have outlined here, equally helping to explain their extension in novel online developments. In this sense, we argue that neoliberalism provides the broader critical frame through which drinking cultures can be read 'symptomatically' as part of a 'conjunctural analysis' (Hall and Jefferson, 2006). A 'symptomatic' reading of drinking cultures entails treating them as reflective of wider social and political changes, rather than solely as reflections of individual motivations or attitudes. A 'conjunctural analysis' entails asking 'why now?', analysing social phenomena in relation to the key 'political, economic and socio-cultural changes of their respective times' (Hall and Jefferson, 2006: xiv). It in this respect that 'neoliberalism' becomes conceptually useful, because it remains our best means for naming, understanding, and critically interrogating the key political, economic and socio-cultural changes that mark out our contemporary societal 'conjuncture', as the current context in which drinking cultures play out in all their complexities. However, using the concept of neoliberalism in this way is not without its pitfalls. As an analytical term, it has been subject to sustained critique, frequently for the very reasons we are suggesting it is potentially advantageous: too often it is ill-defined and yet very broadly applied in analyses that attempt to explain 'everything'. In what follows then, we first outline the major debates over neoliberalism and define what we understand it to mean. Then we seek to show how our definitions of the term can usefully open up avenues of analysis. Ultimately we suggest 'neoliberalism' and 'neoliberal identities' become crucial analytical categories when applied appropriately as part of a symptomatic reading of drinking cultures. That is, these concepts remain extremely helpful for understanding youth drinking practices and their complex, ambivalent relationships to current power relations, identity categories, identity work and digital media.

Neoliberalism, critique and neoliberal identity

Neoliberalism has become one of the most widely invoked critical concepts across a variety of academic disciplines. However, it is often used in ill-defined ways, 'as a sloppy synonym for capitalism itself' (Ferguson, 2010: 171), or is applied in relation to a multitude of competing definitions that are not always reconciled (Bell and Green, 2016; Ferguson, 2010). The term, which has an often unacknowledged and complex history (see Flew, 2012; Phelan, 2014), has therefore attracted significant critique (Barnett, 2005; Flew, 2009; Grossberg, 2010). There is not the space to canvass this history, or the detail of these critiques, here. However, drawing from Phelan's (2014: 26–33) summation of these debates, we would highlight specific aspects of neoliberalism's critique that are particularly pertinent for how we have, in response, structured our argument and analytical approach in this chapter. Neoliberalism can be problematically applied as a monolithic catch-all category that, in analyses which note the elements of a social context that appear neoliberal, go on to attempt to explain 'everything' in neoliberal terms. This tends to ride roughshod over the complexities of differentiated social contexts, while leading to a cookie-cutter approach to analysis which constantly subsumes the particular under the universal. That is, it leads to a tendency to suggest that naming something 'neoliberal' provides a sufficient explanation of all aspects of its nature. At worst, this can eventually lead to empirical phenomena identified as neoliberal being 'cursorily disparaged rather than deemed worthy of additional analysis' (Phelan, 2014: 32). This is a particular issue for our focus on youth cultures and drinking, where power-laden processes of othering, pathologising and marginalising youth practices are already in play. We want to argue that youth drinking cultures are not only contextually differentiated, complex and significant sites worthy of ongoing study, but are also deeply *ambivalent*, being bound up in processes where we see neoliberal forms of power in play but also being places where resistances, evasions and contestations of neoliberal logics are simultaneously enacted.

Critiques of neoliberalism equally suggest it is only useful as an analytical concept when it is applied with a critical self-reflexivity that starts by seeking to establish how neoliberalism plays out in specific contexts, rather than configuring it as a 'fully present structure or agent with the totalizing power to cause, make, determine and act on a variety of social objects and practices' (Phelan, 2014: 32). For us, part of this self-reflexivity involves the recognition that drawing on neoliberalism as our key conceptual category does not exclude other concepts being brought to bear in analysis. We argue our focus on using neoliberalism in a symptomatic reading of drinking cultures can accommodate alternative conceptual understandings. Indeed, concepts such as 'the carnivalesque' (Haydock, 2015a) and 'healthism' (Petersen and Lupton, 1996) have been usefully combined with analyses of neoliberal social formations, and we recognise their ongoing relevance in terms of reading youth drinking cultures symptomatically. Where applicable, we will briefly highlight interconnections with these terms in our analysis. Finally, critiques of neoliberalism suggest explicitly outlining how one intends to define and apply it in specific forms of analysis matters. From the range of applications available, we would highlight two definitions we deem particularly useful to our symptomatic/conjunctural approach.

The first relates to neoliberalism as it is most commonly understood, that is, as an economic ideology, tied to state policy changes, that heralds a process of capitalist restructuring and reform which has occurred globally since the 1970s. Keynesian economics, with its emphasis on state planning and intervention in the economy, and the associated rise of the welfare state, became identified as key impediments to progress in this process (Phelan, 2014). In contrast, neoliberal economics calls for a different set of rationalities to drive the actions of the state. That is, neoliberal reform marks out a series of key conjunctural changes that suggest:

> [T]hat human well-being can best be advanced by liberating individual entrepreneurial freedoms and skills within an institutional framework characterized by strong private property rights, free market, and free trade. The role of the state is to create and preserve an institutional framework appropriate to such practices.
>
> (Harvey, 2005: 2)

Thatcherism in the UK and Reaganism in the USA are often identified as paradigmatic, practical examples of the formation of new neoliberal states. However, a broad range of social democracies including Canada, New Zealand, Australia and Sweden have implemented similar market-centric reforms (Bell and Green, 2016). While the changes enacted since the 1970s have often been drastic in terms of factors such as the extensive roll back of the welfare state, the growing power of global corporations and the subsequent valorising of privatisation and competition, both the political and the corporate elites in Western democracies often refuse to label their actions as neoliberal or even as driven in ideological terms (Phelan, 2014). Rather, neoliberalism is more often positioned in terms of a neutral pragmatism, as simply 'what works' in a globalised economy (Phelan, 2014). Neoliberalism therefore assumes a certain form of invisibility, so that Monbiot (2016) argues it remains ill understood by the general public and is seldom recognised *as* an ideology or as a project consciously enacted. This matters to our argument, as our decision to continue to *name* young people's drinking cultures and associated identity work as profoundly shaped by a 'neoliberal conjuncture', which we conceptualise as the result of a political economic project consciously enacted, takes on a political dimension. That is, we seek to counter its relative anonymity, which is 'both a symptom and cause of its [neoliberalism's] power' (Monbiot, 2016).

Our second conception of neoliberalism, connected closely to the above, builds more directly on its relationship to lived experiences and identity, and relates to how the state reforms enacted through neoliberalism are related to new forms of governmentality (Foucault, 1991). Here neoliberalism refers to a 'highly dispersed' (Ouellette and Hay, 2008: 473) set of techniques and prescriptions, or technologies of the self, that outline how individuals ought to conduct themselves and, above all, take responsibility for their own lives (Lupton, 1999). As Cairns and Johnston (2015) summarise, 'neoliberal governance is not externally imposed onto bodies, but operates *through* the embodied actions of free subjects – often by exercising choice in the market' (p. 155, original emphasis). This notion of the 'free' subject exercising choice is central to a conception of neoliberal governmentality, as such 'freedom' is now increasingly constituted as an obligation, a marker of individual autonomy and distinctive selfhood that must be continually demonstrated and displayed (Cronin, 2000). Rose and colleagues therefore conceptualise freedom as 'a diverse array of invented technologies of the self', where consumption becomes central (Rose et al., 2006: 100). In exercising consumer-based lifestyle choices, the individual is recast as an entrepreneur of the self who becomes responsible for their own fate. Here the concept of risk, and in particular the responsibility placed on the subject for risk avoidance, becomes another key technology of the self with particular resonances for health and well-being (Lupton, 1999). In other words, through practices of consumption, it is the individual who takes on a morally encoded responsibility to exercise self-control, to gain forms of self-knowledge, and to continually enact a regime of self-improvement (Cairns and Johnston, 2015; Lupton, 1999). If one behaves in ways that are seen as excessive, unhealthy, irresponsible or undisciplined, then this is constituted as a moral failure of the self (Croghan et al., 2006). In what follows, we argue these imperatives are particularly pertinent to understanding youth drinking (as a site where 'health risks' are a key factor), the online display of youth drinking cultures, and young people's broader uses of digital technologies. This is, in a dual sense, played out in terms of young people's own social practices/identity work and 'youth drinking' as an increasingly prominent and visible site of neoliberal spectacle.

Neoliberalism and neoliberal identities in young people's drinking cultures: freedoms, constraints and ambivalence

In the previous section we developed a twin focus on neoliberalism as a political economic project that marks out a specific new conjuncture, while simultaneously producing new governmental imperatives in lived experiences. Here we apply these dimensions in a symptomatic reading of young people's drinking cultures. While a critical political economy of the drinks industry is important to an understanding of neoliberalism's conjunctural relationship to youth drinking cultures, alcohol studies have only 'just begun to pay close attention' (Mercille, 2016: 70) to detailed analyses of industry structures and their relationships to government policy. In the context of an extensive push towards increasingly global free trade in Western economies, it is, however, clear that large alcohol corporations now dominate the global marketplace, and are 'increasingly reliant on marketing for their survival' (Jernigan, 2009: 6). Indeed, the 'unfettered expansion of alcohol marketing' (Casswell, 2012: 483) is a key contextual feature of contemporary corporate-driven alcohol consumption across national contexts, one which stands in stark contrast to the comparative controls being placed on other substances such as tobacco. For Mercille (2016) this situation speaks to a broader fundamental re-casting of the role of the state as a facilitator of corporate-led development. In his analysis of Ireland, as a 'prototypical neoliberal state' (p. 61), he suggests that government policies and reforms:

> have supported the drinks industry, including longer opening hours for pubs, the growth of sales through outlets such as off-licences and supermarkets, favourable tax measures, support for voluntary regulatory guidelines and the enactment of weak legal regulations to reduce alcohol consumption.
>
> (p. 70)

Similar legislative and regulatory changes, which in effect actively *encourage* heavy drinking, have been enacted across many Western nations (Gordon et al., 2012). Haydock (2015b) argues this has led to a deeply seated ambivalence in regard to alcohol regulation in England. One the one hand '"responsible" consumption of alcohol has been encouraged for its social, economic and even health benefits' (p. 145). In 'moderation' (p. 145), alcohol consumption is constructed in policy as having a positive impact on economic and social well-being, and the notion of the responsible citizen deserving, or even earning, a drink features centrally. This ties in with the actual enactment of minimal alcohol regulations, as deserving and responsible citizens equally earn an *environment* where alcohol is easily accessible. On the other hand, 'irresponsible' (p. 145) drinking, and in particular the loaded image of 'binge' (p. 145) drinking, is singled out and condemned.

For Haydock (2015b) the concept of the binge is a potential obfuscation, because it is not the *quantity* of alcohol consumed, or even heightened pleasure per se, that is judged. Rather it is a particular *culture* of drinking to get drunk associated with 'little social control' (p. 146) and the subversion of social and identity norms. There is a symbolic violence enacted here, as specific practices (and people) become rebuked. Thus Haydock (2015b) ultimately suggests debates over 'binge drinking' become evocative of the carnivalesque, where both toleration (within defined limits) and unease coincide. It is also here that our two aspects of neoliberalism, as a political economic project and a governmental regime, are bought clearly into play, and it is the concept of identity work which becomes the crucial mediator of this process. Within a deregulated environment that makes alcohol easily accessible, and where it is relentlessly marketed, responsibility is devolved to the individual to develop an appropriate identity and a certain social deportment in relation to alcohol. The swathe of broader regulatory reforms that enact *structural* changes which actively promote alcohol consumption are elided, and moral responsibility for managing behaviour is placed squarely on *individuals* alone. Health promotion policies follow similar logics, devolving responsibility for managing health risks (including those arising from alcohol consumption) to individuals while prioritising good health choices (Ayo, 2012). Indeed, given a reduced role for the state in providing social support and health care, 'healthism' (Crawford, 2006) generally – with the responsibilities it places on individuals to manage health risks and lead healthy lives – becomes central to the broad neoliberal agenda for reform. The emphases on rational choice and individual responsibility that emerge in health promotion can, in particular, have detrimental effects on 'young people living within the contexts of structural disadvantage [e.g. long term unemployment]' (Brown et al., 2013: 333) who are positioned as authors of their own circumstance. In Brown and Gregg's (2012) analysis of Australian alcohol health promotion policies, they highlight young women as particularly subject to judgement from a regulatory gaze. In this sense, profound forms of youth inequality become naturalised within neoliberal social formations.

At the same time as these broader processes are playing out, the deregulation of the alcohol industry has been accompanied by a more specific state and corporate interest in promoting spatially bounded locations for alcohol consumption, as part of fostering a new night-time economy (NTE) central to urban regeneration (Chatterton and Hollands, 2001). These corporately promoted and bounded urban 'wild zones' predominantly target a young adult consumer demographic (Hayward and Hobbs, 2007), and are linked to what Measham and Brain (2005) term a new 'culture of intoxication'. For young people particularly, this extends and heightens the ambivalence at the heart of corporate alcohol promotion and state alcohol policy, as such 'zones' operate with a simultaneous logic of seduction and repression. Young people are seduced into a normalised culture of excessive drinking positively promoted by alcohol corporations and linked to wealth creation in the NTE, while simultaneously risking being pathologised as disordered and disorderly 'binge drinkers' (Szmigin et al., 2008). This encourages young people to exercise a 'calculated hedonism' (Measham, 2004) that combines discourses of discipline, self-knowledge over drinking limits, and self-control alongside pleasure and enjoyment as key categories governing conduct (Measham, 2004). Calculated hedonism, as a 'controlled loss of control', predominantly operates within the boundaries of specific times (the weekend), specific places (a club or bar within the 'wild zone' or a private party), and specific company (young peers and friendship groups) (Measham, 2004). As Cairns and Johnston (2015) point out in relation to a different context (neoliberalism and dieting), there are always different, competing imperatives at work in such forms of neoliberal governmentality, and these must be *actively* negotiated and reconciled by embodied subjects in the complexities of their lived experiences. There is the imperative towards corporeal self-control (Cairns and Johnston, 2015), which in drinking cultures suggests avoiding the embodied experience of being 'out of control' in the overtly and excessively drunken body, but this is *simultaneously experienced* by subjects alongside the 'felt' imperative to consume. In other words, in a 'market-orientated culture that celebrates consumer choice as an expression of freedom, the good (and healthy) citizen cannot be marked solely by restraint' (Cairns and Johnston, 2015: 156). Young people must, therefore, learn when, where and how to indulge in alcohol consumption, not merely forms of self-restraint.

In sum, viewing the complex issues relating to sociality, identity and alcohol consumption through the lens of neoliberalism provides, we argue, a useful analytical stance for symptomatic readings of drinking cultures. It allows us to see productive interconnections between corporate-led development, state policies regarding alcohol regulation and health promotion, urban development, and a series of accompanying governmental imperatives that play out in young people's alcohol-related leisure practices. It also allows us to critique how power relations play out, that is how neoliberalism potentially perpetuates itself through cultural practices. This requires recognition, because the relative invisibility of neoliberalism is compounded here through the production of an immersive neoliberal spectacle that focuses predominantly on young people. The structural changes associated with neoliberal processes of reform that have led to an active promotion of alcohol are elided, fading into the background, as 'binge drinking' becomes located at the level of individualised failings of 'youth' to lead appropriately controlled lives. Recognising this is doubly important because, while neoliberal accounts of the subject suggest the imperative to lead an 'appropriately responsible' life plays out uniformly across populations, neoliberalism in practice tends to 'exacerbate existing social divides' (Cairns and Johnston, 2015: 156) as those suffering *structural* disadvantage are most likely to enact 'failed' subjectivities.

Nevertheless, a fully symptomatic reading of drinking cultures requires greater recognition of the tensions, ambiguities and complexities that emerge in the lived experiences of young people than this potentially totalising account suggests. We must avoid a tendency towards 'theoretical determinism' (Cairns and Johnston, 2015: 157). There is a risk here of viewing young people as ignorant of these processes, or as – simply – thoroughly disciplined subjects. Power here emerges in a more indeterminate form, and also as thoroughly embodied and corporeal and therefore open to forms of subject-driven evasion, contestation and resistance. This suggests an investigative, relatively open stance towards young people's drinking cultures is required, and reminds us that theoretical accounts of neoliberalism do not exhaust the 'reality' of the identity processes in play. For example, the processes of socialisation and associated identity work young people undertake while out drinking have been linked to a strengthened importance for 'friendship groups as sites of collective identity, community, care and support, as well as fun and enjoyment' (Griffin et al., 2009b: 226). Learning to look out for one another while on nights out drinking could help young people avoid, resist or mitigate the effects of the individuating, regulatory nature of neoliberal governmentality and its relationship to the structural forms of inequality they experience. Young people potentially develop self-directed, yet collective forms of group belonging and support and an associated sense of self that disrupts individualisation (Griffin et al., 2009b). Haydock's (2015a, 2015b) insistence on the importance of the 'carnivalesque' to drinking cultures, which suggests a temporary inversion of the social order may at least in part be taking place, are also relevant here.

Equally, young people's collective drunken narratives – so essential to processes of identity formation – often include factors like a loss of consciousness and a lack of rationality that potentially threatens the neoliberal project of the self as a thoroughly rational, calculative effort towards self-responsibility and self-improvement (Griffin et al., 2009a). The very nature of drinking as a sociable, pleasurable, and altered form of embodiment tied to positive affects also suggests it could operate to disrupt the disempowering process whereby structural problems are experienced in neoliberal social orders as private burdens that are routinely *felt* throughout everyday life (Cairns and Johnston, 2015). There is a certain *autonomy* to drinking practices. Somewhat paradoxically, their resistant aspects may be most salient for those who have the greatest difficulty negotiating drinking cultures, such as young women who experience the NTE as a dilemmatic space where they are exhorted to be up for it, sassy, and independent, and yet censured should they drink like men or appear as 'drunken sluts' (Griffin et al., 2013: 184). It is with this sense of complexity in mind that we turn to a symptomatic reading of 'digital life', identity, drinking cultures and their relationship to neoliberalism.

What's going on(line)? Neoliberal identities, drinking and social networking sites

In a strict sense, discussing digital media technologies in a separate section misconstrues their nature. They are thoroughly integrated into young people's lives, and it is no longer possible (if it ever was) to discuss identities in 'online' and 'offline' life as if they were distinct. Yet it is analytically useful here to discuss digital media technologies separately, because – above all – we wish to emphasise that their active appropriation by young people as an integrative part of their drinking cultures extends the deep sense of contradiction, or ambivalence, that we have argued lies at the heart of neoliberalism and neoliberal forms of governmentality. Digital media technologies *simultaneously* enhance the neoliberal, corporate promotion of alcohol in the NTE and the disciplinary dimensions of drinking cultures in novel ways, while providing new avenues and sites of resistance, evasion and contestation. This complexity and ambivalence is central to our argument, and invites a close empirical analysis of young people's actual social practices and identity work online as part of a symptomatic reading of drinking cultures. Despite a spike in recent publications, research work on young people's drinking cultures and digital media technologies is only just beginning. While very little of it currently focuses specifically on neoliberalism, governmentality and identity, there are numerous developments potentially relevant to our discussion (e.g. uses of mobile technologies and smartphones, smartphone app development, and blogging). For the purposes of illustration, and clarity, we will concentrate here on the growing importance of social networking sites (SNS) for young people's drinking cultures.

It is now well established that young people use SNS to share their tastes and preferences, to develop and sustain social connections with friends and their broader peer group, and to perform their identities online (boyd, 2007; Livingstone, 2008). It is perhaps unsurprising, therefore, that a burgeoning literature is now documenting how young people routinely share stories and photos depicting drinking and drunken behaviour on SNS (e.g. Beullens and Schepers, 2013; Egan and Moreno, 2011). Much of this research is conducted within a public health frame, with concern growing that the sheer prevalence of peer-generated alcohol content on SNS profiles is creating 'intoxigenic digital spaces' (Griffiths and Casswell, 2010) – online alcohol promoting environments – potentially damaging to public health (McCreanor et al., 2013). While health concerns are legitimate, it is equally clear that young people have actively appropriated SNS to extend and enhance the socialising and identity work associated with drinking cultures. Young people use SNS like Facebook to anticipate, organise, share and celebrate their pleasurable drinking experiences through status updates, uploading photos, videos, comments, likes and posts (Brown and Gregg, 2012; Hebden et al., 2015; Niland et al., 2014). Digital mobile technologies have enabled young people to engage in these SNS activities while they are preloading (drinking alcohol at private premises before entering the NTE) (Moewaka Barnes et al., 2016) and out in the NTE (Lyons et al., 2014). Such experiences help young people to sustain a collective sense of identification with their peer networks and to solidify close friendship group bonds (Niland et al., 2015).

There is much here to suggest that SNS enable young people to enhance the value of drinking cultures as sites of community, care and support as well as increasing the fun and enjoyment of drinking. These are the very factors that we have argued may well be linked to forms of subject-driven evasion, contestation and resistance to neoliberal regimes. There are novel advantages for young people to be considered here too. SNS allow young people to share drinking content both in real time and asynchronously, to 'store' and re-visit their drinking experiences at will and to enable drinking-related socialising to continue after the fact, in the ensuing 'physical' absence of their peers (Goodwin et al, 2014). Moreover drinking photos are constructed by young people as particularly valuable on SNS like Facebook, as they attract more comments and likes than other forms of content, and therefore *actively* develop social connections (that may not otherwise be made) through making young people far more 'visible' to their peers and 'popular' on the platform (Goodwin et al., 2016).

However, it is precisely because SNS offer young people powerful new forms of 'freedom' (see Rose et al., 2006), in relation to drinking as a central site of consumption, that they reintroduce the question of neoliberal governmentality in social life. Through using SNS extensively, young people potentially come under increasing pressure to perform a self-controlled, responsible and moral self in their drinking practices. This pressure is enhanced through the same technological affordances that augment their socialising, as the ability of SNS software to record searchable and persistent data on young people's activities exposes them to broader 'invisible audiences' potentially watching, such as the police or employers (boyd, 2007; Goodwin et al., 2014). These heightened online visibilities intensify the relationship between young people's drinking cultures and neoliberal spectacle, and introduce *new forms* of 'risk' to be actively managed that relate to 'appropriate' online self-displays. Little is yet understood about how young people negotiate such pressures in drinking cultures. But there is evidence to suggest that they actively manage their online drinking displays through carefully choosing photos to upload, while spending an inordinate amount of time and effort tagging and un-tagging images uploaded by others with their public performance of self in mind (Goodwin et al., 2016). That is, they produce what has been termed carefully managed, 'airbrushed' versions of the self in relation to their SNS displays of drinking practices (Niland et al., 2014). The links increasingly made between alcohol, health and SNS as 'intoxigenic digital spaces' (Griffiths and Casswell, 2010) intensifies these processes further, due to the fundamental connections evident between 'healthism' (Crawford, 2006) and the general neoliberal project of societal reform. The failure to perform a 'healthy', disciplined and self-responsible identity is particularly stigmatised in neoliberal regimes as a moral failure of the self (Croghan et al., 2006). Thus the new 'work' SNS drinking displays require can be conceptualised as a form of disciplinary practice, and young women appear to feel these pressures to perform 'appropriate' online drinking identities most acutely (Lyons et al., 2016).

It is also essential to recognise SNS as environments that have compounded the drive towards wide-ranging, corporate-driven alcohol marketing (McCreanor et al., 2013). Multinational alcohol corporations have been 'well ahead of the curve in developing the potential of SNS for commercial gain' (Goodwin et al., 2014: 62). Nicholls (2012), for example, has documented the extensive use of 'real world tie ins, interactive games, competitions and time-specific suggestions drink'

(p. 486) in corporate SNS alcohol marketing strategies. State legislatures have recognised alcohol brand profile pages as powerful marketing communication tools, but often do little more than apply the weak model of industry self-regulation to online communication (Sven and Carah, 2013). This situation extends the well-established links between the alcohol industry and 'light touch' state regulation, a factor central to neoliberal reform.

Part of this regulatory problem relates to the increasingly sophisticated nature of alcohol SNS marketing strategies. Corporations not only 'mine detailed consumer data that allow them to target advertising to specific audiences', they also exploit SNS sociality in general (Carah et al., 2014: 259). That is, they strategically employ sites like Facebook to manage connections with 'consumer's identity making practices and engage with the mediation of everyday life' (Carah et al., 2014: 259). The brand effectively 'travels' online in a dynamic fashion via young people's online identity performances and the social connections young people make, which blurs clear distinctions between user-generated and commercial content. This also allows corporations to actively manage the 'circulation of affect' around the brand, while 'prompting connections between mediation of drinking and the brand that would not be possible in other media channels' (Carah et al., 2014: 259). This raises fundamental questions about the level and type of autonomy young people enjoy online, while doing nothing to displace the neoliberal notion that it is primarily the 'responsibility' of the *individual* to manage their identity, socialising and alcohol consumption practices. This potentially perpetuates neoliberalism's relative invisibility as a concentrated political project that perpetuates corporate power. At the same time, we may also be witnessing the entrenchment of a *new* form of corporate power, whereby corporations retain ownership of detailed personal information on young people's ostensibly 'private' lives, derived from SNS usage that they can then exploit in a sophisticated manner, while individuals themselves have limited access to their own data (Andrejavic, 2014). It is important to recognise here that SNS alcohol marketing campaigns primarily work because they are *actively* appropriated by young people in their day-to-day lives as part of their own socialising and identity work. Young people themselves are often unconcerned about commercial content on SNS (Goodwin et al., 2016). Nevertheless, the *differential* level of power these marketing models produce, which sees corporations extend and enhance their disproportionate influence in day-to-day life, requires recognition as it arguably supports their central role in sustaining neoliberal social orders.

Young people's digitally mediated drinking cultures, identity and neoliberalism: a symptomatic reading as a critical starting point

In this chapter we have explored the usefulness of neoliberalism as an analytical concept when employed as part of a symptomatic reading of drinking cultures within the frame of a conjunctural analysis (Hall and Jefferson, 2006). In doing so we have sought to occupy a difficult middle ground between what we consider to be two unproductive directions. The first would be, in the face of significant critiques of the term, a failure to apply neoliberalism at all when attempting to understand the complex interconnections between young people's identities, youth drinking cultures and digital media. When carefully defined and judiciously applied as part of a symptomatic reading, we argue neoliberalism becomes critical to gaining important insights into the current conjuncture. Without the concept of neoliberalism, we can fail to fully recognise novel contemporary relationships between alcohol regulation, health policies, corporate-led development and marketing, urban development in the NTE and young people's actual social practices and identity work. Moreover, a symptomatic reading that draws on neoliberalism creates a productive critical space where aspects of the power relations that structure social processes and identity work in youth drinking cultures can be unpacked and interrogated. The second unproductive direction, however, would be to apply neoliberalism in too totalising a manner. That is, to reduce digitally mediated youth drinking cultures to little more than corporately controlled spaces producing thoroughly disciplined subjects. This would fail to recognise the embodied, lived complexities of young people's drinking practices, and would overlook their ties to collective forms of belonging and support that may well be linked to resisting the neoliberal project of the self, and its ties to social inequality. While we do not wish to suggest it is the only critical way forward, we feel our symptomatic approach remains capable of interrogating both these dimensions of contemporary drinking cultures. It creates an investigative, relatively open analytical stance: one that does not anticipate its conclusions before it begins, but remains capable of exploring drinking cultures as open to corporate influence, as overlaid with neoliberal governmental imperatives, while simultaneously being sites of resistance to neoliberal regimes.

References

Andrejavic, M. (2014). *Infoglut: How Too Much Information is Changing the Way We Think and Know*. London: Routledge.

Ayo, N. (2012). Understanding health promotion in a neoliberal climate and the making of health conscious citizens. *Critical Public Health*, *22*(1), 99–105.

Barnett, C. (2005). The consolations of neoliberalism. *Geoforum*, *36*(1), 7–12.

Bell, K., and Green, J. (2016). On the perils of invoking neoliberalism in public health critique. *Critical Public Health*, *26*(3), 239–243.

Beullens, K., and Schepers, A. (2013). Display of alcohol use on Facebook: A content analysis. *Cyberpsychology, Behaviour and Social Networking*, *16*(7), 497–503.

boyd, d. (2007). Why youth (heart) social network sites: The role of networked publics in teenage social life. In D. Buckingham (Ed.), *Youth, Identity and Digital Media Volume* (pp. 119–142, McArthur Foundation Series on Digital Learning). Cambridge, MA: MIT Press.

Brown, R., and Gregg, M. (2012). The pedagogy of regret: Facebook, binge drinking and young women. *Continuum: Journal of Media and Cultural Studies*, *26*(3), 357–369.

Brown, S., Shoveller, J., Chabot, C., and LaMontagne, A. (2013). Risk, resistance and the neoliberal agenda: Young people, health and well-being in the UK, Canada and Australia. *Health, Risk and Society*, *15*(4), 333–346.

Cairns, K., and Johnston, J. (2015). Choosing health: Embodied neoliberalism, postfeminism, and the 'do-diet'. *Theory and Society, 44*(2), 153–175.

Carah, N., Brodmerkel, S., and Hernandez, L. (2014). Brands and sociality: Alcohol branding, drinking culture and Facebook. *Convergence: The Journal of Research into New Media Technologies, 20*(3), 259–275.

Carah, N., Meurk, C., and Hall, W. (2015). Profiling Hello Sunday Morning: Who are the participants? *International Journal of Drug Policy, 26*(2), 214–216.

Casswell, S. (2012). Current status of alcohol marketing policy – an urgent challenge for global governance. *Addiction, 107*, 478–485.

Chatterton, P., and Hollands, R. (2001). *Changing Our 'Toon': Youth, Nightlife and Urban Change in Newcastle*. Newcastle, UK: University of Newcastle upon Tyne.

Crawford, R. (2006). Health as meaningful social practice. *Health, 10*(4), 401–420.

Croghan, R., Griffin, C., Hunter, J., and Pheonix, A. (2006). Style failure: Consumption, identity and social exclusion. *Journal of Youth Studies, 9*(4), 463–478.

Cronin, A. (2000). Consumerism and 'compulsory individuality': Women, will and potential. In S. Ahmed, J. Kilby, C. Lury et al. (Eds.), *Transformations: Thinking Through Feminism* (pp. 273–287). London: Routledge.

Douglas, M. (1987). *Constructive Drinking: Perspectives from Anthropology*. New York: Cambridge University Press.

Egan, K., and Moreno, M. (2011). Alcohol references on undergraduate males' Facebook profiles. *American Journal of Men's Health, 5*(5), 413–420.

Ferguson, J. (2010). The uses of neoliberalism. *Antipode, 41*, 166–184.

Flew, T. (2009). The cultural economy moment? *Cultural Science, 2*(1), http://cultural-science.org/journal/index.php/culturalscience/article/view/23/79.

Flew, T. (2012). Michel Foucault's *The Birth of Biopolitics* and contemporary neo-liberalism debates. *Thesis Eleven, 108*(1), 44–65.

Foucault, M. (1991). Governmentality. In G. Burchell, C. Gordon, and P. Miller (Eds.), *The Foucault Effect: Studies in Governmentality* (pp. 87–104). Chicago: University of Chicago Press.

Goodwin, I., Griffin, C., Lyons, A., McCreanor, T., and Moewaka Barnes, H. (2016). Precarious popularity: Facebook drinking photos, the attention economy, and the regime of the branded self. *Social Media + Society, 2*(1), doi:10.1177/2056305116628889.

Goodwin, I., Lyons, A., Griffin, C., and McCreanor, T. (2014). Ending up online: Interrogating mediated youth drinking cultures. In A. Bennnet and B. Robards (Eds.), *Mediated Youth Cultures: The Internet, Belonging, and New Cultural Configurations.* (pp. 59–74). Basingstoke, UK: Palgrave Macmillan.

Gordon, R., Heim, D., and MacAskill, S. (2012). Rethinking drinking cultures: A review of drinking cultures and a reconstructed dimensional approach. *Public Health, 126*, 3–11.

Griffin, C., Bengry-Howell, A., Hackley, C., Mistral, W., and Szmigin, I. (2009a). 'Every Time I Do It I Absolutely Annihilate Myself': Loss of (self-)consciousness and loss of memory in young people's drinking narratives. *Sociology, 43*(3), 457–476.

Griffin, C., Szmigin, I., Bengry-Howell, A., Hackley, C., and Mistral, W. (2013). Inhabiting the contradictions: Hypersexual femininity and the culture of intoxication among young women in the UK. *Feminism and Psychology, 23*(2), 184–206.

Griffin, C., Szmigin, I., Hackley, C., Mistral, W., and Bengry-Howell, A. (2009b). The allure of belonging: Young people's drinking practices and collective identification. In M. Wetherell (Ed.), *Identity in the 21st Century: New Trends in Changing Times.* London: Palgrave.

Griffiths, R., and Casswell, S. (2010). Intoxigenic Digital Spaces? Youth, Social Networking Sites and Alcohol Marketing. *Drug and Alcohol Review, 29*, 525–530.

Grossberg, L. (2010). *Cultural Studies in the Future Tense.* Durham: Duke University Press.

Hall, S., and Jefferson, T. (2006). Once more around 'Resistance Through Rituals'. In S. Hall and T. Jefferson (Eds.), *Resistance Through Rituals: Youth Sub-cultures and Post War Britain* (2nd edn, pp. vii–xxxv). London: Routledge.

Harvey, D. (2005). *A Brief History of Neoliberalism.* Oxford: Oxford University Press.

Haydock, W. (2015a). The consumption, production and regulation of alcohol in the UK: The relevance of the ambivalence of the carnivalesque. *Sociology,* published online before print September 8, doi: 10.1177/0038038515588460.

Haydock, W. (2015b). Understanding English alcohol policy as a neoliberal condemnation of the carnivalesque. *Drugs: Education, Prevention and Policy, 22*(2), 143–149.

Hayward, K., and Hobbs, D. (2007). Beyond the binge in 'booze Britain': Market-led liminalization and the spectacle of binge drinking. *British Journal of Sociology, 58*(3), 437–456.

Hebden, R., Lyons, A., Goodwin, I., and McCreanor, T. (2015). 'When you add alcohol it gets that much better': University students, alcohol consumption and online drinking cultures. *Journal of Drug Issues, 45*(2), 214–226.

Hutton, F., Griffin, C., Lyons, A., Niland, P., and McCreanor, T. (2016). 'Tragic girls' and 'crack whores': Alcohol, femininity and Facebook. *Feminism and Psychology, 26*(1), 73–93.

Jernigan, D. (2009). The global alcohol industry: An overview. *Addiction, 104*, 6–12.

Kehily, M. (Ed.). (2007). *Understanding Youth: Perspectives, Identities and Practices.* London: Sage.

Livingstone, S. (2008). Taking risky opportunities in youthful content creation: Teenagers' use of SNSs for intimacy, privacy and self-expression. *New Media and Society, 10*(3), 393–411.

Loss, J., Lindacher, V., and Curbach, J. (2014). Online social networking sites—a novel setting for health promotion? *Health and Place, 26*, 161–170.

Lupton, D. (1999). *Risk.* London: Routledge.

Lyons, A., Goodwin, I., Griffin, C., McCreanor, T., and Moewaka Barnes, H. (2016). Facebook and the fun of drinking photos: Reproducing gendered regimes of power. *Social Media and Society,* in press.

Lyons, A., McCreanor, T., Goodwin, I., Griffin, C., Hutton, F., Moewaka Barnes, H., O'Carroll, D., Samu, L., Niland, P., and Vroman, K.-E. (2014). Youth drinking cultures in Aotearoa New Zealand. *Sites: New Series, 11*(2), 78–102.

Lyons, A., and Willott, S. (2008). Alcohol consumption, gender identities and women's changing social positions. *Sex Roles, 59*, 694–712.

MacLean, S. (2016). Alcohol and the constitution of friendship for young adults. *Sociology, 50*(1), 93–108.

McCreanor, T., Lyons, A., Griffin, C., Goodwin, I., Moewaka Barnes, H., and Hutton, F. (2013). Youth drinking cultures, social networking and alcohol marketing: Implications for public health. *Critical Public Health, 23*(1), 110–120.

McCreanor, T., Moewaka Barnes, H., Gregory, A., Kaiwai, H., and Borell, S. (2005). Consuming identities: Alcohol marketing and the comodification of youth. *Addiction Research and Theory, 13*(6), 579–590.

McCreanor, T., Moewaka Barnes, H., Kaiwai, H., Borell, S., and Gregory, A. (2008). Creating intoxigenic environments: Marketing alcohol to young people in Aotearoa New Zealand. *Social Science and Medicine*, *67*(6), 938–946.

Measham, F. (2004). The decline of ecstasy, the rise of 'binge' drinking and the persistence of pleasure. *Probation Journal*, *5*(4), 309–326.

Measham, F., and Brain, K. (2005). 'Binge' drinking, British alcohol policy and the new culture of intoxication. *Crime, Media, Culture*, *1*(3), 262–283.

Mercille, J. (2016). Neoliberalism and the alcohol industry in Ireland. *Space and Polity*, *20*(1), 58–74.

Moewaka Barnes, H., McCreanor, T., Goodwin, I., Lyons, A., Griffin, C., and Hutton, F. (2016). Alcohol and social media: Drinking and drunkenness while online. *Critical Public Health*, *26*(1), 62–76.

Monbiot, G. (2016, 15 April). Neoliberalism – the ideology at the root of all our problems. *The Guardian* 15 April 2016. Retrieved 15 June 2016 from www.theguardian.com/books/2016/apr/15/neoliberalism-ideology-problem-george-monbiot

Nicholls, J. (2012). Everyday, everywhere: Alcohol marketing and social media—current trends. *Alcohol and Alcoholism*, *47*(4), 486–493.

Niland, P., Lyons, A., Goodwin, I., and Hutton, F. (2013). 'Everyone can loosen up and get a bit of a buzz on': Young adults, alcohol and friendship practices. *International Journal of Drug Policy*, *24*(6), 530–537.

Niland, P., Lyons, A., Goodwin, I., and Hutton, F. (2014). 'See it doesn't look pretty does it?' Young adults' airbrushed drinking practices on Facebook. *Psychology and Health*, *29*(8), 877–895.

Niland, P., Lyons, A., Goodwin, I., and Hutton, F. (2015). Friendship work on Facebook: Young adults' understandings and practices of friendship. *Journal of Community and Applied Social Psychology*, *25*(2), 123–137.

Ouellette, L., and Hay, J. (2008). Makeover television, governmentality and the good citizen. *Continuum*, *22*(4), 471–484.

Petersen, A., and Lupton, D. (1996). *The New Public Health: Health and Self in the Age of Risk*. London: Sage.

Phelan, S. (2014). *Neoliberalism, Media, and the Political*. London: Palgrave Macmillan.

Rose, N., O'Malley, P., and Valverde, M. (2006). Governmentality. *Annual Review of Law and Social Science*, *2*, 83–104.

Sheehan, M., and Ridge, D. (2001). 'You become really close … you talk about the silly things you did, and we laugh': The role of binge drinking in female secondary students' lives. *Substance Use and Misuse*, *36*(3), 347–372.

Sven, B., and Carah, N. (2013). Alcohol brands on Facebook: The challenges of regulating brands on social media. *Journal of Public Affairs*, *13*(3), 272–281.

Szmigin, I., Bengry-Howell, A., Griffin, C., Hackley, C., and Mistral, W. (2011). Social marketing, individual responsibility and the 'culture of intoxication'. *European Journal of Marketing*, *45*(5), 759–779.

Szmigin, I., Griffin, C., Mistral, W., Bengry-Howell, A., Weale, L., and Hackley, C. (2008). Re-framing 'binge drinking' as calculated hedonism—Empirical evidence from the UK. *International Journal of Drug Policy*, *19*(5), 359–366.

Weaver, E., Horyniak, D., Jenkinson, R., Dietze, P., and Lim, M. (2013). 'Let's get wasted!' and other apps: Characteristics, acceptability, and use of alcohol-related smartphone applications. *JMIR mHealth uHealth*, *1*(1), e9. doi: 10.2196/mhealth.2709.

2 Social locations

Class, gender and young people's alcohol consumption in a digital world

Lin Bailey and Christine Griffin

Introduction

We provide an overview of how class and gender have been theorised in young people's drinking cultures across different countries. We consider how recent moral panics over young people's public drinking are often highly gendered and class-specific, problematising certain social groups of young people as 'flawed consumers' and 'at risk' groups. At present there is a small yet growing body of research exploring the gendered nature of young people's drinking cultures, but there is very little work exploring how gender intersects with social class. Even fewer studies have explored how gender and class play out in young people's online drinking cultures. We show that recent research is beginning to investigate the classed and gendered dimensions of youth drinking cultures on- and offline.

Theorising class (and gender) in neoliberal times

The concept of class is multifaceted and is generally understood as a means of positioning and classifying (young) people (Furlong and Cartmel, 1997). Youth researchers have drawn on theorists from Marx to Bourdieu to argue that young people's lived experiences and cultural practices in many national contexts are shaped by social class, framing their access to both economic and cultural resources (McCulloch et al., 2006; Reay, 1998; Willis, 1977). With the emergence of neoliberalism and debates over globalisation, social class has increasingly been understood as involving more than a system of stratification. Writers such as Skeggs, Tyler, Lawler, Ringrose and Walkerdine have posited a new cultural perspective, theorising class as profoundly constitutive in the neoliberal order. They see young people's lives as shaped through a process that is simultaneously classed, gendered and racialised, taking different forms in different local and national contexts (Lawler, 2005; Ringrose and Walkerdine, 2008; Skeggs, 2004; Tyler, 2015).

Neoliberalism is generally understood as a form of political and economic rationality characterised by privatisation, deregulation and attempts to 'roll back the state' from many areas of social provision (Hall, 2011). A key element of neoliberalism is the attempt to constitute new forms of subjectivity, especially around a particular form of individualism that has been viewed as a powerful (and new) form of governance (Rose, 1989). In the leisure sphere, it is argued that the neoliberal project involves an obligation to express one's 'true' self, to display oneself as a free and autonomous being, as if unfettered by the constraints of waged work and traditional social expectations (Ringrose and Walkerdine, 2008). Public displays of (bounded) pleasure, (calculated) hedonism and (managed) risk operate as evidence of one's freedom, especially in the context of young people's drinking practices (Griffin et al., 2009a; Szmigin et al., 2008). Behind this mirage of unfettered individualistic hedonism and 'free choice', long-standing patterns of inequality and social exclusion based around class, gender and race remain in force for young people in many parts of the world (Furlong and Cartmel, 1997; Harris, 2004; Nayak and Kehily, 2013; Reay, 1998; Sansone, 1995).

The neoliberal order exhorts subjects to act with moderation as active, rational individuals who are likely to be held responsible and accountable for their actions (Steinberg and Johnson, 2003). In relation to alcohol consumption, young people are called on to 'let go' and 'have fun' within a 'culture of intoxication' in affluent societies across the world (Measham and Brain, 2005). The conditions in which this heavy drinking culture of 'determined drunkenness' have emerged vary in different national and local contexts (Measham, 2006), but it tends to operate through opposing and simultaneous forces of seduction and repression, such that young people are seduced into a culture of normalised heavy drinking, whilst simultaneously being pathologised as disordered and disorderly 'binge drinkers' (Szmigin et al., 2008). McCreanor and colleagues have argued that the marketing of alcohol to young people within this culture of intoxication encourages 'intoxigenic identities' (McCreanor et al., 2005).

Alcohol consumption that is deemed 'inappropriate' in popular media and policy discourses constitutes individuals as 'flawed consumers' in need of regulation (Griffin et al., 2009b; Skeggs, 2004). The ways in which young drinkers are subject to social sanctions and state regulation is also shaped by class, race and gender. Tyler (2008) argues that certain 'social types' become publicly imagined as excessive and caricatured figures that are produced as representative of the working classes. These imagined figures are represented in emotive ways that (re)produce forms of (gendered and racialised) class disgust (Tyler, 2008). Such processes pathologise the alcohol consumption practices of working-class young people, which is most apparent in the ways working-class young women drinkers are frequently represented as excessive, immoral and out of control (Skeggs, 2005).

Working-class young people's drinking practices have been argued to epitomise the fears and fascinations of the middle class. In stark contrast, the middle class are constituted as moral, self-regulating and as ardent yet appropriately restrained consumers, accruing value as 'ideal' neoliberal subjects (Skeggs, 2004). Middle-class culture is constituted as 'right' and 'normal' whereas working-class culture is frequently pathologised as excessive, irresponsible and/or inadequate in comparison. As Lawler has argued in the British context: 'Class is being configured in terms of culture and identity, and "damaged" or "faulty" identities are conferred on working class people by middle class observers' (Lawler, 2005: 803).

Gender, class, religion and race feature in highly uneven, complex and contradictory ways in post-Fordist economies across the world. Reviewing the operation of social relations around youth and gender in relation to social inequalities across a range of countries, Nayak and Kehily (2013) argue that social inequalities are becoming reconfigured within affluent countries in late modernity and enmeshed with gender regulation and gender identities. They consider the ways in which the Western ideas of 'global community' and cosmopolitan citizenship are ambivalent and fragmented, suggesting that 'cultural flows are incorporated into local practices and given new meaning' (Nayak and Kehily, 2013: 160). Thus within the reconfigurations of the local and the cosmopolitan, marginalised young people rework localised identities through global consumption practices. The proliferation of online social networking sites has facilitated the growth of global consumer culture. Social networking sites such as Facebook provide a global system of networked interacting publics, providing tools that shape identities and normative consumption practices (boyd, 2012; van Dijck, 2013).

Griffiths and Casswell (2010) have argued that the widespread and increased marketing of alcohol to young people via social media produces 'intoxigenic digital spaces' which reinforce the pervasive culture of intoxication. Social media platforms now play a central role in many young people's drinking practices and drinking cultures (McCreanor et al., 2013). Many young adults in Western societies regularly engage in heavy drinking episodes with friends and share these practices via digital images and ongoing interactions on social media (Niland et al., 2014). Both alcohol consumption and social media use are valued sites of leisure and pleasure for young people, tied to the formation of identities and the maintenance of sociability (Lyons et al., 2015). Such practices are also gendered and classed, since gendered and classed identities are (re)enacted and (re)created through both alcohol consumption (Griffin et al., 2013) and social media practices (Cook and Hasmath, 2014; Niland et al., 2014). As drinking events and sociability have become routinely mediated through social networking sites, displaying, sharing and commenting on drinking practices between young people have produced novel, evolving negotiations around 'appropriate' and 'inappropriate' masculinities and femininities (Hutton et al., 2016). Relatively few studies have examined the ways in which young people themselves produce and make sense of online portrayals of alcohol consumption, the values and affective dimensions that are involved, and how these are gendered. The ways in which such social media practices are classed, and how they might differ for young people from different social class groups, has scarcely been explored at all, beyond overarching discussions of the 'digital divide' (Norris, 2011).

Moral panics and the problematisation of young drinkers

'Binge drinking': framing working-class youth as excessive drinkers in policy discourses and public health campaigns

Young people are hailed by the alcohol industry through increasingly sophisticated marketing techniques, yet at the same time they are constituted as a problematic group of alcohol consumers, especially in popular media representations, alcohol policies, and health and safety campaigns. Young drinkers are frequently vilified in popular media culture, or portrayed as a grotesque spectacle, fuelling moral panics around 'binge drinking' (Griffin et al., 2009a; Hackley et al., 2008; Hayward and Hobbs, 2007). Media representations of young people's drinking practices are frequently characterised by shock, outrage and intense concern across a range of international contexts (Brown and Gregg, 2012; Fry, 2010; Hackley et al., 2008; Hutton et al., 2013; Peralta et al., 2010). These include voyeuristic TV documentaries, newspaper 'scare stories' and social media sites that focus on representations of young people as excessive and irresponsible 'binge drinkers' (Griffin et al., 2009a).

This focus on problematic 'binge drinkers' is not a neutral process as far as class, gender and race is concerned. The anxieties (re)produced in government alcohol policy documents and health education campaigns are counter-balanced by the widespread representation of drunken working-class youth in structured reality TV shows and documentaries such as *Ibiza Uncovered*, first aired in the UK in the late 1990s, portraying British youth drinking heavily and engaging in hedonistic sexual behaviour on holidays abroad. More recent versions in the USA, such as *The Jersey Shore* which aired from 2009 to 2012, portray young men and women drinking heavily, participating in frequent sexual encounters and physical altercations. Currently on air in Britain is *The Only Way is Marbs*, portraying young people from Essex in South East England holidaying in Marbella in Spain. These shows draw viewers into voyeuristic positions as spectators to scenes of drunken excess and chaos, with predominantly heterosexual, white working-class young people operating as a source of entertainment to be ridiculed, derided and scorned (Wood and Skeggs, 2007).

Such discourses of panic about youth alcohol consumption tend to constitute young working-class people as particularly abject, disordered consumers (Tyler, 2013). As Lawler (2005) argues, this avoids troubling the investments made in middle-class young people as future 'ideal' neoliberal subjects. Kolind (2011) studied youth intoxication amongst 66 young people aged 15–16 years in Denmark and found that middle-class teenagers deliberately drink towards drunkenness in controlled settings where they can safely experiment with drinking. Whereas young people from working-class families engage in risk-taking behaviour within unbounded consumption, a form of consumption engaged in by young people who do not feel included in mainstream society (Kolind, 2011), or who are excluded and prohibited from mainstream consumption (Nayak, 2006). Engaging in unbounded risk taking and valuing excessive unbounded alcohol consumption can create a sense of agency and competence for young people who are in disempowered circumstances. However, the usual outcome is being labelled as an 'at risk' group which only serves to further marginalise these young people (Kolind, 2011).

Working-class cultural practices are constituted as a problem, and rather than considering such activities as products of the pressures of working-class existence, working-class people are criticised for the way they live their lives (Lawler, 2005). Desirable forms of alcohol consumption are linked to being a valuable citizen, and 'irresponsible' drinking constitutes individuals as problematic subjects (Haydock, 2014). Working-class young people's drinking is cast as especially irresponsible, so panics over young people's 'binge drinking' operate to reinforce the view of working-class youth (especially young women) as particularly difficult subjects (Skeggs, 2004, 2005; Tyler, 2008).

British Alcohol Strategy policy documents of 2004 and 2007 and the more recent 'Responsibility Deal' of 2012 oriented government policies around a neoliberal discourse of responsibility. This built on the panic over youthful 'binge drinkers' identified as a particular focus of concern by the then New Labour Prime Minister Tony Blair (Cabinet Office, 2007; Prime Minister's Strategy Unit, 2004). The 2007 Alcohol Strategy policy document 'Safe, Sensible, Social' broadened this discourse of responsibility to include families, schools and other community representatives, such that individuals' drinking behaviour could be attributed to personal responsibility and community obligation (Hackley et al., 2008; Laverty et al., 2015). This obscured the responsibility of the state and of alcohol producers, marketers and retailers, who make considerable financial gain from young people's alcohol consumption. Locating families and community representatives as responsible for young people's drinking constructed those lacking resources as failures, constituting young people and communities in difficult circumstances as the primary perpetrators of problematic drinking.

In the UK context, Haydock has argued that government drinking policies are a key way in which class is constituted (Haydock, 2014). Within the British government's 2012 Alcohol Strategy document, a certain type of drinker is constituted as a 'binge drinker'. Even though 'binge drinking' is discussed as a pervasive problem, it is constituted in classed terms as an activity engaged in by particular social groups. In the case of alcohol regulation different forms of inequality become implicated in 'binge drinking' and drunken behaviour in a way that condemns young working-class people as particularly problematic and irresponsible drinkers (Haydock, 2014). This has striking similarities with National Alcohol Strategies in Australia and New Zealand, where considerable attention is paid to young people as 'excessive' drinkers, focusing on their presumed lack of personal responsibility (Brown and Gregg, 2012; Hutton et al., 2013; Waitt et al., 2011).

The constitution of young people as irresponsible drinkers is also clearly displayed in health education campaigns. For example, the National Binge Drinking Campaign (2008) in Australia represented young people between the ages of 15 and 25 as potentially irresponsible drinkers. The campaign title 'Don't turn a night out into a nightmare' exhorted young people to be responsible consumers, including a series of posters portraying highly intoxicated young people in a variety of disastrous predicaments entitled 'What are you doing to yourself?'. Haydock (2014) points out that these campaigns do not so much focus on crime and risk management or even health risks but rather are designed to engender a sense of reflection and disgust in young drinkers. The intention is to improve young people's self-discipline and reduce their alcohol consumption by drawing on neoliberal discourses of individual self-regulation.

Dimensions of class and gender in contemporary moral panics

The gendered dimensions of contemporary moral panics over youthful drinking are enmeshed with class in manifold ways, since drinking and drunkenness retain their traditional association with hegemonic masculinity, and female drinking, especially to excess, is still constructed as unfeminine (Griffin et al., 2009a; Willott and Lyons, 2012). Women's heavy drinking is linked with working-class femininity, whilst traditional 'hard-drinking' remains associated with working-class masculinity (Bell, 2008; Day et al., 2003, 2004; Griffin et al., 2013; Skeggs, 2005).

The 1990s saw the emergence of the reviled figure of the 'ladette' in British popular culture (Jackson and Tinkler, 2007). These young women were represented as drinking to excess, as (too) independent and distinctly unfeminine, as well as inappropriately masculine. Redden and Brown (2010) have pointed to the classed dimension of this derided figure in their analysis of the UK TV series *Ladette to Lady*. UK newspaper articles have frequently associated young women's drinking with criminal activities, reckless behaviour and a wide range of health problems associated with normative femininity, reinforcing the construction of women's drinking as irresponsible and distasteful (Day et al., 2004; Jackson and Tinkler, 2007).

More recently, young women have been expected to adopt a particular 'look' for going out drinking in the night-time economy (hereafter NTE), involving a form of hyper-sexual femininity, including short revealing outfits, heavy makeup and high-heeled shoes (Bailey, 2012; Bailey et al., 2015; Bell, 2008). Working-class women have generally been associated with such displays of hyper-sexual femininity, which are further condemned when linked with their heavy drinking. Working-class women's femininities are constructed as lacking, abject and 'what not to be', set against the feminine 'ideal' embodied by the normative image of 'respectable' white middle-class femininity (Redden and Brown, 2010; Ringrose and Walkerdine, 2008). Skeggs (1997, 2005) has argued that white and black working-class women have long been constituted as sexual objects, as sexually available and lacking the respectability associated with white middle-class femininity.

Watts et al. (2015) have demonstrated how UK health campaign advertisements blame and shame young women drinkers in particular, exhibiting gendered double standards. The 2008 'Know Your Limits' campaign, funded by the UK Home

Office, had the strap line: 'You wouldn't start a night like this…so why end it that way?' (BBC, 2008). A dominant narrative portrayed a dishevelled young woman covered in vomit, with ripped clothes and smudged makeup (Hackley et al., 2011; Watts et al., 2015). Such images construct drunken young women as transgressing normative femininity and, although not explicitly classed, they resonate with wider circulating discourses in which young white working-class heterosexual women are represented as what Skeggs has termed 'the constitutive limit' of excess (Skeggs, 2004). Likewise gendered double standards are embedded in cautionary tales in Australian campaigns where depictions of drunken young women are often linked to victimised sex, insinuating women's drunkenness is constituted as responsible for actions performed by men (Brown and Gregg, 2012).

Considerable public attention is focused on young women's 'excessive' alcohol consumption, especially online (Dobson, 2014). Websites and social media platforms devoted to representations of drunken celebrities and non-celebrities alike display disproportionately more images of young women compared to young men (Bell, 2008). Young working-class female celebrities such as Kerry Katatona and the late Amy Winehouse appear as scapegoats in moral panics surrounding young women's drinking more generally (Bell, 2008). Perceived lack of morality is inherent in the pathologisation of working-class young women's behaviour and this can be seen clearly in moral judgements concerning young working-class female celebrities whose 'wild excessive' behaviour is frequently constituted as symptomatic of 'mental illness' beyond the bounds of normative, respectable femininity (Bell, 2008). Such representations frequently constitute working-class women who have become celebrities as exemplars of female 'bad behaviour'. Thus 'binge-drinking, vulgarity, sexual excess and single motherhood predominate in the construction of both celebrity and "real life" women as "offensive"' (Tyler and Bennett, 2010: 388).

Linking the older figure of the 'ladette' with more recent concerns over 'hyper sexy girls', Dobson (2014: 253) has argued that moral panics in contemporary popular media discourses about young womanhood are frequently organised in a 'binary-oppositional fashion'. That is, femininity is increasingly constructed around 'notions of (hyper, hetero-normative) "sexiness" … aspects of masculinity, namely sexual hedonism and social, drinking-centred hedonism [that] have conditionally opened up to young women' (p. 253). Dobson argues that while both the figure of the 'sexy girl' and the 'laddish girl' are 'to some extent deplored and constructed as "excessive" and "transgressive" in recent media discourses, they are also both normalised and publicly imag(in)ed through such discourses as central post-feminist paradigms of young womanhood' (Dobson, 2014: 253). Dobson's point is important here. She shows how these two linked representations of unacceptable and inappropriate femininity can be simultaneously derided and operate as normative figures. Alcohol consumption, class and gender form central elements of both the 'sexy girl' and the 'ladette'.

While young working-class women drinkers are frequently represented as a threat to the gender order through exhibiting 'wild' unfeminine behaviour in a perceived masculine domain, young working-class male drinkers have also figured in contemporary moral panics. Drinking to excess is still associated with traditional and working-class forms of masculinity (de Visser and Smith, 2007; Tomsen, 1997) and concerns over working-class young men's drunkenness are linked to wider fears about the state of contemporary society (Thurnell-Read, 2013). As an example, the 'lager lout' emerged from earlier media discourses of anxiety and disgust reflected in moral panics over 'football hooliganism' in the UK during the 1970s and 1980s (Cohen, 2011). Thomas Thurnell-Read (2013) has argued that moral panics centred on the feared figure of the 'lager lout' have shifted to focus on young male 'binge drinkers'.

Such discourses of moral panic have seldom focused on the heavy drinking practices of upper- and upper-middle-class young men such as the public school Oxbridge educated members of the current British Conservative government. Although there is a long history of ritualised drinking to excess amongst upper-class young men, this often takes place in the more secluded spaces of university colleges or private school grounds. In the event of more public displays of drunken excess, this elite group have the money to buy themselves out of trouble (Ronay, 2008). The upper class as a whole is seldom subject to the same level of horrified moral outrage and disgust that has been directed at the drinking practices of white working-class youth (Nayak, 2006).

Violence is frequently represented as an inevitable outcome of rowdy groups of young working-class men out drinking in the NTE. The contribution of those involved in the production, policing and marketing of the NTE remains largely invisible (Hackley et al., 2008; Hobbs et al., 2005). Anxieties around crime and economic displacement have operated to marginalise some young working-class men from mainstream consumption (Nayak, 2006). Young men who engage in excessive drinking within 'street culture' as an alternative to mainstream consumption are aware of their stigmatisation and counteract this by exhibiting localised forms of hegemonic masculinity (McKenzie, 2015; Nayak, 2006). Discourses of fear and anxiety centred around marginalised white and black working-class young men rest on a misrecognition by white middle-class culture of how respect and value are accrued from the exhibition of 'tough', 'street' masculinities (McKenzie, 2015).

Classed and gendered young consumers

Drinking and young femininities and masculinities

Rural pubs have been identified as masculine spaces in which traditional forms of masculinity can be enacted and where young women are particularly unwelcome, as demonstrated by two studies in the UK and New Zealand (Campbell, 2000; Leyshon, 2005). The recent emergence of a metropolitan urban NTE in many affluent societies around the world alongside the widespread culture of drinking to intoxication has been linked to the feminisation of such traditional drinking spaces (Jayne et al., 2008).

There are some local, regional and national variations in the culture of intoxication as a normative form of youth drinking practice. For example, Beccaria and colleagues (2015) demonstrate that drinking to get drunk is not a pervasive norm amongst young drinkers in contemporary Italian society, unlike in many Northern European countries, and in New Zealand, Australia and the USA (Beccaria et al., 2015). Drunkenness is seen as negative, as spoiling one's fun, indicating that young Italians have some resistance to the influence of a global drinking culture. Young Italians see 'binge drinking' as only being 'tipsy', which is viewed as an acceptable form of drinking while maintaining a fairly good level of awareness and control. These terms are used in different ways by their Nordic peers who use the term 'binge drinking' as a synonym for heavier and less acceptable forms of drunkenness. Unfortunately, this study pays little attention to gender or class.

Despite the recent feminisation of the NTE, public spaces are still predominantly masculine domains. Nayak's (2006) study in Newcastle, UK, elucidates how working-class masculine excess is celebrated among working-class young men, especially through circuit drinking as a conspicuous form of consumption in the NTE. De Visser and McDonnell (2012) conducted a mixed methods study with 731 English university students aged 18–25. Across both sets of data, gendered stereotypes for drinking and drunkenness persisted and young men and young women were judgemental of women's 'binge drinking' and drunkenness. Likewise, in a study of young men's drinking in Scotland a gendered double standard was mobilised to stigmatise female 'binge drinkers' and young men also made a specific distinction between their drinking practices and the ways young women drink (Mullen et al., 2007). Furthermore, in Clayton and Humberstone's (2006) study of university football player's talk, young women drinkers were frequently disparaged in particularly negative and sometimes alarmingly derogatory ways.

Research on young women's drinking in South West England found that young white middle-class women construct women drinkers as a heterogeneous group based around classed distinctions (Bailey, 2012; Bailey et al., 2015; Rudolfsdottir and Morgan, 2009). Young women represented as 'problem' drinkers and disparaged for displaying 'excessive' heterosexuality are positioned via coded terms as working class (Bailey, 2012; Bailey et al., 2015; Rudolfsdottir and Morgan, 2009). However, Watts et al. (2015) report that research indicates that young professional women drink more alcohol than working-class young women – and yet working-class young women drinkers are the focus of more intense moral condemnation and concern. In Bailey's (2012) discourse analytic study, 24 women aged 19–24 participated in friendship group discussions. Middle-class young women in this study expressed anxieties over being viewed and treated as working-class young women when out at night drinking, whereas the working-class young women expressed anxieties concerning an awareness of the judgements of others when out drinking in the NTE. Middle-class young women apportioned blame towards working-class young women's drinking practices, deriding their 'unfeminine' behaviour and 'inappropriate' displays of heterosexuality. The ways in which blame was attributed to young working-class women drinkers for men's behaviour towards young middle-class women exonerated men as the perpetrators of disrespectful behaviour.

Attempting to negotiate respectable femininity whilst engaging in heavy drinking in the NTE appears to be creating stronger classed differences among young women (Bailey, 2012). This is linked to the ways in which the high levels of alcohol consumption associated with hedonistic, reckless participation in the NTE situates young women's drinking within postfeminist discourses. Postfeminist discourses of empowerment and liberation are located within a neoliberal ideology of autonomous, compulsory individual consumption (Gill, 2008; McRobbie, 2007). International qualitative research, for example, in Canada (Kovac and Trussel, 2015), Ireland (MacNeela and Bredin, 2010), Australia (Waitt et al., 2011) and the UK (Stepney, 2015), indicates that young women seek to create a desirable self through alcohol consumption, often constituting drunkenness as enabling confidence and boldness. However, this is confounded by the ways in which normative restrained and respectable femininities (Skeggs, 1997) are still constituted as desirable (Kovac and Trussel, 2015; Stepney, 2015). The latter are set in conflict with 'up for it' hypersexual postfeminist femininities. As Griffin and colleagues have argued: 'young women are called on to "have fun" *as if* they are "free" and "liberated" subjects, and *as if* pervasive sexual double standards have faded away' (Griffin et al., 2013: 198, original emphases). Within postfeminist discourse young women are called on to engage in heavy drinking while being hyper-(hetero)sexual, yet still adhere to the norms of respectable femininity. This draws young women into an impossible dilemma in which they risk being condemned whatever they do, as either 'boring' or 'sluttish' (Bailey et al., 2015; Griffin et al., 2013). Ironically alcohol is often used as a tool to attempt to navigate these dilemmas and contradictions (Stepney, 2015).

A recent qualitative study involving 12 young professional women in London aged 21 to 35 found that they viewed drinking high levels of alcohol in relatively positive – and gendered – terms (Watts et al., 2015). Drinking was associated with giving them confidence, strengthening friendships and perceiving oneself as attractive and glamorous. To abstain or drink very little alcohol was represented in negative terms as being 'boring' and 'weak'. Conversely these young women also reported feeling shame about their drinking, and were aware of criticism towards young women's drinking, especially by the media. These young white, middle-class professional women were caught between conflicting media representations, such that alcohol was advertised to women as enabling a desirable self, in contrast to health campaigns that shame women over their drinking. Heavy drinking was seen as a way to attain a form of masculinised power and status. This was located within the culture of intoxication, associated with pressures to drink heavily, reinforcing the notion of drinking as a masculine practice (Watts et al., 2015).

The ability to 'hold' one's drink and retain signs of bodily composure while drunk are associated with traditional hegemonic masculinity (Hunt et al., 2016; Hunt et al., 2005; Peralta, 2007). However, for young men drinking within the culture of intoxication, and especially in relation to initiation or hazing rituals or 'stag tourism', the ties between drinking and maintaining a bounded, controlled male body are not so clear cut (Thurnell-Read, 2013). The ability to 'hold your drink' is often ambiguous within the culture of intoxication, where, in gendered ways, visible displays of drunkenness are accepted as expected behaviour for young women and men on a night out (Mullen et al., 2007). Furthermore, for many young men and women, the loss of control and loss of memory associated with heavy drinking offers a highly valued means of bonding with close friends and a sense of collective identity and belonging (Griffin et al., 2009a).

Class, youth, drinking and sexualisation: a 'spectacle' at home and abroad

Within affluent countries, young people living in constrained economic circumstances and engaging in unbounded drinking are often construed as a threat to civilised society, held up as 'the shame of the nation' and as convenient scapegoats to deflect blame away from government policies and practices that perpetuate inequalities (McKenzie, 2015). The 'shame of the nation' discourse is mobilised in media representations of young people abroad who engage in reckless drinking practices. In the UK, such youth groups are frequently referred to as 'Brits abroad': a term associated with images of predominantly white working-class British youth engaging in heavy drinking, drug use, promiscuity and other risky behaviours, especially whilst on holiday in the Balearic Islands (Briggs and Turner, 2012). Danish party package agencies at Sunny Beach, Bulgaria promote the same type of excessive behaviour that young people engage in when holidaying in Ibiza (Hesse et al., 2008; Tutenges and Sandberg, 2013).

Young people who have the means to afford a holiday abroad represent their hedonistic activities as enabling them to 'be who they want to be' (Briggs and Turner, 2012). They also tend to repackage negative consequences of their activities as exciting adventurous holiday experiences to be displayed and shared on social media and for retrospective retelling when they return home (Briggs and Turner, 2012). According to Tutenges and Sandberg (2013), young Danish holiday makers treat heavy drinking as commonplace, but it is the acts of transgression whilst drinking that become retold as spectacular drinking stories. Tutenges and Sandberg (2013, 2014) argue that drinking stories are no longer male dominated, since young women also engage in retelling stories of drunken abandonment and excess. However, others have countered that it is imperative to consider the gendered and sexualised dimensions within drinking stories of transgression (Griffin, 2014).

Sexual double standards and misogynous practices appear to be taken for granted by young people in the narratives reproduced in Briggs and Turner's (2012) and Tutenges and Sandberg's (2013) studies of British and Danish young people's drinking practices on holiday. This has much in common with recent debates in the UK about so-called 'lad culture'. The latter is associated with 'retro-sexist' behaviours which have been identified in UK student social and sexual lives, especially within the student drinking culture. Within this young and predominantly white and middle-class culture, male students compete to achieve the highest levels of alcohol consumption, to recount the wildest drinking stories and to notch up the highest sexual conquests, whilst representing women as sexually available in highly insulting ways (Phipps and Young, 2015). 'Lad culture' intersects with neoliberal postfeminist femininities in problematic ways, especially as young women are called on to be sexually assertive and hypersexual whilst young men are engaging in misogynist behaviours, mobilising sexual double standards (Phipps and Young, 2015).

The sexualised British NTE, where lap dancing clubs are often located alongside young people's bars and clubs, has been exported to holiday resorts that attract young people thus calling into question the extent to which young women may exercise 'freedom' in these resorts (Measham and Radcliffe, 2014). In Ibiza cheap easily accessible drugs, heavy drinking and sex, including female prostitution, are aggressively promoted and wild transgressive behaviour is condoned (Briggs and Turner, 2012). However, women's transgressive behaviour is treated differently within the accounts in Briggs and Turner's (2012) and Tutenges and Sandberg's (2013) studies. Here women were referred to in terms of sexual body parts while women's sexual behaviour was discussed in highly offensive ways. Women's own accounts pointed towards experiences of sexual groping and abusive behaviour by men.

Young people's classed, gendered drinking and online subjectivities

Youth drinking cultures are now increasingly played out online, in addition to the public spaces of the NTE and the private sphere of the home (McCreanor et al., 2013). Online social networking sites such as Facebook play a powerful role in shaping normative behaviour and providing tools for displaying 'connected' identities (van Dijck, 2013). Relatively few studies have explored the role of young people's drinking practices on social media, but there are some exceptions (e.g. Brown and Gregg, 2012; Lyons et al., 2015; Ridout et al., 2012). The growth of the culture of intoxication has coincided with the rise in the use of social networking sites which have altered traditional patterns of identity construction (Ridout et al., 2012). Promoting and branding the self has also become a normalised, accepted phenomenon (van Dijck, 2013). Drinking identities are carefully displayed and portrayed online by young people (Niland et al., 2014). Thus portraying oneself as a drinker on social networking sites is considered to be important and socially desirable for many young people, contributing to the normalisation of heavy drinking (Ridout et al., 2012). Social networking sites also provide a way for alcohol marketing to infiltrate youth cultures and shape youth identities. Furthermore while young people are enhancing their drinking identities online, they are often unaware that they are being targeted by alcohol companies (Lyons et al., 2015).

Facebook profiles publicly display created selves and lifestyles. On Facebook, tagging is adding a friend's profile name to a photo or status update and young people regularly 'untag' themselves if they do not like how they are depicted in visual and textual alcohol-related content posted by others. This demonstrates an implicit sanctioning of alcohol-related identity placements by others in tagged photos that remain linked to their profile (Ridout et al., 2012). Lyons et al. (2015) found that in terms of drinking practices Facebook photos were carefully managed to portray drinking selves in a positive way. Thus, photos of drunken images are carefully selected to portray drunkenness as sociable and fun, instead of portraying drunkenness as negative and unattractive. However, these 'airbrushed' images normalise and reinforce drinking as always pleasurable without harmful consequences (Lyons et al., 2015; Niland et al., 2014). This is also a highly gendered, racialised and classed practice (Dobson, 2014; Goodwin et al., 2016; Hutton et al., 2016). However, there is a dearth of research exploring these variations in the social locations of users in online drinking cultures.

Brown and Gregg (2012) contribute to addressing the lack of research exploring gendered ways of using online drinking cultures in their study of young women's Facebook use. In particular, young women used Facebook for accounts of mock regret about the previous night's drinking activities, as well as for displaying friendship, belonging, fun and adventurous drinking identities. Facebook also provides a space for engaging with the anticipatory pleasures of the drinking event and the young women routinely used status updates to begin to share the excitement of a night out via anticipatory intent (Brown and Gregg, 2012).

Part of the pleasure of sharing the before, during and after of drinking events online may be concerned with being part of a wider drinking culture, but Brown and Gregg (2012) point out that the gendered social and cultural contexts are also key. It may be that young women respond to circumstances affecting their participation in other sectors of the public sphere through heavy public drinking. Within postfeminist consumer culture, sharing drinking stories and drinking escapades on Facebook is a means for self-marketing using available cultural resources (Goodwin et al., 2016).

Young women's participation in public drinking and their apparent freedom to do so has arisen at the same time as their participation in the paid labour market. However, as Brown and Gregg (2012) argue, the working-class young women especially targeted as cause for concern are those with the least financial capital or chances to succeed, hence displaying drinking on Facebook as a lifestyle choice may be an alternative way of expressing hopes and aspirations. It may be possible that the pleasure working-class young women gain from dramatic and funny drinking episodes and the extended pleasure in re-telling these drinking stories are embedded in a desire to escape from the lack of opportunities and the boredom of their everyday lives (Waitt et al., 2011).

Social networking sites offer ways to extend young people's pleasures around drinking, elucidating the ways in which drinking is far more meaningful for young people than simply as a means of experiencing altered states of intoxication. We have shown that young people make sense of their own drinking practices and the drinking practices of others in classed and gendered ways. The double standards inherent within these understandings are situated within socio-cultural reconfigurations of gender and class and globalised neoliberal ideologies, where young people's drinking is subject to social judgements and moral panic shaped by dimensions of class and gender. Young people's drinking practices take place in a public arena and in the last few years social networking sites have significantly increased the scope of this public arena. The nexus of drinking cultures and social networking use is a vital area for research. However, we have also shown that there is scant research exploring the intersections of gender and class in relation to young people's drinking and online social networking practices.

References

Bailey, L. (2012). Young women and the culture of intoxication: Negotiating classed femininities in the postfeminist context. Unpublished PhD, University of Bath.

Bailey, L., Griffin, C., and Shankar, A. (2015). 'Not a good look': Impossible dilemmas for young women negotiating the culture of intoxication in the United Kingdom. *Substance Use and Misuse, 50*, 747–758.

BBC. (2008, 17 June). Binge-drinking adverts launched. Retrieved 4 April 2014, from http://news.bbc.co.uk/2/hi/uk_news/7457746.stm

Beccaria, F., Petrilli, E., and Rolando, S. (2015). Binge drinking vs drunkenness: The questionable threshold of excess for young Italians. *Journal of Youth Studies, 18*(7–8), 823–838.

Bell, E. (2008). From bad girl to mad girl: British female celebrity, reality products, and the pathologisation of pop-feminism. *Genders, 48*, 1–20.

boyd, d. (2012). Social network sites as networked publics: Affordances, dynamics and implications. In Z. Papacharissi (Ed.), *A Networked Self: Identity, Community and Culture on Social Network Sites* (pp. 119–142). New York: Routledge.

Briggs, D., and Turner, T. (2012). Understanding British youth behaviors on holiday in Ibiza. *International Journal of Culture, Tourism and Hospitality Research, 6*(1), 81–90.

Brown, R., and Gregg, M. (2012). The pedagogy of regret: Facebook, binge drinking and young women. *Continuum: Journal of Media and Cultural Studies, 26*(3), 357–369.

Cabinet Office. (2007). *Safe, Sensible, Social: The Next Steps in the National Alcohol Strategy*. London: HMG Cabinet Office.

Campbell, H. (2000). The glass phallus: Pub(lic) masculinity and drinking in rural New Zealand. *Rural Sociology, 65*(4), 562–581.

Clayton, B., and Humberstone, B. (2006). Men's talk: A (pro)feminist analysis of male university football players' discourse. *International Review for the Sociology of Sport, 41*(3–4), 295–316.

Cohen, S. (2011). *Folk Devils and Moral Panics* (3rd edn). London: Routledge.

Cook, J., and Hasmath, R. (2014). The discursive construction and performance of gendered identity on social media. *Current Sociology, 62*(7), 975–993.

Day, K., Gough, B., and McFadden, M. (2003). Women who drink and fight: A discourse analysis of working-class women's talk. *Feminism and Psychology, 13*(2), 141–158.

Day, K., Gough, B., and McFadden, M. (2004). 'Warning! Alcohol can seriously damage your feminine health': A discourse analysis of recent British newspaper coverage of women and drinking. *Feminist Media Studies, 4*(2), 165–183.

de Visser, R., and McDonnell, E. (2012). 'That's OK. He's a guy': A mixed-methods study of gender double-standards for alcohol use. *Psychology and Health, 27*(5), 618–639.

de Visser, R., and Smith, J. (2007). Young men's ambivalence toward alcohol. *Social Science and Medicine, 64*(2), 350–362.

Dobson, A. (2014). 'Sexy' and 'laddish' girls: Unpacking complicity between two cultural imag(inations)es of young femininity. *Feminist Media Studies, 14*(2), 253–269.

Fry, M. (2010). Countering consumption in a culture of intoxication. *Journal of Marketing Management, 26*(13–14), 1279–1294.

Furlong, A., and Cartmel, F. (1997). *Young People and Social Change: Individualization and Risk in Late Modernity*. Buckingham: Open University Press.

Gill, R. (2008). Culture and subjectivity in neoliberal and postfeminist times. *Subjectivity, 25*, 432–445.

Goodwin, I., Griffin, C., Lyons, A., McCreanor, T., and Moewaka Barnes, H. (2016). Precarious popularity: Facebook drinking photos, the attention economy, and the regime of the branded self. *Social Media + Society, 2*(1).

Griffin, C. (2014). Significant absences: The luxury of being less critical. *International Journal of Drug Policy, 25*, 354–355.

Griffin, C., Bengry-Howell, A., Hackley, C., Mistral, W., and Szmigin, I. (2009a). 'Every Time I Do It I Absolutely Annihilate Myself': Loss of (self-)consciousness and loss of memory in young people's drinking narratives. *Sociology, 43*(3), 457–476.

Griffin, C., Szmigin, I., Bengry-Howell, A., Hackley, C., and Mistral, W. (2013). Inhabiting the contradictions: Hypersexual femininity and the culture of intoxication among young women in the UK. *Feminism and Psychology, 23*(2), 184–206.

Griffin, C., Szmigin, I., Hackley, C., Mistral, W., and Bengry-Howell, A. (2009b). The allure of belonging: Young people's drinking practices and collective identification. In M. Wetherell (Ed.), *Identity in the 21st Century: New Trends in Changing Times* (pp. 213–230). London: Palgrave.

Griffiths, R., and Casswell, S. (2010). Intoxigenic digital spaces? Youth, social networking sites and alcohol marketing. *Drug and Alcohol Review, 29*, 525–530.

Hackley, C., Bengry-Howell, A., Griffin, C., Mistral, W., and Szmigin, I. (2011). Young people's binge drinking constituted as a deficit of individual self-control in UK government alcohol policy. In C. Candlin and J. Crichton (Eds.), *Discourses of Deficit* (pp. 293–310). London: Palgrave Macmillan.

Hackley, C., Griffin, C., Szmigin, I., Mistral, W., and Bengry-Howell, A. (2008). The discursive constitution of the UK alcohol problem in Safe, Sensible, Social: A discussion of policy implications. *Drugs: Education, Prevention and Policy, 15*(S1), 65–78.

Hall, S. (2011). The neo-liberal revolution. *Cultural Studies, 25*(6), 705–728.

Harris, A. (2004). *Future Girl: Young Women in the Twenty-first Century*. London: Routledge.

Haydock, W. (2014). '20 tins of Stella for a fiver': The making of class through Labour and coalition government alcohol policy. *Capital and Class, 38*(3), 583–600.

Hayward, K., and Hobbs, D. (2007). Beyond the binge in 'booze Britain': Market-led liminalization and the spectacle of binge drinking. *British Journal of Sociology, 58*(3), 437–456.

Hesse, M., Tutenges, S., Schliewe, S., and Reinholdt, T. (2008). Party package travel: Alcohol use and related problems in a holiday resort: A mixed methods study. *BMC Public Health, 8*(1), 351–359.

Hobbs, D., Winlow, S., Hadfield, P., and Lister, S. (2005). Violent hypocrisy: Governance and the night-time economy. *European Journal of Criminology, 2*(2), 161–183.

Hunt, G., Antin, T., Bjonness, J., and Ettorre, E. (2016). The increasing visibility of gender in the alcohol and drugs fields. In T. Kolind, B Thome and Geoffrey Hunt (Eds), *The Handbook of Drug and Alcohol Studies: Social Science Approaches* (in press). London: Sage.

Hunt, G., MacKenzie, K., and Joe-Laidler, K. (2005). Alcohol and masculinity: The case of ethnic youth gangs. In T. Wilson (Ed.), *Drinking Cultures: Alcohol and Identity* (pp. 225–254). Oxford: Berg.

Hutton, F., Griffin, C., Lyons, A., Niland, P., and McCreanor, T. (2016). 'Tragic girls' and 'crack whores': Alcohol, femininity and Facebook. *Feminism and Psychology*, *26*(1), 73–93.

Hutton, F., Wright, S., and Saunders, E. (2013). Cultures of intoxication: Young women, alcohol, and harm reduction. *Contemporary Drug Problems*, *40*, 451–480.

Jackson, C., and Tinkler, P. (2007). 'Ladettes' and 'modern girls': 'Troublesome' young femininities. *The Sociological Review*, *55*(2), 251–272.

Jayne, M., Valentine, G., and Holloway, S. (2008). Fluid boundaries-British binge drinking and European civility: Alcohol and the production and consumption of public space. *Space and Polity*, *12*(1), 81–100.

Kolind, T. (2011). Young people, drinking and social class. Mainstream and counterculture in the everyday practice of Danish adolescents. *Journal of Youth Studies*, *14*(3), 295–314.

Kovac, L., and Trussel, D. (2015). 'Classy and never trashy': Young women's experiences of nightclubs and the construction of gender and sexuality. *Leisure Sciences*, *37*(3), 195–209.

Laverty, L., Robinson, J., and Holdsworth, C. (2015). Gendered forms of responsibility and control in teenagers' views of alcohol. *Journal of Youth Studies*, *18*(6), 794–808.

Lawler, S. (2005). Introduction: Class, culture and identity. *Sociology*, *39*(5), 797–806.

Leyshon, M. (2005). No place for a girl: Rural youth, pubs and the performance of masculinity. In J. Little and C. Morris (Eds.), *Critical Studies in Rural Gender Issues* (pp. 104–122). Aldershot: Ashgate.

Lyons, A., Goodwin, I., McCreanor, T., and Griffin, C. (2015). Social networking and young adults' drinking practices: Innovative qualitative methods for health behavior research. *Health Psychology*, *34*(4), 293–302.

MacNeela, P., and Bredin, O. (2010). Keeping your balance: Freedom and regulation in female university students' drinking practices. *Journal of Health Psychology*, *16*(2), 284–293.

McCreanor, T., Lyons, A., Griffin, C., Goodwin, I., Moewaka Barnes, H., and Hutton, F. (2013). Youth drinking cultures, social networking and alcohol marketing: Implications for public health. *Critical Public Health*, *23*(1), 110–120.

McCreanor, T., Moewaka Barnes, H., Gregory, A., Kaiwai, H., and Borell, S. (2005). Consuming identities: Alcohol marketing and the comodification of youth. *Addiction Research and Theory*, *13*(6), 579–590.

McCulloch, A., Stewart, A., and Lovegreen, N. (2006). 'We just hang out together': Youth cultures and social class. *Journal of Youth Studies*, *9*(5), 539–556.

McKenzie, L. (2015). *Getting By: Estates, Class and Culture in Austerity Britain*. Bristol: Policy Press.

McRobbie, A. (2007). Top girls? Young women and the post-feminist sexual contract. *Cultural Studies*, *21*(4–5), 718–737.

Measham, F. (2006). The new policy mix: Alcohol, harm minimisation, and determined drunkenness in contemporary society. *International Journal of Drug Policy*, *17*, 258–268.

Measham, F., and Brain, K. (2005). 'Binge' drinking, British alcohol policy and the new culture of intoxication. *Crime, Media, Culture*, *1*(3), 262–283.

Measham, F., and Radcliffe, P. (2014). Repositioning the cultural: Intoxicating stories in social context. *International Journal of Drug Policy, 25*, 346–347.

Mullen, K., Watson, J., Swift, J., and Black, D. (2007). Young men, masculinity and alcohol. *Drugs, Education, Prevention and Policy, 14*(2), 151–165.

Nayak, A. (2006). Displaced masculinities: Chavs, youth and class in the post industrial city. *Sociology, 40*(5), 813–831.

Nayak, A., and Kehily, J. (2013). *Gender, Youth and Culture: Global Masculinities and Femininities* (2nd edn). London: Palgrave Macmilan.

Niland, P., Lyons, A., Goodwin, I., and Hutton, F. (2014). 'See it doesn't look pretty does it?' Young adults' airbrushed drinking practices on Facebook. *Psychology and Health, 29*(8), 877–895.

Norris, P. (2011). *Digital Divide: Civic Engagement, Information Poverty, and the Internet Worldwide*. Cambridge: Cambridge University Press.

Peralta, R. (2007). College alcohol use and the embodiment of hegemonic masculinity among European college men. *Sex Roles, 56*(11), 741–756.

Peralta, R., Steele, J., Nofziger, S., and Rickles, M. (2010). The impact of gender on binge drinking behaviour among U.S. college students attending a midwestern university: An analysis of two gender measures. *Feminist Criminology, 5*(4), 355–379.

Phipps, A., and Young, I. (2015). Neoliberalisation and 'lad cultures' in higher education. *Sociology, 49*(2), 305–322.

Prime Minister's Strategy Unit. (2004). *Alcohol Harm Reduction Strategy for England*. London: Prime Minister's Strategy Unit, Cabinet Office. www.strategy.gov.uk/files/pdf/al04SU.pdf.

Reay, D. (1998). Rethinking social class: Qualitative perspectives on class and gender. *Sociology, 32*(2), 259–275.

Redden, G., and Brown, R. (2010). From binging booze bird to gilded cage: Teaching girls gender and class on Ladette to Lady. *Critical Studies in Education, 51*(3), 237–249.

Ridout, B., Campbell, A., and Ellis, L. (2012). 'Off your Face(book)': Alcohol in online social identity construction and its relation to problem drinking in university students. *Drug and Alcohol Review, 31*(1), 20–26.

Ringrose, J., and Walkerdine, V. (2008). Regulating the abject: The TV makeover as a site of neo-liberal reinvention toward bourgeois femininity. *Feminist Media Studies, 8*(3), 227–246.

Ronay, B. (2008, 9 May). Young, rich and drunk. *The Guardian*. Retrieved 5 April 2016, from www.theguardian.com/education/2008/may/09/oxbridgeandelitism.higher education

Rose, N. (1989). *Governing the Soul: The Shaping of the Private Self*. London: Routledge.

Rudolfsdottir, A., and Morgan, P. (2009). 'Alcohol is my friend': Young middle class women discuss their relationship with alcohol. *Journal of Community and Applied Social Psychology, 19*, 492–505.

Sansone, L. (1995). The making of black youth culture: Lower class young men of Surinames origin in Amsterdam. In V. Amit-Talai and H. Wulf (Eds.), *Youth Cultures: A Cross-Cultural Perspective* (pp. 114–143). London: Routledge.

Skeggs, B. (1997). *Formations of Class and Gender: Becoming Respectable*. London: Sage.

Skeggs, B. (2004). *Class, Self, Culture*. London: Routledge.

Skeggs, B. (2005). The making of class and gender through visualizing moral subject formation. *Sociology, 39*(5), 965–982.

Steinberg, D., and Johnson, R. (Eds.). (2003). *Blairism and the War of Persuasion: Labour's Passive Revolution.* London: Lawrence and Wishart.

Stepney, M. (2015). The challenge of hyper-sexual femininity and binge drinking: A feminist psychoanalytic response. *Subjectivity, 8*(1), 57–73.

Szmigin, I., Griffin, C., Mistral, W., Bengry-Howell, A., Weale, L., and Hackley, C. (2008). Re-framing 'binge drinking' as calculated hedonism—Empirical evidence from the UK. *International Journal of Drug Policy, 19*(5), 359–366.

Thurnell-Read, T. (2013). 'Yobs' and 'snobs': Embodying drink and the problematic male drinking body. *Sociological Research Online, 18*(2), 3–12.

Tomsen, S. (1997). A top night: Social protest, masculinity and the culture of drinking violence. *British Journal of Criminology, 37*(1), 90–102.

Tutenges, S., and Sandberg, S. (2013). Intoxicating stories: The characteristics contexts and implications of drinking stories among Danish youth. *International Journal of Drug Policy, 24*, 538–544.

Tutenges, S., and Sandberg, S. (2014). Bad boys telling stories. *International Journal of Drug Policy, 25*, 348–349.

Tyler, I. (2008). 'Chav mum, chav scum': Class disgust in contemporary Britain. *Feminist Media Studies, 8*(1), 17–34.

Tyler, I. (2013). *Revolting Subjects: Social Abjection and Resistance in Neoliberal Britain.* London: Zed.

Tyler, I. (2015). Classificatory struggles: Class, culture and struggle in neoliberal times. *Sociological Review, 63*, 493–511.

Tyler, I., and Bennett, B. (2010). 'Celebrity chav': Fame, femininity and social class. *European Journal of Cultural Studies, 13*(3), 375–393.

van Dijck, J. (2013). 'You have one identity': Performing the self on Facebook and Linkedin. *Media, Culture and Society, 35*(2), 199–215.

Waitt, G., Jessop, L., and Gorman-Murray, A. (2011). 'The guys in there just expect to be laid': Embodied and gendered socio-spatial practices of a 'night out; in Wollongong, Australia. *Gender, Place and Culture, 18*(2), 255–275.

Watts, R., Linke, S., Murray, E., and Barker, C. (2015). Calling the shots: Young professional women's relationship with alcohol. *Feminism and Psychology, 25*(2), 219–234.

Willis, P. (1977). *Learning to Labour: How Working Class Kids Get Working Class Jobs.* Farnborough: Saxon House.

Willott, S., and Lyons, A. (2012). Consuming male identities: Masculinities and alcohol consumption in Aotearoa New Zealand. *Journal of Community and Applied Social Psychology, 22*, 330–345.

Wood, H., and Skeggs, B. (2007). Spectacular morality: 'Reality' television, individualisation and the remaking of the working class. In D. Hesmondhalgh and J. Toynbee (Eds.), *The Media and Social Theory* (pp. 177–193). London: Routledge.

3 Curating identity

Drinking, young women, femininities and social media practices

Jo Lindsay and Sian Supski

Introduction

In this chapter we explore the connections between alcohol consumption, social media practices and identity construction for young women. We argue that social network sites (SNS) provide a new and expanded public drinking space which interweaves online and offline experience to provide a platform for fun, social belonging and the curation of identity. The changed spatiality and temporality of young women's drinking has implications for identity construction and gender relations most visibly in understandings of femininity. The enactment of femininity and consumption now extends across physical and virtual space. Young women are avid users of social network sites and use them more often and in different ways to young men (cf. Brown and Gregg, 2012; Haferkamp et al., 2012; Hutton et al., 2016; Moewaka Barnes et al., 2016; Niland et al., 2014).

We draw together recent scholarship on young women's drinking, femininity and their online practices. We outline the contradictory social terrain young women negotiate as they drink with friends and the corporate interests of alcohol companies and advertisers who view young women as an increasingly important market segment. We explore the nuances of contemporary gender performance online and argue that women are carefully curating their identities: as feminine and sometimes hyper-feminine, as 'free' and therefore intoxicated, as networked and popular as they socialise with friends, and as sexual, sometimes shamelessly so. We end by discussing the implications for women's liberation or power in 'intoxigenic digital spaces' and suggest that social realities for most young women are more heterogenous than the stereotypes and moral panics suggest.

Changing gender relations and alcohol

The relationship between femininity and alcohol consumption has been markedly reconfigured over two generations. For much of the twentieth century, women's drinking was frowned upon, regarded as 'unfeminine' and the province of working-class women in developed nations such as the UK, New Zealand and Australia. There were particular spaces that allowed women some freedom from the male gaze and were accepted as places women could drink – for middle class women the home was seen as most appropriate (cf. Holloway et al., 2009). For working-class women in Australia, the 'Ladies Lounge' in the pub was a space set aside exclusively for women, which was the only acceptable place for them to drink (unless of course they worked behind the public bar) (Kirkby, 1997; Wright, 2003). With the rise of second-wave feminism in the 1960s–1970s, as women's rights and roles began to irrevocably change, new opportunities for public drinking also opened up for young women. There is no longer the strict spatial demarcation between women's and men's drinking spaces (except perhaps in rural areas), although a spatial element to women's drinking remains. Young women's drinking is now accepted, and even promoted in the twenty-first century, but social anxieties about young women consuming alcohol in public continue, and there are ongoing moral panics regarding respectability, femininity and safety. Young women's drinking is performed in physical space and enhanced through social network sites – through the organisation of nights out, uploading and sharing of photos, telling and re-telling of drinking stories and alcohol marketing (Moewaka Barnes et al., 2016).

We suggest that the movement from the 'ladies lounge' to the 'online lounge' needs to be taken into consideration when thinking through young women's drinking and gendered use of online networks. Tracing women's historical relationship to drinking is important, as it indicates that women's drinking is always relational – it has always been set against men's drinking and within a patriarchal framework (cf. Lyons and Willott, 2008). Even within the changing nature of gender relations, how women represent themselves in physical and online space is subject to moral censure. Social anxieties about appropriate behaviour for young women are nothing new. For example, researchers such as Jackson and Tinkler (2007) and Watts et al. (2015) have shown that the moral panic over young women's increased drinking, as in those surrounding 'ladette' femininity and drinking in the 2000s, have historical precedents in the 'modern girl' identities of the early twentieth century. Watts et al. (2015: 220) suggest that, 'Indignation at women's drinking has continued: Jackson and Tinkler (2007) discuss the parallels in media outbursts in response to the "modern girl" of the 1920s, and the "ladette" of the 2000s, both defined by youth, boisterously assertive behaviour, and drinking.' As Lyons and Willott (2008) contend, women's social position has changed over time, giving them greater access to employment and leisure activities traditionally regarded as men's domain, including drinking. Young women have become a new target market for the alcohol industry in the night-time economy and they now have more opportunities to drink and consequently drink more alcohol.

Alcohol marketing and the creation of intoxigenic digital spaces

In the 1990s, researchers began to chart fundamental changes in the regulation of the night-time economy (NTE) where a multitude of spaces and opportunities for young people to drink were created. One of the distinguishing features of the development of the night-time economy in urban centres around the world is that young women were welcomed as active participants and public drinking became feminised (Chatterton and Hollands, 2001; Griffin et al., 2013: 187; cf. Lyons and Willott, 2008).

Bailey et al. (2015: 756) define the night-time economy as:

> The transformation of city-centers through the development of licensed leisure spaces, especially bars and clubs for 18–35-year-old consumers. The development of the NTE is designed to produce hedonistic consumption and coincides with the deregulation of … licensing laws.

The transformation of the night-time economy in developed countries, including Australia, the UK and New Zealand, includes changes to alcohol advertising, marketing and retail trade, and an opening up of 'female-friendly' (Szmigin et al., 2008) spaces for young women to drink. Young women are now free to actively engage with the night-time economy: their consumption and the frequency of nights out have increased and the strength and type of drinks they consume have also risen (Australian Institute of Health and Welfare, 2014; Griffin et al., 2013). Further, alcohol was re-developed as the drug of choice for young people as the night-time economy developed (Measham and Brain, 2005). There is now an 'everydayness' associated with young people's drinking which has become 'an all but compulsory aspect' of young people's lives in the UK, as well as in other developed nations (Griffin et al., 2009b: 226; Lindsay, 2012; Lyons and Willott, 2008). In turn this has led to the 'regular normative practice of drinking to intoxication' (Griffin et al., 2013: 187). Multinational alcohol companies have pursued the new market of young women with gusto, creating new fashionable drinks for them particularly with white spirits and marketing products heavily to young female audiences both online and offline (Carah et al., 2014; Griffiths and Casswell, 2010; McCreanor et al., 2008).

McCreanor et al. (2008) develop the idea of 'intoxigenic social environments', which brings together alcohol marketing, young people and drinking to intoxication to describe this all pervasive phenomenon. They define intoxigenic social environments as 'the discursive social practices that engage with and utilise pro-intoxication talk to create and maintain expectations, norms and behaviours around alcohol consumption' (McCreanor et al., 2008: 939). Of particular importance is the impact of alcohol marketing on young people's drinking behaviours. They suggest that the sophistication of alcohol marketing operates implicitly and explicitly. Explicitly, 'young people trust and value industry-given knowledge and messages presented in important domains of youth culture', as well as being 'critically reflexive readers' of the alcohol and alcohol marketing environments they inhabit (McCreanor et al., 2008: 939, 949), which also includes the online environment. Implicitly, they contend that young people are 'so immersed' in the intoxigenic social environment that alcohol marketing is 'under the radar' and taken for granted (McCreanor et al., 2008: 945). The taken-for-grantedness of the availability and presence of alcohol builds the idea of the normalisation of youth drinking in everyday lives.

Griffiths and Casswell (2010) build on McCreanor et al.'s (2008) earlier research by focusing on the ways in which young people's use of SNS has extended the reach of intoxigenic social environments to create 'intoxigenic digital spaces'. Specifically, they suggest that young people's sharing of information on SNS – organising nights out, posting photos of themselves drinking, partying, having fun – are integral to the creation of both 'intoxigenic social identities' and 'intoxigenic digital spaces'. This new spatial frontier allows young people to (co)-construct their identity by sharing their nights out, through photos and stories being told and re-told, as well as being used in subtle and sophisticated ways by alcohol marketers. Through online quizzes and association with alcohol brands, the extension of drinking spaces operates to reinforce normative intoxication while also building group belonging. Intoxigenic digital spaces serve to expand the sites of young people's drinking by 'normalising heavy drinking and increasing exposure to commercial interests' (Moewaka Barnes et al., 2016: 63).

Changes in drinking behaviours – increased alcohol consumption, feminisation of the NTE, online drinking, everydayness of drinking, drinking to intoxication – have created public anxiety, especially surrounding young women's health and, importantly, questions of identity, in particular, femininity and what it means to be a young woman in a heavy drinking context. Much recent research on young women's drinking has focused on examining the links between femininity and drinking, especially through the lens of 'gender as performance' and the discourse of postfeminism to which we turn now (Bailey et al., 2015; Griffin et al., 2013; Hutton et al., 2016; Lyons and Willott, 2008; Waitt et al., 2011).

Gender performance in a post-feminist context

Recent scholarship on young women's drinking notes that questions of femininity are central to understanding the changes in women's alcohol consumption (Bailey et al., 2015; Brown and Gregg, 2012; Dobson, 2014a, 2014b; Griffin et al., 2013; Hutton et al., 2016; Lyons and Willott, 2008; Stepney, 2015; Waitt et al., 2011). There are two useful cultural-social theoretical frameworks which scholars draw upon to explore intoxicated femininities (Butler, 1990; Gill, 2008; McRobbie, 2007). In recent years, postfeminist understandings of young women's relationship to alcohol have gained more traction. Both of these frames will be discussed below.

Lyons and Willott (2008) draw on Butler's work on 'gender as performative', which opens the possibility for women to enact multiple femininities. Perhaps this is the key to understanding young women's relationship to alcohol consumption, gender and women's identities. In thinking of gender as performance, 'masculinities and femininities are continuously (re)created' (Lyons and Willott, 2008: 694). In the continuous (re)creation of femininities, young women must negotiate on a daily basis (or on each night out) different femininities if not simultaneously, then serially (cf. Renold and Ringrose, 2011). Choosing and managing modes of feminine performance is a challenge because some modes are more (or less) acceptable and some face greater sanctions than others, particularly around bodily comportment. Much research and media discussion has been concerned with the way in which drunken young women no longer appear 'feminine'. They use their bodies in ways which interrupt normative understandings of femininity – yelling, vomiting, falling over, waving arms and legs, using 'big movements and risk-taking' (Waitt et al., 2011: 271). However, Waitt et al. (2011: 271), drawing on Iris Marion Young's (1990) work on women's gendered embodiment, suggest that women's drinking to intoxication 'should perhaps be considered in terms of asserting an alternative femininity that embraces the risks of drinking and drunkenness'.

The question remains, however, are young women able to position themselves differently and if so, how might they do this? Waitt et al.'s (2011) research indicates that the way in which women use space whilst drinking might offer fleeting moments of respite from gendered discourses. This momentary respite might be found in 'private spaces' women create in pubs and clubs – away from the main bar occupied by men. Waitt et al. (2011: 272) contend that the way in which women 'territorialise a space' and 'sustain a space of privacy in pubs/clubs suggests drinking and drunkenness are grounded in belonging and the assertion of feminine identities'. In this interpretation, women's use of space carves out a niche that is not relational to men or men's drinking – it is a women's only space in which the pleasure of drinking and getting drunk is also a way of 'doing' femininity. To extrapolate this argument, performance space might also be gained through the use of SNS. Although women's online representation is a source of debate and speculation, the way in which they choose to represent themselves through the photos they post can be understood as a means of asserting feminine identities (cf. Dobson, 2014a, 2014b).

Other theorists suggest that this argument incorporates elements of postfeminist understandings of femininity. In using a postfeminist lens to think through the phenomena of young women and drinking, researchers have begun to unpack the many dilemmas that young women face. Young women must negotiate the contradictions and ambiguities of femininity, in what Bailey et al. (2015: 747) describe as an 'impossible dilemma'. This dilemma is one in which the juxtaposition of 'hypersexual femininity and the culture of intoxication' forces young women to make choices between 'achiev(ing) the "right" form of hypersexual femininity and an "optimum" level of drunkenness'. Griffin et al. (2013: 184) in earlier research argue that this 'dilemmatic space' is one which places young women in a contradictory relationship with alcohol and femininity. Thus, as Skeggs (1997) and Bailey et al. (2015: 748) contend, young women are 'called on to drink heavily within a pervasive culture of intoxication of "extreme drinking," while simultaneously inhabiting [a] hypersexual form of femininity'.

Feminist researchers have analysed the strengthening connection between hypersexual femininity and young women's alcohol consumption. For the purposes of this chapter we follow an understanding of postfeminism as outlined by Gill (2008). Postfeminist discourse is:

(a) way of constructing an image of contemporary femininity. This discourse situates the representation of contemporary femininity as stylishly groomed, youthful, bold, 'sassy,' and 'sexually knowing'. Postfeminism incorporates the shift from objectification to subjectification and integrates a focus on self-transformation through consumption.

(cited in Bailey et al., 2015: 756)

In effect postfeminism acknowledges and celebrates women's agency, subjectivity and individualisation whilst recognising that identity is constructed through consumption – of fashion, beauty products, technology and alcohol, among other things. Much of the research on young women's drinking positions them within a postfeminist context, but acknowledges that this is a contradictory discourse which incorporates understandings of postfeminist femininity whilst simultaneously holding onto traditional notions of femininity that rely on well-worn understandings of how women should behave, what they should wear and where they can be seen. Race and class are also configured within postfeminist discourse so that white and middle-class expressions of femininity are predominant (Dobson, 2014a, 2014b; Jackson and Tinkler, 2007). Working-class women and women of colour must 'abide' by standards, which draw on white, middle-class ideals of femininity (cf. Skeggs, 1997).

Further, the connection between postfeminism and consumption (explored in depth by Angela McRobbie, 2007, 2009) shows a persistent representation of femininity, which simultaneously asks young women to negotiate 'acceptable femininities' and an adventurous 'up for it' attitude (Bailey, 2012; Hutton et al., 2016). Notions of respectability further complicate this 'tight-rope' walk. Young women must also remain 'respectable' in the midst of heavy drinking cultures. Hutton et al. (2016: 74) suggest that young women are 'invited to engage in drunkenness and "fun" without relinquishing their claims to "decency", "desirability" and "respectability" (Gill, 2008; Hutton et al., 2013). Within this postfeminist, neo-liberal context young female drinkers are entangled in these competing and contradictory discourses as they negotiate their drinking practices.' Thus, young women must navigate this tension. They must maintain respectability and a particular kind of femininity whilst being drunk and having fun. Stepney (2015: 57–58) suggests that this tension creates a 'fundamental dispute':

> *on the one hand*, there is the view that women's participation in the night-time economy is associated with a 'new' form of femininity, that of liberation and social progress which may be equated with (sexual) empowerment, choice and female achievement (Walter, 1998; Laurie et al, 1999; Power, 2009; Baker, 2010); *on the other hand*, there is the view that this represents a breakdown of traditional values that have been replaced by permissiveness and irresponsibility, associated with social deviance, disorder and moral anarchy (Lyons, 2006).

(Authors' emphasis)

Dobson (2014b: 99) provides another view. She contends that there are four discourses in which femininity is positioned within a Western neoliberal socio-cultural context:

1   protectionist/moralist discourses about girls ... and young women and their ... 'sexualisation';

2   continuation of heavy female body ... commodification in post-feminist Western visual culture;

3   convergence of girl-power discourses with neo-liberalist ideals of girls as the ultimate late-modern capitalist success stories; and

4   institutionalisation of ... 'gender melancholia' and the psycho-pathologisation of femininity.

Renold and Ringrose (2011) describe the dilemma young women face within this postfeminist discourse as a '"schizoid" discourse of femininity'. Class and race are further layered within this 'schizoid' understanding. Griffin et al. (2013: 185) suggest that postfeminism has created:

> new forms of classed and racialised femininity in which young white middle class women are constituted as the vanguard of a new form of neo-liberal subjectivity (Walkerdine, 2003), and young (white) working class women are condemned as feckless, disordered and excessive consumers. (Redden and Brown, 2010; Skeggs, 2004).

Thus, young women are betwixt and between with seemingly multiple femininities to choose from, or at least the appearance of choice, within a patriarchal understanding of 'acceptable' and respectable femininity. The outlining of the 'impossible dilemma' that young women face allows a richer understanding of why young women may present themselves as 'hypersexual' or 'hyperfeminine' in physical and online space and opens a space which does not 'obscur[e] the messy realities of lived sexual subjectivities and how girls may be positioned in these ways simultaneously' (Renold and Ringrose, 2011: 392). We discuss this further below.

Curating an online identity

Social networking sites have in effect become new 'public' spaces for women to perform, create and maintain their feminine identities and their friendships. Haferkamp et al. (2012: 98) contend that the use of SNS is gendered, suggesting that women 'reveal a more hedonistic use – that is, they concentrate on entertainment and self presentation – while men focus on the pragmatic functions of SNS'. In particular, they argue that young women use SNS to 'compare themselves with others' and to find information, whilst men tend to 'look at other people's profiles to find friends' (Haferkamp et al., 2012: 91). Although there are many SNS, such as Instagram, Twitter and Pinterest, as well as MySpace and Bebo, and country-specific sites such as StudiVZ (in Germany), most of the research on young people and alcohol has centred on Facebook, the predominant global SNS (cf. Brown and Gregg, 2012; cf. for Bebo, Griffiths and Casswell, 2010; cf. for Studi VZ, Haferkamp et al., 2012; Hutton et al., 2016; McCreanor et al., 2008; Niland et al., 2014; Ridout et al., 2012).

Recent research has shown that social network sites have become increasingly important in most people's everyday lives, particularly for young people. In Australia nearly 50% of people access some form of social media every day, with the rate increasing to 79% for young people (18–29 years) (Sensis, 2015). Those connecting to Facebook 'spend the equivalent of a full working day on Facebook each week, averaging 8.5 hours on the site' (Sensis, 2015: 2). These figures confirm that SNS have become pervasive in our everyday lives and influence how we interact with each other. For young people, research has shown that SNS are particularly important for maintaining friendships, in the 'real' sense (as well as online 'friends') and that, in particular, the ability to post photos, make comments, organise nights out and re-live them the next day is integral to these relationships (Brown and Gregg, 2012; Hutton et al., 2016; Niland et al., 2014). Further, many of the photos uploaded to Facebook tell visual stories and with accompanying text young people construct identities in specific ways. For young women the connection between the display of photos (on SNS) and alcohol is, as a number of researchers suggest, a 'feminine activity' (Brown and Gregg, 2012; Niland et al., 2014; Waitt et al., 2011). A dominant theme throughout recent research has acknowledged an 'airbrushing' effect of photos, particularly in relation to photos connected to nights out and drinking which serve to reinforce the acceptability of some drinking behaviours. For example, Niland et al. (2014: 889–890) demonstrate that only certain drinking photos are posted, therefore, 'airbrushing' the negative aspects of young people's drinking, which, in turn, 'normalise(s) and reinforce(s) drinking as always pleasurable without harmful consequences'.

Brown and Gregg (2012: 357) argue that the connection between young women, SNS and drinking is one which draws on prosaic, and routine uses of Facebook. In particular:

> Ordinary and mundane uses of Facebook – status updates anticipating the weekend, mobile posts in the midst of intoxication, photo uploading and album dissemination the morning after – reveal the anticipatory pleasures, everyday preparations and retrospective bonding involved in hedonistic and risky alcohol consumption. This demonstrates the fundamentally social dimensions accompanying young women's drinking. The enjoyment derived from sharing the 'risky' and 'regrettable' experience on Facebook is part of ongoing narratives between girls.

In part this 'ongoing narrative' is constructed through the unique features which allow easy access for users as well as 'friends' to post images, comments and status updates. Depending on the privacy settings chosen by each user, a Facebook profile can be viewed by the public, only 'friends' or a mixture of both. Ridout et al. (2012: 21) suggest that the 'wall' function of Facebook serves as a place where users and their 'friends' can actively create (and co-create) their online identity:

> By allowing both self- and other generated information as well as textual information, the full process of identity construction can be observed ... This

also increases the objectivity and validity of SNS profiles, as third-party information is considered more reliable than self-disclosed claims. (Walther et al., 2008).

The importance of self and other generated identity construction on SNS is important particularly in relation to young women's drinking because young women actively 'curate' their online selves. They select, edit and post photos which show how their identities collide with the new drinking culture afforded them – often they portray themselves as intoxicated, 'messy', 'rowdy', but also as confident, strong and sexy young women. They curate their online selves to show their engagement with drinking and fun nights out, but they also actively 'airbrush' their photos to 'minimize the appearance of intoxication for known and unknown audiences' (Hutton et al., 2016: 73). One way of curating their identity is to 'untag' themselves from photos posted by friends or others. Young women actively check their friends Facebook pages and remove their names from photos that show them in a disparaging light, such as showing them as very drunk or in compromising ways (Hutton et al., 2016; Niland et al., 2014).

Social network sites allow young women the freedom to project an image of self, which is at once agentic in the sense that they curate their online presence, but this curation must also adhere to gendered norms of respectability and femininity. Identity is thus actively constructed and curated through the presentation of photos on Facebook. The (un)tagging and airbrushing of drinking photos has become integral to nights out, 'drinking in the right way' (Harrison et al., 2011: 472) and 'displaying a good time and a sexy persona on Facebook' (Hutton et al., 2016: 76). When examined together these elements also build 'social capital', in particular ways – young women want to be seen to be having 'drunken fun' with friends, but in ways that reinforce belonging and acceptable forms of femininity. Young women must ensure that the 'right' drunken photos are posted, thereby 'airbrushing' their identity and ensuring that their performance of femininity is not 'labelled as promiscuous or disreputable' (Hutton et al., 2016: 76; Niland et al., 2014).

Performing femininity, heterosexuality and intoxication

Hypersexuality or hyperfemininity are terms used by a number of researchers in the field (Bailey, 2012; Bailey et al., 2015; Gill, 2008; Griffin et al., 2013; Hutton et al., 2016; Skeggs, 1997; Stepney, 2015) to describe the way in which young women present themselves on 'nights out'. Hypersexuality can be defined as 'high heels, short skirts, low-cut tops, fake tan, long, straight and (bottle) blonde hair, smooth bare legs in all climates, lots of make-up and a buxom slimness' (Griffin et al., 2013: 194). Thus, hypersexuality is a distinct form of heterosexual femininity which Bailey et al. (2016) and Skeggs (1997) suggest 'presents a precarious combination of hedonistic, bold and heterosexually attractive hyperfemininity which unsettles traditional forms of respectable femininity' (Bailey et al., 2015: 748; Skeggs, 1997). This is also a classed and racialised phenomenon in which white, working-class women challenge middle-class notions of respectability thereby increasing social anxieties about young women's performance of femininity.

In relation to young women's drinking, hypersexuality presents a potential problem. Young women must negotiate contradictory desires on nights out – to have fun and enjoy being with friends whilst avoiding potential risks associated with excessive drinking and drunkenness. An underlying gendered discourse pervades young women's new engagement in the night-time economy and drinking – there is an expectation that young women will drink like 'one of the boys' while at the same time adhering to notions of respectability, as well as behaving in a hypersexualised way.

Young women's engagement with the night-time economy, including dressing in a hypersexual way (which in some cases risks censure because of 'unfeminine' or 'unrespectable' behaviour), must also be understood as one which is essentially about young women's pleasure. For example, Szmigin et al. (2008) discuss the 'calculated hedonism' of young people's drinking in which young people identify nights out and drinking excessively as a pleasurable activity. In relation to young women, Lyons and Willott (2008: 709) note that 'linking the pursuit of pleasure with female empowerment is a difficult place for women to occupy, given that it seems to empower but also simultaneously borders on "unrespectability"'.

Further, Griffin et al. (2013: 188) suggest that young women's drinking to intoxication aids in pleasure-seeking, having fun, enabling self-confidence and boosting sociability, but it does so at the risk of contravening 'respectable' femininities. They contend that young women enacting a hypersexual femininity are required to 'look and act as agentically sexy within a pornified nighttime economy pervaded by "cheap deals" on alcohol, but to somehow distance themselves from the troubling figure of the 'drunken slut' (de Visser and McDonnell, 2012; Griffin et al., 2013: 187). In effect, young women are encouraged to 'drink like one of the boys' but if they go too far they are at risk of being labelled 'drunken sluts'. Thus, the question of women's identity is constantly brought into focus – and always in relation to men's drinking. Young women must negotiate contradictory discourses of what it means to be a woman in a postfeminist context.

The choices young women are required to make in a postfeminist context about their self-identity, in the end, are highly circumscribed. Postfeminist discourse offers young women an escape from the 'boring constraints of respectable femininity' through an illusory promise of freedom and sexual empowerment while simultaneously creating 'paralyzing anxieties' about how to appear and behave (Griffin et al., 2013: 199).

The idea of an 'anxious politics' can be used to describe the many dilemmas and contradictions that young women must navigate, around safety, engaging with the night-time economy, dressing up, femininities and consuming alcohol (cf. Stepney, 2015). SNS, such as Facebook, also raise anxieties because of the challenge of managing multiple audiences, including family, friends, school peers and prospective and current employers. In particular, an 'anxious politics' can be exemplified in the regular moral panics around young women and drinking. As

Stepney (2015: 58) and others contend, hypersexuality and binge drinking have become the focus of moral panics over the last two decades (Lyons and Willott, 2008). Holloway et al. (2009: 822), in discussing the UK context, state that the media representations of 'ladettes' out on the town, drinking heavily, having riotous fun and dressing in a hypersexual way coincided with public health messages about the harm of excessive drinking to women's health and the risk of male violence. Such moral panics further entrench gendered discourses about women's 'proper' role in society, that is, as mothers and carers. For many young women, dressing in a hypersexual way provides an outlet from the 'gendered moralities' that women must negotiate (Holloway et al., 2009).

Displaying a hypersexualised femininity also offers young women a pathway to recognition. Stepney's (2015: 69) research with Dutch and British young women highlights a contradiction of hypersexual femininity in the night-time economy whereby dressing in a particular way is at once liberating as well as damning:

> Alcohol plays an important role in this conflict offering participants a route to recognition. Narratives were replete with ambivalences about the female identity at night – wearing particular clothes, such as a short skirt, was seen as both empowering and sexually attractive while at the same time shameful and shocking. Admiration – 'good for her' – was accompanied by social censure on the grounds that such dressing was 'slutty', 'indecent', 'common' and 'asking for trouble'. The fun 'top girl' who chooses to dress how she pleases and be drunk must not be seen to be having too much fun – she must remain, in part, contained and in control.

Thus, young women know that they have the freedom to dress and drink in particular ways, but they also know that their 'femininity' will be called into question if they drink excessively or dress in overtly sexual ways. For some young women the self-identity that drinking and a hypersexualised femininity offers them is 'a way of obtaining social capital and recognition when other avenues of economic and cultural capital are not equally open to them' (cf. Brown and Gregg, 2012; Stepney, 2015: 69).

Within a postfeminist discourse such crafting of identity also allows for the possibility of autonomy and empowerment. For example, Gill (2008) suggests that the way in which young women engage with consumption, particularly in relation to clothing and their appearance, does offer opportunities for empowerment. However, the overarching gendered discourse is one which continues to rely on 'sexual double standards around heterosexual attractiveness and the importance of respectable femininity' (Bailey et al., 2015: 748; cf. McRobbie, 2007; Skeggs, 1997).

Going too far: performative shamelessness

In a contradictory 'impossible' context comprising the patriarchal gaze, moral panics, neoliberal individualisation and sexualisation, it is challenging to 'get it right' and curate a risk-taking but socially acceptable performance of drunk femininity in offline and online contexts (Bailey et al., 2015; Brown and Gregg, 2012; Dobson, 2014a, 2014b; Hutton et al., 2016; Niland et al., 2014).

The young women in the UK study conducted by Bailey and colleagues (2015) talked about creating a particular 'look' and their preferences for high heels and skimpy clothes. Yet the women also drew on judgemental discourses to talk about other young women's clothing. As Carrie reported, 'they all had fake tan on and high-heels and um they had their bums literally hanging out of their clothes and I think, oh no, it's not a good look' (Bailey et al., 2015: 752). The women were also aware of the necessity of self-management while out drinking as quotes from the focus group illustrate: 'Yeah with girls, they need to be able to handle themselves' and 'know when to stop' to avoid judgement. As Nancy said, 'It's quite disgusting, drinking and getting drunk like that' (Bailey et al., 2015: 753).

Dobson (2014b) develops the idea of 'performative shamelessness' to describe how young women represent their drunken selves on SNS such as MySpace and Facebook. Her idea is useful as it draws together three main discourses – femininity, postfeminism and neoliberalism – and focuses attention on how these interplay with young women's drinking to produce new understandings of gender performativity. Further, she shows how young women embody or 'play with' notions of gender. Specifically, young women are often portrayed as displaying masculine drinking habits, indicated by terms such as 'ladette'. The way in which Dobson (2014a: 142) frames this behaviour is to suggest that rather than feminists (or the broader population) seeing this as a negative identity construction, it is in fact one of 'few options available to young women wishing to maintain a sense of self definition in the face of intense social and cultural scrutinising, and often sexually objectifying, gazes'. Further, Dobson (2014a: 144) understands young women's gender performativity as more than reproduction, resistance or subversion of traditionally masculine traits, such as 'laddishness', and suggests that the way in which they represent themselves online with images of drinking and drunkenness is 'a way for young women to maintain a sense of self-definition by performatively inviting the (masculinized and heterosexualizing) gaze'. In doing so, Dobson (2014a: 160) contends that 'performative shamelessness' may be an 'agentic urge' in which young women 'pre-emptively defend themselves, by deploying signals of pride and pleasure, against scrutinizing, sexualizing and pathologizing gazes of which they are often made well aware in public discourse'.

However, Dobson does make clear that such a feminist reading is also highly political. Although young women enact and perform 'laddish' drinking habits, extreme in some cases and often in a hypersexualised manner, she is making a case for thinking about this behaviour in ways that are not linear or binary, either/ or feminine or masculine. That, in fact, young women are embodying a gender fluidity that does not reproduce traditional patriarchal understandings of masculinity and femininity but offers a more open, agentic understanding of feminine pleasure and sexuality. In doing so, young women are viewed as exercising autonomy through appropriating traditionally masculine domains and manipulating them to bring about a different 'demystified' understanding of young women's (re)presentation (Dobson, 2014a: 159).

In contrast to Dobson's (2014a, 2014b) analysis of 'laddishness online' and 'performative shamelessness', Hutton et al. (2016: 86) contend that the images young women post on Facebook (mostly) adhere to 'notions of "respectable" femininity'. They suggest that there is a difference between 'drinking femininities' and 'drunken femininities', with the latter identity less acceptable. The difference between these two representations can be characterised as identities which remain within the realm of respectability (drinking femininities) and those that do not (drunken femininities). 'Drinking femininities' acknowledges that young women enthusiastically consume alcohol, enjoy the night-time economy, dress up, gain pleasure from drinking and sharing time with friends, and posting photos of nights out on SNS. 'Drunken femininities', as Lyons and Willott (2008) suggest are contradictory; 'difficult to imagine and enact'. The key difference in these terms is that one acknowledges that young women are consuming alcohol and that it is a part of what it means to be a young woman in the twenty-first century, but that drunkenness is unacceptable and constitutes a breach of traditional understandings of femininity. Furthermore, the curation of identity is itself gendered, producing double standards. Young women spend a great deal of time and effort curating their online performances to 'get it right' and manoeuvre through contradictory representations of femininity. Young men have more freedom in their online representation and are not subject to the same social scrutiny and opprobrium.

Thus, young women enact different drinking femininities depending on circumstances. Their curation of identity relies on gendered discourses which offer agency and empowerment but must be done so within the realms of feminine respectability. The transgression of accepted forms of femininity results in public censure. However, there are other ways in which young women can curate their identities, which we discuss below.

Recognising diversity in social network use and alcohol consumption

The connections we have discussed in this chapter between drinking, feminine performance and social networking sites are apparent across developed nations, but there are important national differences too. Young people's drinking cultures in the UK display a greater commitment to extreme drinking (Griffin et al., 2009a) and classed modes of feminine performance are also more pronounced than in former British colonies such as Australia and New Zealand. Furthermore, ethnicity and culture are particularly relevant in postcolonial societies, where drinking patterns among indigenous populations (including young people) differ to other groups, and meanings of alcohol and drinking also vary across cultural and ethnic groups.

Before closing this chapter we would like to sound a note of caution in focusing too heavily on the stereotype of the culturally troubling figure of the hypersexual (heterosexual) drunk girl on Facebook. Young women are, of course, diverse, and alternative and multifaceted modes of femininity are enacted on social networking sites including by religious women such as young Muslims (Bayat and Herrera, 2010), sportswomen such as roller derby girls (Pavlidis and Fullagar, 2012) and lesbian, gay and bisexual women (Lincoln and Robards, 2014). Moreover, though alcohol consumption has colonised online socialising among some groups of young women, there is considerable diversity in ways of engaging with social networking (cf. Lincoln and Robards, 2014). There is also considerable diversity in alcohol consumption patterns. Young women have always drunk less than men, and though the gap is closing, young women continue to drink less and suffer less of the harms associated with excessive drinking such as alcohol-related violence (Lindsay, 2012). Indeed, many young women continue to prefer shopping to drinking when they socialise with friends (Lindsay, 2003). Finally, there is evidence that alcohol consumption among young people is beginning to decline overall and that young people are becoming more polarised in terms of their commitment to extreme drinking and abstinence (Hutton et al., 2013; Livingston, 2014).

Conclusion

Consuming alcohol and using social network sites are intensely pleasurable social and relational activities for contemporary young women. Young women actively create and perform friendships through drinking together in physical space and extending and enhancing this in new public drinking spaces online. Young women use SNS such as Facebook to curate their identities for multiple audiences and they take opportunities to play with and transgress traditional gender roles. Yet just as old stereotypes have given way, new modes of feminine conformity have been created and these are always enacted in relation to masculine dominance (Budgeon, 2013). Young women being sexually 'up for it', or 'shameless' or without regret is at once a resistance to traditional notions of feminine respectability and passivity, but also a new constraint to be negotiated in a postfeminist context where hypersexual and hyperfeminine modes of presentation are simultaneously encouraged and harshly judged.

Finally, there is an anxious politics around young women's drinking, their sexuality and their social networking. Young women have gained freedom to drink in public, to be sexy and to create and dominate 'public' spaces on social network sites but new constraints have evolved rapidly from these freedoms. Among some groups of young women, social network sites reinforce the dominance of heavy alcohol consumption and a particular version of hypersexual femininity. Yet a sexual double standard remains in place and young women, in particular working-class young women in the UK, are judged and stigmatised. This is indeed an impossible, contradictory context for young women to negotiate (Bailey et al., 2015; Dobson, 2014a, 2014b). But beyond the new stereotype of drunken femininity, we suggest that there are more diverse performances of gender identity and less drunk modes of femininity available to young women curating their identities in virtual and physical spaces.

References

Australian Institute of Health and Welfare. (2014). Alcohol use in the general population. *National Drug Strategy Household Survey 2013*. Retrieved 11 March 2016, from www. aihw.gov.au/alcohol-and-other-drugs/ndshs-2013/ch4/

Bailey, L. (2012). Young women and the culture of intoxication: Negotiating classed femininities in the postfeminist context. Unpublished PhD, University of Bath.

Bailey, L., Griffin, C., and Shankar, A. (2015). 'Not a good look': Impossible dilemmas for young women negotiating the culture of intoxication in the United Kingdom. *Substance Use and Misuse, 50*, 747–758.

Bayat, A., and Herrera, L. (Eds.). (2010). *Being Young and Muslim: New Cultural Politics in the Global South and North.* Oxford: Oxford University Press.

Brown, R., and Gregg, M. (2012). The pedagogy of regret: Facebook, binge drinking and young women. *Continuum: Journal of Media and Cultural Studies, 26*(3), 357–369.

Budgeon, S. (2013). The dynamics of gender hegemony: Femininities, masculinities and social change. *Sociology*, published online before print July 18, doi: 10.1177/0038038513490358.

Butler, J. (1990). *Gender Trouble: Feminism and the Subversion of Identity.* New York: Routledge.

Carah, N., Brodmerkel, S., and Hernandez, L. (2014). Brands and sociality: Alcohol branding, drinking culture and Facebook. *Convergence: The Journal of Research into New Media Technologies, 20*(3), 259–275.

Chatterton, P., and Hollands, R. (2001). *Changing Our 'Toon': Youth, Nightlife and Urban Change in Newcastle.* Newcastle, UK: University of Newcastle upon Tyne.

de Visser, R., and McDonnell, E. (2012). 'That's OK. He's a guy': A mixed-methods study of gender double-standards for alcohol use. *Psychology and Health, 27*(5), 618–639.

Dobson, A. (2014a). Laddishness online: The possible significations and significance of 'performative shamelessness' for young women in the postfeminist context. *Cultural Studies, 28*(1), 142–164.

Dobson, A. (2014b). Performative shamelessness on young women's social network sites: Shielding the self and resisting gender melancholia. *Feminism and Psychology, 24*(1), 97–114.

Gill, R. (2008). Culture and subjectivity in neoliberal and postfeminist times. *Subjectivity, 25*, 432–445.

Griffin, C., Bengry-Howell, A., Hackley, C., Mistral, W., and Szmigin, I. (2009a). 'Every time I do it I absolutely annihilate myself': Loss of (self)-consciousness and loss of memory in young people's drinking narratives. *Sociology, 43*, 457–476.

Griffin, C., Bengry-Howell, A., Hackley, C., Mistral, W., and Szmigin, I. (2009b). The allure of belonging: Young people's drinking practices and collective identification. In M. Wetherell (Ed.), *Identity in the 21st Century: New Trends in Changing Times* (pp. 213–230). Basingstoke, UK: Palgrave Macmillan.

Griffin, C., Szmigin, I., Bengry-Howell, A., Hackley, C., and Mistral, W. (2013). Inhabiting the contradictions: Hypersexual femininity and the culture of intoxication among young women in the UK. *Feminism and Psychology, 23*(2), 184–206.

Griffiths, R., and Casswell, S. (2010). Intoxigenic digital spaces? Youth, social networking sites and alcohol marketing. *Drug and Alcohol Review, 29*, 525–530.

Haferkamp, N., Eimler, S., Papadakis, A., and Kruck, J. (2012). Men are from Mars, women are from Venus? Examining gender differences in self-presentation on social networking sites. *Cyberpsychology, Behavior, and Social Networking, 15*(2), 91–98.

Harrison, L., Kelly, P., Lindsay, J., Advocat, J., and Hickey, C. (2011). 'I don't know anyone who has two drinks a day': Young people, alcohol and the government of pleasure. *Health, Risk and Society, 13*(5), 469–486.

Holloway, S., Valentine, G., and Jayne, M. (2009). Masculinities, femininities and the geographies of public and private drinking landscapes. *Geoforum, 40*(5), 821–831.

Hutton, F., Griffin, C., Lyons, A., Niland, P., and McCreanor, T. (2016). 'Tragic girls' and 'crack whores': Alcohol, femininity and Facebook. *Feminism and Psychology, 26*(1), 73–93.

Hutton, F., Wright, S., and Saunders, E. (2013). Cultures of intoxication: Young women, alcohol, and harm reduction. *Contemporary Drug Problems, 40*, 451–480.

Jackson, C., and Tinkler, P. (2007). 'Ladettes' and 'modern girls': 'Troublesome' young femininities. *The Sociological Review, 55*(2), 251–272.

Kirkby, D. (1997). *Barmaids: A History of Women's Work in Pubs*. Melbourne: Cambridge University Press.

Lincoln, S., and Robards, B. (2014). 10 years of Facebook. *New Media and Society, 16*(7), 1047–1050.

Lindsay, J. (2003). 'Partying hard', 'partying sometimes' or 'shopping': Young workers' socializing patterns and sexual, alcohol and illicit drug risk taking'. *Critical Public Health, 13*(1), 1–14.

Lindsay, J. (2012). The gendered trouble with alcohol: Young people managing alcohol related violence. *International Journal of Drug Policy, 23*, 236–241.

Livingston, M. (2014). Trends in non-drinking among Australian adolescents. *Addiction, 109*(6), 922–929.

Lyons, A., and Willott, S. (2008). Alcohol consumption, gender identities and women's changing social positions. *Sex Roles, 59*, 694–712.

McCreanor, T., Moewaka Barnes, H., Kaiwai, H., Borell, S., and Gregory, A. (2008). Creating intoxigenic environments: Marketing alcohol to young people in Aotearoa New Zealand. *Social Science and Medicine, 67*(6), 938–946.

McRobbie, A. (2007). Top girls? Young women and the post-feminist sexual contract. *Cultural Studies, 21*(4–5), 718–737.

McRobbie, A. (2009). *The Aftermath of Feminism: Gender, Culture and Social Change*. Los Angeles: Sage.

Measham, F., and Brain, K. (2005). 'Binge' drinking, British alcohol policy and the new culture of intoxication. *Crime, Media, Culture, 1*(3), 262–283.

Moewaka Barnes, H., McCreanor, T., Goodwin, I., Lyons, A., Griffin, C., and Hutton, F. (2016). Alcohol and social media: Drinking and drunkenness while online. *Critical Public Health, 26*(1), 62–76.

Niland, P., Lyons, A., Goodwin, I., and Hutton, F. (2014). 'See it doesn't look pretty does it?' Young adults' airbrushed drinking practices on Facebook. *Psychology and Health, 29*(8), 877–895.

Pavlidis, A., and Fullagar, S. (2012). Becoming roller derby grrrls: Exploring the gendered play of affect in mediated sport cultures. *International Review for the Sociology of Sport*, published online before print 5 June, doi: 10.1177/1012690212446451.

Renold, E., and Ringrose, J. (2011). Schizoid subjectivities? Re-theorizing teen girls' sexual cultures in an era of 'sexualization'. *Journal of Sociology, 47*(4), 389–409.

Ridout, B., Campbell, A., and Ellis, L. (2012). 'Off your Face(book)': Alcohol in online social identity construction and its relation to problem drinking in university students. *Drug and Alcohol Review, 31*(1), 20–26.

Sensis. (2015). Sensis social media report May 2015: How Australian people and businesses are using social media. Retrieved 2 March 2016, from www.sensis.com.au/assets/PDFdirectory/Sensis_Social_Media_Report_2015.pdf

Skeggs, B. (1997). *Formations of Class and Gender: Becoming Respectable.* London: Sage.

Stepney, M. (2015). The challenge of hyper-sexual femininity and binge drinking: A feminist psychoanalytic response. *Subjectivity, 8*(1), 57–73.

Szmigin, I., Griffin, C., Mistral, W., Bengry-Howell, A., Weale, L., and Hackley, C. (2008). Re-framing 'binge drinking' as calculated hedonism—Empirical evidence from the UK. *International Journal of Drug Policy, 19*(5), 359–366.

Waitt, G., Jessop, L., and Gorman-Murray, A. (2011). 'The guys in there just expect to be laid': Embodied and gendered socio-spatial practices of a night out in Wollongong, Australia. *Gender, Place and Culture, 18*(2), 255–275.

Walther, J., Van Der Heide, B., Kim, S.-Y., Westerman, D., and Tong, S. (2008). The role of friends' appearance and behavior on evaluations of individuals on Facebook: Are we known by the company we keep? *Human Communication Research, 34*, 28–49.

Watts, R., Linke, S., Murray, E., and Barker, C. (2015). Calling the shots: Young professional women's relationship with alcohol. *Feminism and Psychology, 25*(2), 219–234.

Wright, C. (2003). *Beyond the Ladies Lounge: Australia's Female Publicans.* Melbourne: Melbourne University Publishing.

Young, I. M. (1990). *Throwing Like a Girl and Other Essays in Feminist Philosophy and Social Theory.* Bloomington: Indiana University Press.

4   Masculinities, alcohol consumption and social networking

Antonia C. Lyons and Brendan Gough

Men consume alcohol more often and more heavily than women internationally (Rahav et al., 2006). Drinking and drunkenness have traditionally been masculine practices linked to masculine identities (Lemle and Mishkind, 1989) and to socially constructed ideals of masculinity, such as autonomy, independence, bodily composure, control, self-discipline and strength (Thurnell-Read, 2013). Research has drawn on Connell's concept of hegemonic masculinity to explore men's consumption of alcohol, particularly in Western contexts. In many Western societies night-time economies provide a range of opportunities for (especially young) adults to drink, with alcohol available for purchase during most of the night and vast numbers of alcoholic products on offer. Drinking excessively, drinking primarily beer and drinking in public are ways in which men demonstrate hegemonic masculinity (Peralta, 2007; Willott and Lyons, 2012). Hegemonic masculinity is a dominant position that is constructed in relation to femininities and subordinated masculinities (Connell, 1995). It is concerned 'with the maintenance of power within and between social configurations of gender' (Matthews, 2016: 5). It is dynamic, and while most men do not embody it, it is a context-bound form of masculinity that many men aspire to. In this way it is distinguished from other local masculinities, particularly subordinated masculinities, and functions to legitimate patriarchal social relations (Connell and Messerschmidt, 2005). For example, drinking (lots of) beer as opposed to, say, gin, is a conventional way of distinguishing 'real' men from women, gay men and so on.

In reviewing the research in this area, Willott and Lyons (2012) have noted that 'the relationship between traditional masculine identities and alcohol (particularly beer) seems to be alive and strong in some contexts, whereas in other contexts, resistant or alternative ways of constructing gender identities in relation to alcohol consumption are evident' (pp. 332–333). With changes in drinking cultures over the previous three decades, including the rise in women's public drinking (Lyons and Willott, 2008), the diversity of drinking locations and products, and the increase in accessibility and availability of alcohol, it may not be surprising that masculinity is being redefined around alcohol use. Additionally, more diverse forms of alcohol use may still define traditional masculinities. For example, the increase in 'craft beer' consumption in recent years may be linked to changing masculine identities in (older) middle-class men, a way for them to distinguish themselves from (younger) working-class lager drinkers. There may also be alternative ways that men are constructing their gender identities, particularly in relation to femininities and to recent increases in women's consumption (Lyons, 2009). Research in Scotland has demonstrated the rapidly changing contexts of young men's drinking practices, and suggests that young men have a plurality of masculine identities now available in relation to alcohol consumption (Mullen et al., 2007). In the UK, young men have been found to demonstrate masculine identities in various ways, including traditional ways of drinking alcohol (in the USA too, see Peralta, 2007). However, as de Visser and Smith (2007) show, young men also trade in masculine drinking competence with a display of competence in other behavioural domains (such as sports) to define a masculine identity. In other words, not drinking on a Friday night may be acceptable if a young man is the captain of the rugby team with a game the following day; more generally, doing something unmanly or feminised can be construed as a sign of heroic masculine autonomy, strength and/or bravery. As one of de Visser and McDonnell's (2013) participants noted, 'You can't remove your masculinity by having a feminine trait. It doesn't damage your masculinity, it just adds femininity to your character' (p. 11). Men also drink more diverse alcoholic products than previously (not solely beer), although in focus group research males appear to be required to justify drinking wine or other drinks, which they do through emphasising the context in which the alcohol is consumed (e.g. at home, with clients, at a restaurant, with female partners) (e.g. Emslie et al., 2013; Willott and Lyons, 2012).

One key feature of drinking to demonstrate hegemonic masculinity is the ability to tolerate alcohol (Peralta, 2007). Alcohol consumption is 'inherently and inescapably an embodied action' (Thurnell-Read, 2013) with physiological effects. Hegemonic masculinity has been linked to controlling the embodied drunkenness that occurs following excessive alcohol consumption. This resonates with broader historically valued notions of rational and disembodied masculinity (Seidler, 1994). Thus, it has been important for men to 'hold' one's drink, and effects such as slurring, stumbling, and passing out are seen as signs of weakness (Thurnell-Read, 2013). Campbell's (2000) work on male drinking practices in rural pubs in New Zealand highlights the importance of being in control of the male body while drinking, through maintaining composure and urinating infrequently.

However, more recent research has questioned the links between consuming alcohol, idealised forms of masculinity and retaining control over the male body. Heavy drinking, drunkenness and the ensuing loss of bodily control are celebrated by some young men. Research highlights how young men celebrate their drunken loss of bodily control across different contexts, such as when they are away on stag weekends in Europe (Thurnell-Read, 2011), partying at twenty-first birthdays in the USA (Kimmel, 2008), and drinking after rugby sessions in New Zealand (Willott and Lyons, 2012). Furthermore, research in the UK (Griffin et al., 2009) and New Zealand (Lyons et al., 2014) highlights that many young people, both men and women, socialise and drink together with the explicit aim of getting drunk and losing bodily control (and memory).

Thurnell-Read (2011, 2013) suggests that drinking and drunkenness are appealing for (young) men because they allow for a pleasurable release from the ongoing, everyday imperative to control the male body. Drunkenness has also been found to provide young women with a 'break' or 'release' from everyday embodied gender norms (Stepney, 2015; Waitt et al., 2011). Idealised men's bodies are controlled, rational, autonomous and independent, and drinking and drunkenness may allow men a sought-after escape from such embodied performances. As Robertson (2006, 2007) has demonstrated, (young) men may need to negotiate the control/release dichotomy; while drinking as a release can be viewed as masculine, there is an increasing (neoliberal) requirement for individuals to be health-conscious and responsible. In practice this might mean being sensible (controlled, e.g. working out at the gym etc.) during the week and letting go and getting drunk at weekends.

Drinking alcohol also enables men to engage with aspects of embodiment that are traditionally denied in idealised masculinity, such as experiencing and expressing emotion, pain and friendship. Scottish men viewed their drinking in the pub as an 'act of friendship' which allowed them to explicitly display and discuss emotions and mental health (Emslie et al., 2013). In the USA, Peralta (2008) reported how alcohol enabled young men and women to transgress gender boundaries, with young men discussing how alcohol created a context that allowed them to engage in behaviours considered non-masculine (e.g. crying, being emotional) or that were homosexual (see also Scoats, 2015). Drinking therefore may allow men to transgress notions of everyday idealised (heterosexual) masculinity and its embodiment, and engage in gender performances that go against proscribed gender practices (Peralta, 2008).

The advent and rapid ascent of social media, particularly social networking sites (SNS), has seen drinking practices and cultures move into online spaces. Popular SNS platforms include Facebook, Twitter, Instagram and YouTube. People use SNS to connect with other people, explicitly articulating their social networks and making them visible (boyd and Ellison, 2007). Young people are high users of SNS, sharing their drinking events, experiences and practices through posts, status updates, checking in, likes, photos and videos (e.g. see Moreno and Whitehill, 2016; Ridout, 2016; Westgate and Holliday, 2016 for overviews). Research has demonstrated that sharing drinking events, experiences and alcohol-related content on Facebook functions to solidify friendship bonds (Niland et al., 2013), create drinking cultures that are 'airbrushed', minimise the visibility of negative consequences (Niland et al., 2014), and also enables (gendered) identity work to take place (Lyons, et al., 2014). It additionally intensifies the normalisation of alcohol and drinking to intoxication (Niland et al., 2014; Ridout et al., 2012) and provides a fertile (unregulated) context for the marketing and branding of alcohol products (such as SNS brand pages, events, and competitions that encourage user interaction with the brand (e.g. see Critchlow et al., 2016; Michaelidou and Moraes, 2016).

Gender, masculinities and social networking sites

Young people use SNS to share their tastes and preferences, stay connected with friends and broader peer-groups, display social connections and perform social identities (boyd, 2007; Livingstone, 2008). Social media use is a gendered activity, and SNS have always been employed by users to construct and perform gendered identities (Cook and Hasmath, 2014). Technology has historically been identified with masculinity and masculine competencies, and gendered stereotypes about computing continue (Pechtelidis et al., 2015). Gendered assumptions about technology (Kelan, 2007) may mean that, for example, women distance themselves from technology as a way to construct feminine identities while men appropriate technology to 'do masculinity' (Kelan, 2007). However, Light (2013) has argued that such simplistic alignments of masculinities with technology may become more complicated with the rise of social networking technologies.

Researchers have examined online gender performances on SNS and have generally found that they reflect traditional notions of masculinity and femininity (e.g. Haferkamp et al., 2012; Kapidzic and Herring, 2014). Early research with MySpace users found that self-presentation mirrored stereotypical gender norms, such that women portrayed themselves as attractive and affiliative, and men as embodying strength and power (Manago et al., 2008). Further, females were found to have more friends and be more interested in using MySpace for friendship, while males were more interested in using it for dating (Thelwall, 2008). Female MySpace users were also found to both give and receive more positive comments than male users (with no difference for negative comments), leading researchers to conclude that 'females are more successful social network site users partly because of their greater ability to textually harness positive affect' (Thelwall et al., 2010: 190).

A body of literature has developed exploring the performance of femininity on SNS. Much of this work has focused on the ways in which young women negotiate postfeminist expectations of online gender performances that position them as successful, popular and authentic. These performances require highly sexualised public displays of femininity, including posting sexualised pictures and content (Bailey et al., 2013; Cook and Hasmath, 2014; Dobson, 2014a, 2014b, 2014c). Girls have also been found to construct identities that involve sexualised femininity (Ringrose and Barajas, 2011). Much less research attention has focused on the performance of masculinity on SNS, and what has been conducted has primarily dealt with gay, bisexual and queer men's masculinities (Light, 2013). Light (2013) suggests this focus on masculinities, sexuality and sexual practice has perhaps arisen because researchers want to challenge heteronormative assumptions, but argues that we need to broaden our scope and 'men need to be gendered beyond the sexual when it comes to our understandings of digital media' (p. 249). In terms of SNS, these sites provide a high degree of 'publicness' in which men can perform and validate their masculinity, although comparatively little work has examined heterosexual masculinities and SNS (Light, 2013). One exception is a study with teenage boys in London. This found that boys amassed cultural capital through sharing images of consumer objects that signify wealth (e.g. sunglasses, shoes) on SNS. These enabled them to embody masculine 'swagger' and popularity through likes and comments, thus performing desirable forms of youth masculinity which circulated through digital networks (Harvey et al., 2013).

Siibak (2010) analysed visual self-presentations of men on Rate, a popular Estonian SNS. She specifically studied young men on the Rate community 'Damn I'm Beautiful', and found that these young men used photos to predominantly portray themselves as sexual or romantic objects. The posing techniques employed were similar to those in the advertising industry, and can be seen as self-marketing strategies that are more sexual and in some ways considered more feminine and metrosexual than previously, emphasising hairstyles and fashion trends. Since the 1980s there has been greater visibility, idealisation and eroticisation of male bodies as well as a more general notion that the male body can be a source of cultural capital and identity (Gough et al., 2014). This may be linked to consumption shifting from a feminised activity to one that is appropriate and suitable for men (Moore, 1989), as well as a societal shift to a focus on the body (Turner, 1996), and using bodies as key resources to create and recreate identities (Gough et al., 2014).

Hall and colleagues (2012) explored the performance of metrosexual masculinities on SNS by analysing a YouTube video tutorial created by a young man teaching peers how to apply makeup and the online responses by other men. Results demonstrated that while men were able to identify themselves as interested in clothes, cosmetics and appearance, their online identify performances were constructed to ward off being positioned as gay and emphasised their heterosexuality. Other research has explored the online forums in which young men provide information regarding their use of appearance-enhancing substances, such as ephedrine (for weight loss: Hall et al., 2015a) and synthol (to make muscles appear larger: Hall et al., 2015b). This work shows that young men provide each other with support online, downplay health concerns and accentuate the benefits of the substances (when they are used by insider, experienced community members). Other research has analysed masculinities on YouTube. Morris and Anderson (2015) analysed the video-blogging of Britain's most popular 'vloggers' on YouTube, namely Charlie McDonnell (*Charlieissocoollike*), Dan Howell (*Danisnotonfire*) and Jack and Finn Harries (*JacksGap*). They concluded that these vloggers are performing a new form of modern masculinity that is softer and without homophobia, misogyny and aggression. They theorise this in terms of 'inclusive masculinity theory' (Anderson, 2009) and suggest these young YouTubers embody this more inclusive masculinity, which suggests a shift in dominant youth culture. However, inclusive masculinity theory has been strongly critiqued for its ignorance of gender and power relations in a postfeminist context, and its lack of attention to structural aspects of people's lives such as class (Nagel and Mora, 2010; O'Neill, 2015). It appears to be derived from research with primarily white, heterosexual, middle-class and privileged young men.

Hybrid masculinity may be a more useful conceptual framework to help understand the ways in which white, heterosexual (elite) men have appropriated ideals and practices from 'other' communities, such as women (e.g. cosmetics), gay men (e.g. fashion) and black men (e.g. gangsta rap styles) while retaining their hegemonic status. From this perspective, masculinity is repackaged and modernised without any loss of power or status (Bridges and Pascoe, 2014). Atkinson's (2011) notion of pastiche masculinity may also be useful here. Matthews (2016) has used this idea to explore how the hegemony of certain men continues to exist, despite changes in understandings around masculinity and men's lives. Matthews draws on Atkinson (2011) to argue that power is based on being able to change and reform masculine identities, and realign them with (previously) marginalised identities (such as those that are racialised or working class) to:

> make one appear as culturally progressive, cool, sensitive, moral, genuine, correct, or liberal in one context or another; each of these becomes techniques for achieving power in a liquid modern, reflexive identity-based society.
>
> (Atkinson, 2011: 41)

Therefore power comes about at the intersection of multiple processes, and as changes occur, there are possibilities for new forms of power to arise (Matthews, 2016).

These studies suggest that in the context of SNS, we may have seen a shift in ideals of masculinity. However, as Manago's (2013) case study of a US male undergraduate's MySpace profile highlights, 'these new masculine ideals employ irony to maintain power and superiority over homosexuality and femininity' (p. 493). Manago suggests that irony and parody are employed on SNS in a similar way to men's magazines promoting metrosexuality, namely to portray a sexualised display while retaining power and avoiding vulnerability or exploitation. This is similar to Benwell's (2004) analysis of men's lifestyle magazines, in which she demonstrated the deployment of irony as a way of inoculating performances of hegemonic masculinity against charges of sexism. Irony functioned 'both to give voice to reactionary and antifeminist sentiments and to continually destabilize the notion of a coherent and visible masculinity' (p. 3).

Masculinities, drinking cultures and social networking sites

As noted previously, SNS are also crucially implicated in many young people's drinking practices, where the sharing and consuming of both self-produced and commercial images of female and male drinking is central (Hebden et al., 2015; Lyons, et al., 2014). Sharing photos is an important affordance of many SNS, allowing users not just to share but also to comment and communicate with their networks about specific photos (Lobinger, 2016). Digital mobile technologies have allowed young people to connect on SNS, upload photos, comment and interact while they are drinking alcohol when preloading (drinking alcohol at private premises before going out into town, to bars and clubs) (McCreanor et al., 2015) and when out in the night-time economy (Lyons et al., 2014). Some research highlights that the displaying, sharing, and commenting on drinking photos on social media sites is where notions of appropriate and inappropriate masculinities and femininities are negotiated (Brown and Gregg, 2012; Dobson, 2014a).

Mendelson and Papacharissi (2010) examined the photos in male and female US college students' personal Facebook photo galleries and found gender differences in the types of photos and poses employed. Most photos were taken at parties, with alcohol a key feature. Photos were posted by many different people, so the galleries were constantly changing. To manage this, people untagged themselves from photos they did not want on their gallery. Women had more casual photos, and more flirtatious and sexy poses in their photos, than men. Men were likely to only have photos taken at more formal (compared to casual) events, emphasising the importance of 'drinking buddies' to their sociality on Facebook. The authors concluded that posting and sharing drinking and socialising photos were ways to show bonds between friends, highlight leisure activities and perform gendered identities (Mendelson and Papacharissi, 2010).

Goodwin and colleagues' (2016) research in New Zealand highlighted the ways in which drinking photos on Facebook act as discursive resources among friendship groups, through being commented on, shared, 'liked', discussed, tagged, untagged and so on. These authors argue that 'drinking photos facilitate valued forms of "amplified", "authentic" sociality, visibility, and popularity' (p. 1) but that the risks and opportunities within such contexts are uneven due to structural power relations, including gender. The practices around taking and uploading photos, checking, tagging and untagging were gendered, and more intensely engaged in by young women (see also Lyons et al., 2016). These differences can be understood as practices embedded within 'sexual power relations that constitute young women as subject to gendered regulatory scrutiny' (Goodwin et al., 2016: 6). There were also other intersectional complexities identified, including those around class and ethnicity. For example, Māori (indigenous population of Aotearoa New Zealand) participants were much more reluctant to engage in photo-taking and uploading within the night-time economy and they avoided night-time photographers and sometimes going out altogether. As the authors note, 'these young Māori participants' reticence to engage in online [drinking] display cannot be disentangled from broader, problematic representations of Māori in general' (p. 8).

Lyons and colleagues (2016) focused on the gendered nature of photo-taking practices in young people's drinking cultures in the same New Zealand sample. They found that male participants did not describe engaging in the same level of photo-taking, posing for photos, self-surveillance while out drinking, constant checking of Facebook photos, or tagging and untagging in photos as the female participants. In group discussions (in both same- and mixed-sex groups) male participants were often heavily disparaging of these practices, defining them as feminine, excessive and frivolous, with a focus on appearance rather than (the more important task of) drinking and getting drunk with friends. Nevertheless, in individual interviews in which male participants took the researcher on a tour around their Facebook pages and showed and discussed their drinking photos, it was clear that their drinking photos were highly valued both individually and within their peer groups. These photos often led to ongoing online interactions with friends and the recounting of humorous stories. Perhaps the common view that men are not as concerned about their online identities as women, and therefore put less effort into them, is a myth (Manago et al., 2008). Manago and colleagues (2008) suggest that this may be a way for (young) men to shore up hegemonic (and particularly heterosexual) masculine power.

In the UK, Scoats (2015) analysed over 1000 photographs from the Facebook profiles of 44 heterosexual, white males studying at a British university. As might be expected within this group, many (just over half) of the photographs were taken at pubs, clubs and parties, and more involved drinking and alcohol outside of these settings. Scoats' analysis demonstrated that the photos overwhelmingly displayed homosocial behaviours, such as men touching, kissing and dancing with each other, and he argued that this provides evidence for wider cultural shifts in gender norms towards 'inclusive masculinity', which involves decreasing levels of homophobia (see Anderson, 2009). The 18 photos of men kissing were all taken in clubs, bars or at parties with the implied presence of alcohol, suggesting alcohol was a key contextual feature for this particular behaviour. Others have argued that alcohol enables heterosexual men to transgress gender boundaries in this way (de Visser and Smith, 2007; Peralta, 2008), something that has occurred over many previous generations as media accounts of powerful people's drinking attest to (such as media stories of David Cameron's university drinking days). Inclusive masculinity theory has been said to erase sexual politics and outlines a cultural shift that may only be apparent in a particular sub-group of classed (privileged) young men (O'Neill, 2015).

However, what has changed is that these transgressions are now photographed and posted online on Facebook pages in a way that the young men involved appear not to be concerned about. Without talking to the men in the photographs we cannot know what the photo means to them, why they include it in their photo gallery, or indeed who took and who posted the image. It may be an indicator of reducing homohysteria within young men's peer culture, as Scoats claims. However, as Manago (2013) shows, young men use irony to include gender transgressions within online identity performances, while at the same time reinforcing dominant forms of masculinity and gendered power relations.

Although it has been argued that 'social networking sites, such as Facebook, offer relatively accurate representations of the identities that people wish to portray' (Scoats, 2015: 7), as researchers we need to be very careful about assuming we can take material from SNS, including photos, and 'read off' their meanings at face value. A range of research highlights that the meanings that (drinking) photos hold for young people cannot be taken at face value, and can function to represent situations that are implied or only known about by people who were present, or those who are part of the friend group (e.g. Hebden et al., 2015; Niland et al., 2014; Tonks et al., 2015). In other words, the meanings surrounding the identity performance are invisible for those outside the friendship group. Similarly, Manago (2013) and McCormack (2012) demonstrate that men can use photos in an ironic way, which functions to present non-traditional masculine practices that are understood as humorous within peer groups, rather than as evidence of shifting cultural norms. Similarly, recent research highlights the issues of sexual politics and gendered power relations in practices around sharing drinking images on social networking sites (e.g. see Dobson, 2014c; Hutton et al., 2016; Lyons et al., 2016) that can be overlooked by focusing solely on image content without considering why and how the images function for the user, and what meanings they have. The findings from Scoats' (2015) study demonstrate the privilege that young, white, university male students have, a privilege that 'enables these men to engage in homoerotic, homosexual, and effeminate behaviours with impunity' (Nagel and Mora, 2010: 110). Intersections of class, ethnicity and sexuality are all involved in gendered power relations and cannot be ignored or overlooked in online analyses of gender and drinking cultures.

Conclusions

Certain types of drinking practices, and certain types of social media usage, become gendered through their association with notions of masculinity or femininity. Masculinities are produced and reproduced through engagement in drinking cultures as well as their online representations, and the practices involved in creating these representations. With the ubiquity of mobile technologies, there are 'new and intensified ways for value to circulate within young people's peer networks' (Harvey et al., 2013: 7). Research demonstrates that popularity, authenticity and attention are important in young people's displays of their engagements in the culture of intoxication (Goodwin et al., 2016). Furthermore, 'sexual displays are an efficient attention-getting tactic on SNS' (Manago, 2013: 489) for both men and women. However, most of the research has been conducted with heterosexual young adults, and little work has explored sexuality, social networking and drinking cultures. De Ridder and Van Bauwel (2013, 2015) highlight how gender and sexualities are negotiated on social networking sites by young people. There is also a dearth of research exploring men, masculinities, drinking practices and virtual intoxigenic identities. Additionally, we know little about if and how marketing on social media plays a role in the (re)creation and maintenance of these identities, although it has been argued as actively at work in conventional media (Towns et al., 2012). Furthermore, few studies have examined whether young men's creation of, and engagement with, drinking photos differ from young women's practices, and why virtual displays of drinking or drunk bodies are important for young men in particular contexts. This is an area of research that is important, timely and ripe for exploration.

References

Anderson, E. (2009). *Inclusive Masculinity: The Changing Nature of Masculinities.* London: Routledge.

Atkinson, M. (2011). *Deconstructing Men and Masculinities*. Oxford: Oxford University Press.

Bailey, J., Steeves, V., Burkell, J., and Regan, P. (2013). Negotiating with gender stereotypes in social networking sites: From 'bicycle face' to Facebook. *Journal of Communication Inquiry, 37*(2), 91–112.

Benwell, B. (2004). Ironic discourse: Evasive masculinity in British men's lifestyle magazines. *Men and Masculinities, 7*(1), 3–21.

boyd, d. (2007). Why youth (heart) social network sites: The role of networked publics in teenage social life. In D. Buckingham (Ed.), *Youth, Identity and Digital Media Volume* (pp. 119–142, McArthur Foundation Series on Digital Learning). Cambridge, MA: MIT Press.

boyd, d., and Ellison, N. (2007). Social network sites: Definition, history, and scholarship. *Journal of Computer-Mediated Communication, 13*(1), 210–230.

Bridges, T., and Pascoe, C. (2014). Hybrid masculinities: New directions in the sociology of men and masculinities. *Sociology Compass, 8*(3), 246–258.

Brown, R., and Gregg, M. (2012). The pedagogy of regret: Facebook, binge drinking and young women. *Continuum: Journal of Media and Cultural Studies, 26*(3), 357–369.

Campbell, H. (2000). The glass phallus: Pub(lic) masculinity and drinking in rural New Zealand. *Rural Sociology, 65*(4), 562–581.

Connell, R. (1995). *Masculinities*. Cambridge: Polity Press.

Connell, R., and Messerschmidt, J. (2005). Hegemonic masculinity rethinking the concept. *Gender and Society, 19*(6), 829–859.

Cook, J., and Hasmath, R. (2014). The discursive construction and performance of gendered identity on social media. *Current Sociology, 62*(7), 975–993.

Critchlow, N., Moodie, C., Bauld, L., Bonner, A., and Hastings, G. (2016). Awareness of, and participation with, digital alcohol marketing, and the association with frequency of high episodic drinking among young adults. *Drugs: Education, Prevention and Policy,* published online 26 January, doi: 10.3109/09687637.09682015.01119247.

De Ridder, S., and Van Bauwel, S. (2013). Commenting on pictures: Teens negotiating gender and sexualities on social networking sites. *Sexualities, 16*(5–6), 565–586.

De Ridder, S., and Van Bauwel, S. (2015). The discursive construction of gay teenagers in times of mediatization: Youth's reflections on intimate storytelling, queer shame and realness in popular social media places. *Journal of Youth Studies, 18*(6), 777–793.

de Visser, R., and McDonnell, E. (2013). 'Man points': Masculine capital and young men's health. *Health Psychology, 32*(1), 5–14.

de Visser, R., and Smith, J. (2007). Alcohol consumption and masculine identity among young men. *Psychology and Health, 22*(5), 595–614.

Dobson, A. (2014a). Laddishness online: The possible significations and significance of 'performative shamelessness' for young women in the postfeminist context. *Cultural Studies, 28*(1), 142–164.

Dobson, A. (2014b). 'Sexy' and 'laddish' girls: Unpacking complicity between two cultural imag(inations)es of young femininity. *Feminist Media Studies, 14*(2), 253–269.

Dobson, A. (2014c). Performative shamelessness on young women's social network sites: Shielding the self and resisting gender melancholia. *Feminism and Psychology, 24*(1), 97–114.

Emslie, C., Hunt, K., and Lyons, A. (2013). The role of alcohol in forging and maintaining friendships amongst Scottish men in midlife. *Health Psychology, 32*(1), 33–41.

Goodwin, I., Griffin, C., Lyons, A., McCreanor, T., and Moewaka Barnes, H. (2016). Precarious popularity: Facebook drinking photos, the attention economy, and the regime of the branded self. *Social Media + Society, 2*(1), doi: 10.1177/2056305116628889.

Gough, B., Hall, M., and Seymour-Smith, S. (2014). Straight guys do wear make-up: Contemporary masculinities and investment in appearance. In S. Roberts (Ed.), *Debating Modern Masculinities: Change, Continuity, Crisis?* (pp. 106–124). Basingstoke: Palgrave.

Griffin, C., Bengry-Howell, A., Hackley, C., Mistral, W., and Szmigin, I. (2009). 'Every time I do it I absolutely annihilate myself': Loss of (self)-consciousness and loss of memory in young people's drinking narratives. *Sociology, 43*, 457–476.

Haferkamp, N., Eimler, S., Papadakis, A., and Kruck, J. (2012). Men are from Mars, women are from Venus? Examining gender differences in self-presentation on social networking sites. *Cyberpsychology, Behavior, and Social Networking, 15*(2), 91–98.

Hall, M., Gough, B., and Seymour-Smith, S. (2012). 'I'm METRO, NOT Gay!': A discursive analysis of men's accounts of makeup use on YouTube. *Journal of Men's Studies, 20*(3), 209–226.

Hall, M., Grogan, S., and Gough, B. (2015a). 'It is safe to use if you are healthy': A discursive analysis of men's online accounts of ephedrine use. *Psychology and Health, 30*(7), 770–782.

Hall, M., Grogan, S., and Gough, B. (2015b). Bodybuilders' accounts of synthol use: The construction of lay expertise online. *Journal of Health Psychology*, published online February 2, doi:10.1177/1359105314568579.

Harvey, L., Ringrose, J., and Gill, R. (2013). Swagger, ratings and masculinity: Theorising the circulation of social and cultural value in teenage boys' digital peer networks. *Sociological Research Online, 18*(4), Article 9. www.socres-online.org.uk/18/14/19.html

Hebden, R., Lyons, A., Goodwin, I., and McCreanor, T. (2015). 'When you add alcohol it gets that much better': University students, alcohol consumption and online drinking cultures. *Journal of Drug Issues, 45*(2), 214–226.

Hutton, F., Griffin, C., Lyons, A., Niland, P., and McCreanor, T. (2016). 'Tragic girls' and 'crack whores': Alcohol, femininity and Facebook. *Feminism and Psychology, 26*(1), 73–93.

Kapidzic, S., and Herring, S. (2014). Race, gender, and self-presentation in teen profile photographs. *New Media and Society, 17*(6), 958–976.

Kelan, W. (2007). Tools and toys: Communicating gendered positions towards technology. *Information, Communication and Society, 10*(3), 358–383.

Kimmel, M. (2008). *Guyland: The Perilous World Where Boys Become Men: Understanding the Critical Years Between 16 and 26.* New York: Harper Collins.

Lemle, R., and Mishkind, M. (1989). Alcohol and masculinity. *Journal of Substance Abuse Treatment, 6*(4), 213–222.

Light, B. (2013). Networked masculinities and social networking sites: A call for the analysis of men and contemporary digital media. *Masculinities and Social Change, 2*(3), 245–265.

Livingstone, S. (2008). Taking risky opportunities in youthful content creation: Teenagers' use of SNSs for intimacy, privacy and self-expression. *New Media and Society, 10*(3), 393–411.

Lobinger, K. (2016). Photographs as things – photographs of things. A text-material perspective on photo-sharing practices. *Information, Communication and Society, 19*(4), 475–488.

Lyons, A. (2009). Masculinities, femininities, behaviour and health. *Social and Personality Psychology Compass*, *3*(4), 394–412.

Lyons, A., Goodwin, I., Griffin, C., McCreanor, T., and Moewaka Barnes, H. (2016). Facebook and the fun of drinking photos: Reproducing gendered regimes of power. *Social Media and Society*, *1–13*. DOI: 10.1177/2056305116672888.

Lyons, A., McCreanor, T., Goodwin, I., Griffin, C., Hutton, F., Moewaka Barnes, H., O'Carroll, D., Samu, L., Niland, P., and Vroman, K.-E. (2014). Youth drinking cultures in Aotearoa New Zealand. *Sites: New Series*, *11*(2), 78–102.

Lyons, A., and Willott, S. (2008). Alcohol consumption, gender identities and women's changing social positions. *Sex Roles*, *59*, 694–712.

Manago, A. (2013). Negotiating a sexy masculinity on social networking sites. *Feminism and Psychology*, *23*(4), 478–497.

Manago, A., Graham, M., Greenfield, P., and Salimkhan, G. (2008). Self-presentation and gender on MySpace. *Journal of Applied Developmental Psychology*, *29*(6), 446–458.

Matthews, C. R. (2016). Exploring the pastiche hegemony of men. *Palgrave Communications*, *2*, 16022. doi: 10.1057/palcomms.2016.22.

McCormack, M. (2012). *The Declining Significance of Homophobia*. Oxford: Oxford University Press.

McCreanor, T., Lyons, A., Moewaka Barnes, H., Hutton, F., Goodwin, I., and Griffin, C. (2015). 'Drink a twelve box before you go'*: Pre-loading among young people in Aotearoa New Zealand. *Kotuitui*, published online: 9 Jun 2015.

Mendelson, A., and Papacharissi, Z. (2010). Look at us: Collective narcissism in college student Facebook photo galleries. In Z. Papacharissi (Ed.), *The Networked Self: Identity, Community and Culture on Social Network Sites* (pp. 251–273). Abingdon: Routledge.

Michaelidou, N., and Moraes, C. (2016). How companies use Facebook to promote alcohol brands to young adults. In C. Campbell and J. Ma (Eds.), *Looking Forward, Looking Back: Drawing on the Past to Shape the Future of Marketing* (pp. 487–490). New York: Springer.

Moore, S. (1989). Getting a bit of the other – the pimps of postmodernism. In R. Chapman and J. Rutherford (Eds), *Male Order: Unwrapping Masculinity* (pp. 165–192). London: Lawrence & Wishart.

Moreno, M., and Whitehill, J. (2016). # Wasted: the intersection of substance use behaviors and social media in adolescents and young adults. *Current Opinion in Psychology*, *9*, 72–76.

Morris, M., and Anderson, E. (2015). 'Charlie is so cool like': Authenticity, popularity and inclusive masculinity on YouTube. *Sociology*, published online before print February 6, doi: 10.1177/0038038514562852.

Mullen, K., Watson, J., Swift, J., and Black, D. (2007). Young men, masculinity and alcohol. *Drugs, Education, Prevention and Policy*, *14*(2), 151–165.

Nagel, E., and Mora, R. (2010). Inclusive Masculinity: The Changing Nature of Masculinities by Eric Anderson. New York and London, Routledge, 2009, 190 pp [Book Review]. *Journal of Men's Studies*, *18*(1), 109–110.

Niland, P., Lyons, A., Goodwin, I., and Hutton, F. (2013). 'Everyone can loosen up and get a bit of a buzz on': Young adults, alcohol and friendship practices. *International Journal of Drug Policy*, *24*(6), 530–537.

Niland, P., Lyons, A., Goodwin, I., and Hutton, F. (2014). 'See it doesn't look pretty does it?' Young adults' airbrushed drinking practices on Facebook. *Psychology and Health*, *29*(8), 877–895.

O'Neill, R. (2015). Whither critical masculinity studies? Notes on inclusive masculinity theory, postfeminism, and sexual politics. *Men and Masculinities, 18*(1), 100–120.

Pechtelidis, Y., Kosma, Y., and Chronaki, A. (2015). Between a rock and a hard place: Women and computer technology. *Gender and Education, 27*(2), 164–182.

Peralta, R. (2007). College alcohol use and the embodiment of hegemonic masculinity among European college men. *Sex Roles, 56*(11), 741–756.

Peralta, R. (2008). 'Alcohol allows you to not be yourself': Toward a structured understanding of alcohol use and gender difference among gay, lesbian, and heterosexual youth. *Journal of Drug Issues, 38*(2), 373–399.

Rahav, G., Wilsnack, R., Bloomfield, K., Gmel, G., and Kuntsche, S. (2006). The influence of societal level factors on men's and women's alcohol consumption and alcohol problems. *Alcohol and Alcoholism, 41,* 147–155.

Ridout, B. (2016). Facebook, social media and its application to problem drinking among college students. *Current Opinion in Psychology, 9,* 83–87.

Ridout, B., Campbell, A., and Ellis, L. (2012). 'Off your Face(book)': Alcohol in online social identity construction and its relation to problem drinking in university students. *Drug and Alcohol Review, 31*(1), 20–26.

Ringrose, J., and Barajas, K. (2011). Gendered risks and opportunities? Exploring teen girls' digitized sexual identities in postfeminist media contexts. *International Journal of Media and Cultural Politics, 7*(2), 121–138.

Robertson, S. (2006). 'I've been like a coiled spring this last week': Embodied masculinity and health. *Sociology of Health and Illness, 28*(4), 433–456.

Robertson, S. (2007). *Understanding Men and Health: Masculinities, Identity and Wellbeing.* Maidenhead, Berkshire: McGraw-Hill Education.

Scoats, R. (2015). Inclusive masculinity and Facebook photographs among early emerging adults at a British university. *Journal of Adolescent Research,* published online before print September 23, doi: 10.1177/0743558415607059.

Seidler, V. (1994). *Unreasonable Men: Masculinity and Social Theory.* London: Routledge.

Siibak, A. (2010). Constructing masculinity on a social networking site: The case-study of visual self-presentations of young men on the profile images of SNS Rate. *Young Nordic Journal of Youth Research, 18*(4), 403–425.

Stepney, M. (2015). The challenge of hyper-sexual femininity and binge drinking: A feminist psychoanalytic response. *Subjectivity, 8*(1), 57–73.

Thelwall, M. (2008). Social networks, gender, and friending: An analysis of MySpace member profiles. *Journal of the American Society for Information Science and Technology, 59*(8), 1321–1330.

Thelwall, M., Wilkinson, D., and Uppal, S. (2010). Data mining emotion in social network communication: Gender differences in MySpace. *Journal of the American Society for Information Science and Technology, 61*(1), 190–199.

Thurnell-Read, T. (2011). Off the leash and out of control: Masculinities and embodiment in Eastern European stag tourism. *Sociology, 45*(6), 977–991.

Thurnell-Read, T. (2013). 'Yobs' and 'snobs': Embodying drink and the problematic male drinking body. *Sociological Research Online, 18*(2), www.socresonline.org. uk/18/12/13.html

Tonks, A., Lyons, A., and Goodwin, I. (2015). Researching online visual displays on social networking sites: Methodologies and meanings. *Qualitative Research in Psychology, 12*(3), 326–339.

Towns, A., Parker, C., and Chase, P. (2012). Constructions of masculinity in alcohol advertising: Implications for the prevention of domestic violence. *Addiction Research and Theory*, 20(5), 389–401.

Turner, B. (1996). *The Body and Society: Explorations in Social Theory* (2nd edn). London: Sage.

Waitt, G., Jessop, L., and Gorman-Murray, A. (2011). 'The guys in there just expect to be laid': Embodied and gendered socio-spatial practices of a night out; in Wollongong, Australia. *Gender, Place and Culture*, 18(2), 255–275.

Westgate, E., and Holliday, J. (2016). Identity, influence, and intervention: The roles of social media in alcohol use. *Current Opinion in Psychology*, 9, 27–32.

Willott, S., and Lyons, A. (2012). Consuming male identities: Masculinities and alcohol consumption in Aotearoa New Zealand. *Journal of Community and Applied Social Psychology*, 22, 330–345.

5   Ethnicity/culture, alcohol and social media

Helen Moewaka Barnes, Patricia Niland, Lina Samu, Acushla Deanne Sciascia and Tim McCreanor

In Aotearoa New Zealand there are key differences in the ways in which different ethnic groups use alcohol (Ministry of Health, 2015). Pākehā populations drink more than Māori or Pasifika populations but in more regular and controlled ways that incur less harm.

This situation is not uncommon internationally as shown in studies in other countries where European colonisation has displaced indigenous peoples and used racist migration policies that create marginalised minority immigrant populations (Saggers and Gray, 1998). Multiple studies in the United States, Australia and elsewhere show indigenous or minority group drinkers experience harms at higher levels than white populations with similar levels of consumption (Duff et al., 2011; Malone et al., 2012; Pascal et al., 2009; Spillane and Smith, 2007; Wilson et al., 2010; Yan et al., 2008).

As many chapters in this volume and elsewhere argue, consumption is strongly influenced by alcohol marketing and marketing is increasingly moving to include social media in its toolkit. In New Zealand and elsewhere, research is showing use of social media rapidly approaching saturation throughout the population (Gibson et al., 2013; Smith et al., 2010).

This chapter reports data from a qualitative study of this emerging area of concern (Lyons et al., 2014b) and aims to explore the dynamics and tensions thrown up at the intersection of alcohol and social media as it plays out for young adult members of three key ethnic groupings in Aotearoa New Zealand – Māori, Pasifika and Pākehā. In this setting Māori are the indigenous people of Aotearoa who have been colonised over 175 years by Pākehā settler groups largely from western Europe. Pasifika peoples are more recent immigrants to this country from diverse Pacific islands especially Samoa, the Cook Islands and Tonga.

In the context of substance use, Oetting et al. (1998) articulate a theory of primary socialisation in which ethnicity is 'perceived membership of a cultural group' and cultural identity is 'strength of identification with a group' (p. 2075); this complex is seen as pivotal to the ways in which individuals respond to exposure to substances. While we are aware of the influences of gender and socio-economic status, the main focus here is on ways in which this ethnic/cultural complex plays out in the dynamics in the convergence of alcohol and social media. Gender and class are clearly part of the complex, as we have argued elsewhere

(Hutton et al., 2016; Lyons et al., 2014a) but, for this analysis, they are not foregrounded as we work with broad, inclusive notions of ethnicity and the associated aspects of culture to make sense of data gathered from focus groups constituted in this frame.

In this country, young people in all their diversity meet, mingle and interact, in schools, workplaces, sport and many other domains, but their life chances, experiences and relationships are structured by fundamental variations in social inclusion and exclusion (Spoonley et al., 1996). In this nominally bicultural democracy, the legacy of colonisation (primarily by the British from 1840 onwards) is visible in patterns of privilege and discrimination favouring European settler populations over indigenous Māori people and Pasifika migrants (Spoonley et al., 2004). Commitments to indigenous sovereignty promised by the Treaty of Waitangi have been severely breached through the entrenchment of an unreconstituted colonial state and minimally redressed, leaving deep divisions between Māori and Pākehā (Belich, 2007; Walker, 2004). Narratives of national identity stress unity, but there are deeply entrenched ethnic, gender and class disparities in health, education and socio-economic status (Ministry of Social Development, 2010). For instance, life expectancy data show a current gap of 7.1 years between Māori and Pākehā and slightly smaller discrepancies between Pasifika and Pākehā (Statistics New Zealand, 2013a, 2013b). In the 18–24-year-old age range, Pākehā make up 74% of the population, Māori 15% and Pasifika 7% with the balance made up of largely Indian and Chinese (Statistics New Zealand, 2013a).

Colonial context

Berry's (1992, 2006) modelling of acculturation strategies by dominant and non-dominant social groups, along the dimensions of intergroup relationships and preservation of culture and identity, leads to acculturation stress for all cultural groups. This includes the dominant group that, in various ways, polices and maintains the acculturation process; however, non-dominant groups are both more vulnerable and face larger challenges and changes to identity and culture (Berry, 2006). Here, we argue that these dynamics are at work in cultural patterning in the understandings and practices articulated by the young people who participated in the project as they navigate the challenging territory at the confluence of alcohol and social media use, in a steadily liberalising policy environment.

Within the colonial/bicultural context sketched above, it is possible to suggest some broad cultural dynamics that are at work in young adults' experiences with alcohol and social media (Lyons et al., 2014a). For example Pasifika cultures in Aotearoa, while as diverse as the homelands they hail from, often reflect characteristics of the social structures, language, practices and beliefs of the parent cultures. These are generally relational, communitarian, church-oriented and location specific so Pasifika cultures, broadly speaking, are networked, family-based, religious and imbued with pride in their homeland, language and culture

(Anae, 2001). Some of these characteristics are attenuating as the generations turn from the cultures of their immigrant parents and grandparents and become increasingly bi- or multicultural as they acculturate to life in New Zealand society (Fairbairn-Dunlop and Makisi, 2003).

Māori, as the indigenous peoples of Aotearoa, are also deeply communitarian, working from tribal, kin-group and family groupings to resist the processes of colonisation that for many have alienated their land, resources and language and have eroded cultural practices and institutions (Walker, 2004). While migration to large cities has contributed to the disruption of Māori society, this urban diaspora has also injected new ideas, resources and approaches into efforts towards aspirational autonomy and sovereignty. Partial restitutions for colonial harm and loss achieved through the Waitangi Tribunal are allowing Māori to slowly rebuild economic prosperity (Te Puni Kokiri, 2012) supporting a growing cultural renaissance.

Pākehā as beneficiaries of the colonial process are set in a Western mould now heavily inflected by neoliberal values. This has seen individualised, meritocratic capitalism, marketisation and deregulation (Kelsey, 2002) elevating economic development at the expense of social, cultural and environmental sustainability. For many this is manifest in a deep-seated, but often glossed or denied, sense of superiority that persists over Māori (McCreanor, 2010; Wetherell and Potter, 1992), in particular but over Pasifika and other more recent migrants in general, manifesting in victim-blaming of those experiencing difficulties and an overarching sense of privileged entitlement (Moewaka Barnes et al., 2014).

At the interface of these diverse populations, culture is contested, dynamic and evolving. Mutual reciprocities, influences and changes are evident for all groups and political, economic and demographic power is a key driver in trajectories of national identity. In Berry's (2006: 290) acculturation model, Pākehā are the fully acculturated 'dominant group', indigenous Māori are colonised and acculturated but resistant, with cultural traditions, homelands and possessions intact or renascent, and Pasifika are more recent (1950s) immigrants, first- and second-generation settlers with strong parent cultures in home islands, whose acculturation status is at an earlier stage than Māori.

Policy environment

The focus on the convergence of drinking cultures and social media use requires some contextualising to alcohol and media policy in Aotearoa New Zealand. The policy environments surrounding both are largely determined by a major swing in the politics of this country commencing in 1984 that saw the entrenchment of radical neoliberalism through the 1990s and early twenty-first century (Kelsey, 1995, 2002).

Alcohol policy was reformed via the Sale of Liquor Act (SOLA) 1989 that liberalised the criteria for granting licenses, extended licencing arrangements, allowing a proliferation and range of outlets including supermarkets and sports clubs (Hill and Stewart, 1998). Further SOLA reforms lowered the legal age of purchase from 20 to 18 in 1999 (Huckle et al., 2006). Changes to legislation in 1992 permitted alcohol promotion and marketing in broadcast media, resulting in a proliferation of advertisements on radio and television (Habgood et al., 2001; Hill and Casswell, 2004). As the internet became increasingly accessible in the mid-2000s, this new broadcast alcohol marketing culture migrated and took powerful root via online social media platforms. In combination these developments resulted in increased youth access to alcohol and led to higher exposure of young people to digital alcohol marketing (Lyons et al., 2014b). Studies suggest that exposure to alcohol marketing via digital media at an early age increases young people's chances of becoming a drinker in adolescence (Griffiths and Casswell, 2010; Lin et al., 2012).

Alcohol consumption

For various reasons much quantitative alcohol research has focused on dominant populations, with adequate samples of smaller population groups not always feasible or prioritised. Literature examining alcohol consumption and ethnicity largely focuses on disparities and problems, highlighting concerns about, for example, 'high risk' drinking in indigenous and other ethnic minorities (Chartier and Caetano, 2010; Jones-Webb et al., 1995).

Qualitative research indicates that we might expect convergences in meanings and motivations around drinking practices in young adults across ethnic groups given the globalising nature of what has been termed a culture of intoxication (Järvinen and Room, 2007; Measham and Brain, 2005) in Western countries. This is characterised as entailing widespread determined drunkenness (Measham, 2006) and routine hedonistic practices around 'controlled loss of control' (Measham and Brain, 2005: 273), supported by peer approval, pro-drinking meaning-making and lively discourses around extreme intoxication that circulate as marks of honour within peer groups (Griffin et al., 2009; Szmigin et al., 2008).

Consistent with international findings from similar societies, survey data in Aotearoa New Zealand show that consumption patterns of young people are broadly in line with notions of a culture of intoxication (Babor et al., 2010; Järvinen and Room, 2007; Rehm et al., 2009; Wicki et al., 2010). The New Zealand Health Survey (Ministry of Health, 2015) showed that more than 40% of 15–17 year olds reported starting drinking before age 15; a higher percentage than any other age band, suggesting that the age of recruitment to alcohol consumption is falling.

More widely, the survey reports that 85% of 20–24 year olds drank alcohol in the past year (more than any other age-band), with females less likely to have done so than males. Pākehā and Māori were considerably more likely to have consumed alcohol in the past year (85% and 80% respectively) than Pasifika (at 56%). Of the drinkers, 80% of 20–24 year olds consumed enough to feel drunk at least once in the past 12 months and nearly 20% drank to intoxication at least once a week. The survey showed that this group experience the greatest levels of biomedical, psychological and physical injury harms and that the distribution of these impacts were heavily negatively inflected by ethnicity and level of social deprivation (Ministry of Health, 2015).

Social media use

In this country 95% of people under the age of 30 use social media and Facebook is predominant (Gibson et al., 2013). Most young people have entrenched the use of social media, increasingly on mobile technologies, into their cultures as a means to circulate information and images that they value through their networks (Harvey et al., 2013; Lyons et al., 2015; Niland et al., 2013; O'Carroll, 2013). These online social networks confound distinctions between user and consumer, identity and persona (Hearn, 2008), public and private space (Papacharissi, 2009) and entail diverse pleasures or benefits as well as threats and risks (Brown and Gregg, 2012; Goodwin et al., 2016).

The convergence of drinking cultures and web-based social media use made it almost inevitable that representations of drinking – photographs, video, postings – as expressions of value and interest (Goodwin et al., 2016; Niland et al., 2013) would begin to appear online. The affordances of the new technologies – liking, sharing, tagging and commenting – make this information available to both its intended audiences (friend networks) and to wider unidentified groups and interests such as public authorities, employers and commercial marketers including those selling alcohol (McCreanor et al., 2013).

This chapter draws on focus group data from participants in each of the ethnic groupings referred to above in an effort to chart similarities and differences in some of their experiences as alcohol use and social media intersect. We collected data from 34 friendship focus groups of 18–25 year olds, in three ethnic strands, recording and transcribing their discussions about alcohol and social media in their lives (Lyons et al., 2015). These data have been explored using thematic analysis (Braun and Clarke, 2006) and a range of findings described (Lyons et al., 2014a; Moewaka Barnes et al., 2016). The intention is to document drivers, motivations and implications of this conjunction. We previously argued that there are subtle but significant differences in the meanings that different ethnic groups of young adults attach to alcohol use (Lyons et al., 2014a). Here we move to consider the particular meanings and experiences they discuss that are at the confluence of alcohol and social media use.

Alcohol and social media

A number of commentators argue that key to understandings young people have of social media is their experience of the excitement, utility and restraints of social media platforms (Brown and Gregg, 2012; Goodwin et al., 2016; Niland et al., 2013) while others worry over the potential and actual commercial exploitation of the facilities (Griffiths and Casswell, 2010; Jernigan and Rushman, 2014; McCreanor et al., 2013; Nicholls, 2012). We present qualitative data where both elements are under discussion within each of the social groups, to shed light on particular experiences and meanings participants shared in relation to alcohol and social media.

Pasifika participants

A common thread in the talk by Pasifika participants was the way in which the central communality of their cultures meant that their profiles in social media were always public property. As such, relationships, drug use, religion, language and culture were often implicitly measured against the standards of the dominant Pākehā culture, and were understood by participants as always available for community critique. Alcohol in particular is ambiguously proscribed for Pasifika people.

Although there was a strong sense of drinking being highly valued, it was also more widely understood as transgressive of Pasifika cultural norms, with dominant culture surveillance, intergenerational consequences and sensitivities presented as significant controls. In relation to young Pasifika and visible alcohol use, Atamai put it this way:

> ATAMAI: I think cos we're Pacific Islanders ... it's knowing that every time your name gets called out – you're not representing yourself, you're representing your family, your village.
>
> (Pasifika FG 10)

While drinking at clubs/bars, local pubs and domestic settings was enjoyed by many Pasifika participants, some of whom made strenuous efforts to hide their consumption from family and church members in particular, there were others who told us they did not drink at all.

Pasifika participants often identified and named their culture as salient to the ways they are seen on social media. Multiple data excerpts relate specifically to social media postings about the use of alcohol.

> KALETI: Like sometimes you're on such a buzz it's like 'oh my gosh, nice night out tonight it was funny as when you got drunk did duh da duh...' And then you forgot you added your Aunty 'Oh I didn't know you started drinking Kaleti'.
>
> PENITA: oops.
>
> ALAN: uh oh.
>
> (Pasifika FG 1)

The strength of networks within Pasifika communities makes the work of managing the intergenerational contexts around alcohol challenging. This is evident in this excerpt where a post on social media inflected with articulations of pleasure and fun intended for the peer group draws an imagined questioning response from an older relative that is recognised as disciplinary by the others in the group. In Kaleti's scenario, his self-monitoring of alcohol-related posts slip to the point where the older generations can view such posts. Penita and Alan note the unknown consequences and suggest expectations of censure.

Other participants talked about their efforts to pre-empt such difficulties by hiding (photographic) evidence of consumption.

> ANNA: We try not to take photos with alcohol.
> CHERIE: Or when we're with Terina, we hide our alcohol but when it's me and this one (to Anna) we're like
> INT: 'cheers to the freakin' weekend I'll drink to that'
> CHERIE: but when we're standing with Terina it's gonna be on her FB we're like 'cover up'
> INT: Book of Mormon stories
> TERINA: Exactly! 'Terina where were you last night? Are you sure you were at home'?
>
> (Pasifika FG 2)

In this group Terina is a non-drinker with strong church affiliations so her friends Cherie and Anna, who do drink, take extra care to avoid taking pictures that might implicate her in drinking. Although Cherie and Anna are more relaxed about how they themselves are portrayed, elsewhere in the transcript they also report removing photos and untagging others that do show alcohol or inappropriate behaviours, knowing that such images will produce religious parental reactions of the kind that Terina imagines in her final comment.

There was also a common perception that the peer group was under surveillance around alcohol and other behaviours, in direct and indirect ways.

> LESIELI: I never used to be really concerned about it until people in church that I'm not really close with knew things about me that I didn't really tell them. Stuff like that like freaks me out so ah yeah but I haven't changed my privacy, but I intend to but
> LAGI: Me too like I used to not care what um people thought of the photos and stuff like that but then I've realised you know cos we've graduated now, and we're like going into an industry where professional people are gonna look like at your page and like employ, future employers or current employers will look at your page, just to see what you're up to. So you don't want photos of you, at a party like going like this [looking intoxicated] cos [it] changes a lot of people's view of you.
>
> (Pasifika FG 3)

In this excerpt two young men describe parallel experiences of coming to the realisation that their social media pages were more public than they had perhaps envisaged. Church networks were used as evidence of actual outsider use of their pages and the ways in which images might be read by other professionals or employers were seen as potential problems.

There was also widespread concern that what is posted on social media is often outside of individual control and in some instances even awareness.

> LENNOX: when it's a photo of something you weren't even aware of, let's just say you were drinking with your friends and somebody took a photo, it's uploaded and they'll tag you on there, it's bad because
> GINO: All your friends can see
> LENNOX: Hello what if you're working at, working at Vodafone your boss could see that, you know or if you're in school, your parents, my worst one is parents …
>
> (Pasifika FG 10)

This excerpt distils many of the concerns that Pasifika participants and others expressed in their discussions of life at the interface of drinking and social media. Lennox articulates the dynamic of images being spread via activities such as posting and tagging by others intent on fun and/or mischief; this can occur deliberately or unthinkingly in drinking (and other) settings. These practices contribute to a blurring of public and private space as representations of behaviours occurring in specific contexts with particular groups of people become available to wider, largely unknown audiences. Gino and Lennox co-construct a range of such viewers illustrating how problematic this can be.

Concerns about loss of privacy and scrutiny by unwanted others, were reiterated by other participants.

> NANCY: I remember there was one in my last year of Uni, I liked it cos it was so true they were like 'Look, I'm looking at your FB and all you do is drink' and this group was like, the group was something along the lines of 'no I'm not always drinking I just don't always take photos when I'm studying'.
>
> (Pasifika FG 5)

Here Nancy, with almost palpable frustration at the scrutiny she has experienced, reports a collective measure that was taken to push back against an oppressive sense of criticism of student representations on social media. The ironic tone is characteristic perhaps of Pasifika students who out of respect for parents and elders are more likely to make such diplomatic manoeuvres than their Palagi (Pākehā) peers whose reactions to parental criticism are generally more abrasive and defiant.

Māori participants

In most Māori participants' talk, the cultural identity politics in play was either assumed or left implicit in the domain where alcohol and social media interact. However there were some instances in which the politics were spelled out.

INT: So you sort of screen them?

TARA: Yeah. Make sure that they're PG [laughs].

INT: Wow, yeah I guess you've gotta maintain a certain image as that in your school.

TARA: And cos' there's two head girls and so like, I'm the Māori one, and she's the Pākehā one and so I didn't want to make it look like Māoris were bad.

(Māori FG10)

In this excerpt about alcohol-related socialising, the discussion of managing social media photographs is co-constructed with the interviewer as a selection process whose aim is to ensure a certain image is produced. This is described as 'PG' (a reference to the acronym of the censor's cinema category 'parental guidance required') that in this instance, with gentle irony means 'suitable for parents to view'. A second imperative is explicitly cultural in intent and openly in comparison to her Pākehā counterpart, since in her role as a student leader she is determined not to show images that could be seen as evidence that 'Māoris were bad'.

Other strategies were used by some participants, particularly when they had broader social goals than managing family relations and social status.

TANIA: Like you never know who you're going to meet or where [laughter] so what if someone comes across your page it's like [clicks fingers] damn cos' I don't want to see no tragic photos up there. Just if I don't want my parents to see or my brothers and sisters, cos' my brother came back from Australia and was like 'your photos are a bit crazy' and I was like 'I can't really help that, I have a good time, what can I say?'

(Māori FG3)

Tania explains earlier that she works on her social media profile to ensure that alcohol is not present in every image she posts, which is evidently a challenge given her active social life. The general caution she offers about who may view her pages has distilled into a practice of eliminating 'tragic' photos, but spills into specific concerns about reaction from her immediate family. Her brother in particular seems to have challenged her quite strongly evoking a defensive reaction. Her somewhat defiant – 'what can I say?' – in the face of her public image appears to arise from the seamless association of drinking and social media.

There was some talk about the ubiquity and addictiveness of FB, and about it being the default setting for keeping in touch. This excerpt comes from a resident advisor within a university hostel.

TUI: Yeah so because I am an Resident Advisor now I find that there is a lot more parties and a lot more people … all the different personalities, genres, people in there all with cameras all taking photos, all with Facebook the next day. That was the other thing like after those big parties a lot of people will be on the [hall of residence] page like 'oh mean night last night' or um 'repeat this Thursday' and things like that.

(Māori FG12)

The convergence with social media via photography and the subsequent enthusiastic online approval and 'hyping up' (Goodwin et al., 2016) of the party scene underscores the ways in which social media and drinking cultures complement each other.

Multiple groups and participants made comments on the general understanding that diverse audiences should not be exposed to information and images about their drinking behaviours or plans in social media.

WHITI: We can't put up 'are we all on the piss tonight?'
CONNIE: Yeah nah.
WHITI: Cos' bro we don't do that stuff but like … we don't do that.
CONNIE: Yeah hard out.
HARIATA: Not in the public…
WHITI: Not when you're telling kids like drinking is bad.

(Māori FG5)

In this instance the problematic is that to post such materials would present inconsistencies with their role model status among the young people they work with as youth workers. In this context, to share drinking information could be seen as projecting a double standard that would reduce their effectiveness with clients and possibly put their employment in jeopardy.

Another common discussion was around strategies to manage one's public profile in social media.

VICTORIA: I didn't actually realise that me and one of my friends had alcohol in our hands, and it wasn't until a week later that I realised my profile picture had alcohol in it, and I'm like 'Mira, I don't really like having alcohol in my pictures'. I still haven't taken it down cos' I've just realised.
INT: Why don't you like it?
VICTORIA: I don't know it's just, if you wanna drink alcohol, that's all your business you don't have to really sorta chuck it all out on Facebook I know I'm like of age now, but it still sort of gives off the wrong image, yeah drunk.
MIRA: Yeah tragic.

(Māori FG9)

Two women who are members of a kapahaka (customary performance) group discuss the challenge of managing their public face in relation to alcohol on social media. The idea that socialising with alcohol is the commonplace subject of photographs and posts is taken for granted but the reality that undesirable images can appear unheralded is a problem cast as projecting the 'wrong image … drunk

... tragic' (Hutton et al., 2016). In this instance the difficulty has arisen from a breakdown in Victoria's monitoring of her Facebook pages and a failure to notice that the photograph in question shows alcohol. This is significant enough that a remedy is planned in terms of removing the problem item. The final turns discuss the point that although the participants are not breaking any law, the social sanction makes being seen drinking on social media inappropriate. This discussion is followed by a longer consideration about protecting the image of their kapahaka group and the use of other strategies such as obscuring drinks when photographs are being taken to avoid the posting of problematic images.

Pākehā participants

Among Pākehā participants there were few dissenters from the pervasive trope of drinking as a pleasurable, naturalised, accepted, routine activity within peer social events in the diverse settings of everyday leisure-time experience. In this focus group excerpt, flatmates signal their approval of drunkenness, giving a glimpse of how their drinking culture operates:

> CATHY: That's like what I like about you Andy. You set the atmosphere...
> ANDY: [laughs]
> CATHY: ...Music's on and you're already like half-pissed and I'm like 'yes! [hits couch arm] I'm getting a glass of wine [hits her knee]. It is all go.'
> (Pākehā FG11)

Data from some marginalised segments of the community such as young solo mothers signal anxiety about surveillance of their drinking by government agencies. However, overall the Pākehā corpus gives little sense of sanction beyond knowing personal limits, aligning with a status quo where consumption is seen as a matter of personal responsibility that speaks to, and reflects individual choice. Leah considers living with deregulated consumption:

> LEAH: Some nights I just get that pissed that I can't walk properly and I can't, I don't know, I don't remember what I've done the next day and stuff like that.
>
> (Pākehā FG3)

The hegemonic understanding that Pākehā participants articulated was that they were established drinkers in a regime that was a central and valued part of adult life and identity, which did not entail any consideration of their own ethnicity or whiteness. While there is caution about representations of alcohol in social media and active management of their profiles, there is also a strong sense that, as well as being very useful and a source of excitement and fun, the dangers are minimal.

Both of these notions are represented in this first excerpt:

JAN: A lot of my photos have me [laughs] with a glass of wine in my hand. But in an appropriate way. Not a argh leaning up against a wall but [Pam laughs] like a lot of my soc... a lot of our socialising does involve having a glass of wine.

EVA: Yeah.

PAM: Yeah.

EVA: Yeah and we don't. And you don't post a photo because you're boozing it up you know, you post it because you happen to be at an event with alcohol and you're posting photos of the event rather than of you drinking.

JAN: No. Yeah. Just happened to have. Yeah.

PAM: Well. [laughs]

JAN: Do tell! [laughing]

PAM: I'm slightly different because I reckon I. Well it's probably the three year age difference. Potentially. But I will go out drinking into town and I'll just take photos on my iPhone like lots of photos of us in clubs drinking.

(Pākehā FG6)

These women create an age-linked distinction in the ways in which they choose to represent their drinking in social media. While Pam constructs an image of unfettered drinking in commercial premises, Jan and Eva articulate a more restrained approach that can depict 'appropriate' drinking but not open displays of intoxication, a balancing act more commonly applied to women. Indeed the basis for appropriate social media use in this regard is founded on a fundamental difference between drinking practices where for Jan and Eva alcohol is incidental and related posts are intended to signal occasions, rather than what is seen in the discursively disapproving term as, 'boozing', a term generally used for heavy male drinking. However, for Pam, with her laughing interruption 'I'm slightly different...', it is implied that her interest is very much in the drinking and the representation of this in social media that it is central to the socialising that she engages in.

Many participants in other focus groups make points similar to those raised by Jan and Eva, where the reasons for taking this approach to depictions of drinking are spelled out.

CARLA: Things like I would never want my patients to ever see me drinking with my friends, like in that light, because you do [it] like completely outside of work and you have a certain image at work, which is for work and then you have a separate life.

(Pākehā FG 10)

Carla seeks to manage her social media presence so that it does not impact in problematic ways on her professional status as a dentist. She hints that her 'drinking with friends' may undermine this status and so she works at the separation of personal and professional life in social media. Other participants spoke of similar practices to avoid complications with parents, employers, law enforcement and in one instance a potential landlord, worrying that particular photographs or posts may bring controversy, trouble or retribution.

There was, however, a distinct and somewhat dominant strand of talk among Pākehā participants that was more closely aligned with Pam's understandings, reinforcing this view and discounting concerns about possible repercussions.

> FRED: One of my tutors um his son posted a bunch of photos of him[self] at a party and [the tutor] told him that he didn't like him doing that. Like binge drinking and going out with those sort of people. Going with that crowd. And then um his son pulled up a few pictures of his dad when he was his age [laughs] from the internet.
>
> T: Oh funny.
>
> JILL: Oooh.

(Pākehā FG 12)

Fred's anecdote serves to counter the parental criticism of the younger generation's drinking practices, by highlighting the hypocrisy of criticising the son for practices that the father had perhaps engaged in himself. Interestingly, given that the father is now in a position of authority, the story also suggests that such behaviours are likely to be dismissed as youthful indiscretion, possibly pointing to a male rite of passage, rather than a serious impediment to a career trajectory.

Other contributions were even more direct in their dismissal of potential repercussions.

> DES: Heaps of the older generation read the news, complain about Facebook you know taking over the world, have got data images of all of us and all this crap and I'm just like [pause] get over it. It's happened. It's. They're not going to do anything bad with it.

(Pākehā FG 2)

Without necessarily denying the power and reach of social media, Des is openly contemptuous of the concerns that social media, through control of personal data, can have any serious impact on people's lives. The somewhat fatalistic tone is leavened with an expression of trust in social media corporations that no harm will come from ongoing engagement with their platforms.

This combination of active management of social media representations and belief in negligible risk flows through the Pākehā data to produce a broad sense of the confidence that participants felt in relation to alcohol and social media in their lives. This ambience was not nearly so obvious in the discussions among Pasifika and Māori participants.

Ethnicity/culture, alcohol and social media

This study showed the expected convergences in meanings and motivations around drinking practices in young adults across the three ethnic/cultural groups.

Participants in all groups described peer approval, pro-drinking meaning-making and provided lively discourses around intoxication; however, there were also divergences. Pākehā, as the least reflective of ethnicity as a consideration or concern and the most acculturated group, appear to have less at stake and fewer adaptive changes to make to fully engage in the emerging phenomena at the confluence of drinking and social media cultures. Equally findings pointed to a corollary in which Māori and Pasifika participants would have more work to do to manage and protect their identities and practices in such environments.

Although alcohol was seen as important in socialising with peers, for some, particularly Pasifika participants, alcohol consumption did not feature in their talk about their lives. Overall the data from the Pākehā corpus showed participants concerned with knowing personal limits and not having internet images of their intoxication impact negatively on their work or professional standing. Although these were concerns for all participants, the marginalised status of both Māori and Pasifika seemed salient as they spent more energy discussing concerns and sanctions. Beyond this, they actively reflected on their ethnicity/culture and the negative connotations and shame that could be attached to them as members of particular groups with a collective sense of identity at stake, when social media identified them drinking.

While parental scrutiny was mentioned by some Pākehā participants this appeared to have little bearing on the kinds of materials they might post. There was some suggestion that representations of alcohol consumption could be dismissed as youthful indiscretion. For Māori and Pasifika there was more of a sense that the responses of elders mattered and this was manifest in efforts to minimise the evidence of drinking in social media.

Alcohol use came across as more widely understood as transgressive of Pasifika cultural norms, with elder scrutiny seen as a significant control. Concerns about criticism from church and family were expressed, with the surveillance available through social media arguably producing a protective effect; however, this may not deflect the effects of alcohol marketing through social media. As the generations turn, with new cohorts growing up within a strong culture of intoxication and an increasingly secular society, it is likely that any such protections will lessen.

Concerns about drinking images in social media echoed across the data, with various nuances by gender and ethnicity. Women, might for example be concerned about the extent to which alcohol is seen as central to representations of socialising and how drunkenness might transgress acceptable female behaviours, while males may be more concerned with maintaining images of masculinity and their ability to handle alcohol. One key difference noted here is that Pasifika and Māori named their ethnicities, with their images seen to represent their community both within and beyond it. Māori talked about managing social media images for school, work, family and kapahaka while Pasifika were also concerned with their communities, particularly the church. Pākehā rarely reflected on their culture and were far more likely to interpret their actions as individual mistakes rather than as reflections on the family or community groups.

A key point, 'between the lines', of the empirical work offered here is that the normalised Western sense of identity evident in the Pākehā data is coded into Facebook's architecture and is a critical element of the differences reported here. Such technological, 'baked in' affordances in social media make using and appropriating these tools more complex and risky for young Māori and Pasifika people. The very notion of a 'user profile' *assumes* an individuated subjectivity is always the most salient and that the subject is not representative of a group in any sense.

Beyond the specificities of ethnicity/culture explored here, the nuances wrought within the drinking cultures of young adults in the relatively close-knit, interwoven society in Aotearoa New Zealand are also inflected with gender and specificities of socio-economic status that are not explored for want of space. We suggest that our study highlights the importance of factoring culture into efforts to understand the significance of the growing interplay between drinking cultures and social media.

While the research is yet to be done at the confluence of ethnicity/culture and alcohol in social media in many countries, we expect that these broad findings reported from Aotearoa New Zealand will be of interest to those concerned about patterns of alcohol consumption, particularly in colonial societies. There may be relevance also to other settings where exploitative immigration policies and resultant marginalisation of minority groups are at play. We reiterate that these differences are intersected with the effects of gender and class as well as patterns of privilege and power that demarcate diverse social locations.

Along with other pivotal influences including gender, class and age, Oetting et al. (1998) have proposed that the ethnicity/culture complex is an important determinant of responses to exposure to intoxicant substances. Alcohol use, particularly with its escalating promotion via social media, is a potential source of confusion and harm to many groups given the implacable globalisation of societies, the relentless commercialisation of social orders and the humanitarian disasters arising from war and climate change. For marginalised and migrant ethnic/cultural groups these stresses are particularly acute as they attempt to acculturate to alien norms and practices around alcohol in new or contested social settings and where social media images may serve to reinforce prejudice.

References

Anae, M. (2001). The new 'Vikings of the sunrise': New Zealand-borns in the information age. In C. Macpherson, P. Spoonley and M. Anae (Eds.), *Tangata o te Moana Nui: The Evolving Identities of Pacific Peoples in Aotearoa New Zealand* (pp. 101–122). Palmerston North: Dunmore Press.

Babor, T., Caetano, R., Casswell, S., Edwards, G., Giesbrecht, N., Graham, K., Grube, J., Hill, L., Holder, H., Homel, R., Livingston, M., Osterberg, E., Rehm, J., Room, R., and Rossow, I. (2010). *Alcohol: No Ordinary Commodity Research and Public Policy* (2nd edn). Oxford: Oxford University Press.

Belich, J. (2007). *Making Peoples: A History of the New Zealanders from Polynesian Settlement to the End of the Nineteenth Century*. Auckland: Penguin.

Berry, J. (1992). Acculturation and adaptation in a new society. *International Migration, 30*, 69–85.

Berry, J. (2006). Acculturative stress. In P. Wong and L. Wong (Eds.), *Handbook of Multicultural Perspective on Stress and Coping* (pp. 287–298). New York: Springer.

Braun, V., and Clarke, V. (2006). Using thematic analysis in psychology. *Qualitative Research in Psychology, 3*(2), 77–101.

Brown, R., and Gregg, M. (2012). The pedagogy of regret: Facebook, binge drinking and young women. *Continuum: Journal of Media and Cultural Studies, 26*(3), 357–369.

Chartier, K., and Caetano, R. (2010). Ethnicity and health disparities in alcohol research. *Alcohol Research and Health, 33*(1–2), 152–160. http://pubs.niaaa.nih.gov/publications/arh40/152–160.htm

Duff, C., Puri, A., and Chow, C. (2011). Ethno-cultural differences in the use of alcohol and other drugs: Evidence from the Vancouver Youth Drug Reporting System. *Journal of Ethnicity in Substance Abuse, 10*(1), 2–23.

Fairbairn-Dunlop, P., and Makisi, G. (Eds.). (2003). *Making Our Place: Growing Up PI In New Zealand.* Palmerston North: Dunmore Press.

Gibson, A., Miller, M., Smith, P., Bell, A., and Crothers, C. (2013). *The Internet in New Zealand 2013.* Auckland: Institute of Culture Discourse and Communication, Auckland University of Technology.

Goodwin, I., Griffin, C., Lyons, A., McCreanor, T., and Moewaka Barnes, H. (2016). Precarious popularity: Facebook drinking photos, the attention economy, and the regime of the branded self. *Social Media + Society, 2*(1), doi: 10.1177/2056305116628889.

Griffin, C., Bengry-Howell, A., Hackley, C., Mistral, W., and Szmigin, I. (2009). 'Every time I do it I absolutely annihilate myself': Loss of (self)-consciousness and loss of memory in young people's drinking narratives. *Sociology, 43*, 457–476.

Griffiths, R., and Casswell, S. (2010). Intoxigenic digital spaces? Youth, social networking sites and alcohol marketing. *Drug and Alcohol Review, 29*, 525–530.

Habgood, R., Casswell, S., Pledger, M., and Bhatta, K. (2001). *Drinking in New Zealand: National Surveys Comparison 1995 and 2000.* Auckland: Alcohol and Public Health Research Unit, University of Auckland.

Harvey, L., Ringrose, J., and Gill, R. (2013). Swagger, ratings and masculinity: Theorising the circulation of social and cultural value in teenage boys' digital peer networks. *Sociological Research Online, 18*(4), Article 9. www.socres-online.org.uk/18/14/19.html

Hearn, A. (2008). 'Meat, mask, burden': Probing the contours of the branded self. *Journal of Consumer Culture, 8*(2), 197–217.

Hill, L., and Casswell, S. (2004). Alcohol advertising and sponsorship: Commercial freedom or control in the public interest? In N. Heather and T. Stockwell (Eds.), *The Essential Handbook of Treatment and Prevention of Alcohol Problems* (pp. 339–359). Chichester: John Wiley and Sons.

Hill, L., and Stewart, L. (1998). 'Responsive regulation' theory and the Sale of Liquor Act. *Social Policy Journal of New Zealand, 11*, 49–65.

Huckle, T., Pledger, M., and Casswell, S. (2006). Trends in alcohol-related harms and offences in a liberalized alcohol environment. *Addiction, 101*(2), 232–240.

Hutton, F., Griffin, C., Lyons, A., Niland, P., and McCreanor, T. (2016). 'Tragic girls' and 'crack whores': Alcohol, femininity and Facebook. *Feminism and Psychology, 26*(1), 73–93.

Järvinen, M., and Room, R. (Eds.). (2007). *Youth Drinking Cultures. European Experiences.* Aldershot: Ashgate.

Jernigan, D., and Rushman, A. (2014). Measuring youth exposure to alcohol marketing on social networking sites: Challenges and prospects. *Journal of Public Health Policy*, *35*(1), 91–104.

Jones-Webb, R., Hsiao, C., and Hannan, P. (1995). Relationships between socioeconomic status and drinking problems among Black and White men. *Alcoholism: Clinical and Experimental Research*, *19*(3), 623–627.

Kelsey, J. (1995). *The New Zealand Experiment: A World Model for Structural Adjustment?* Auckland: Bridget Williams and Auckland University Press.

Kelsey, J. (2002). *At the Crossroads: Three Essays*. Wellington: Bridget Williams Books.

Lin, E.-Y., Casswell, S., You, R. Q., and Huckle, T. (2012). Engagement with alcohol marketing and early brand allegiance in relation to early years of drinking. *Addiction Research and Theory*, *20*(4), 329–338.

Lyons, A., Goodwin, I., McCreanor, T., and Griffin, C. (2015). Social networking and young adults' drinking practices: Innovative qualitative methods for health behavior research. *Health Psychology*, *34*(4), 293–302.

Lyons, A., McCreanor, T., Goodwin, I., Griffin, C., Hutton, F., Moewaka Barnes, H., O'Carroll, D., Samu, L., Niland, P., and Vroman, K.-E. (2014a). Youth drinking cultures in Aotearoa New Zealand. *Sites: New Series*, *11*(2), 78–102.

Lyons, A., McCreanor, T., Hutton, F., Goodwin, I., Moewaka Barnes, H., Griffin, C., Vroman, K.-E., O'Carroll, A. D., Niland, P., and Samu, L. (2014b). *Flaunting it on Facebook: Young Adults, Drinking Stories and the Cult of Celebrity*. Wellington, New Zealand: School of Psychology, Massey University. http://mro.massey.ac.nz/handle/10179/5187

Malone, P., Northrup, T., Masyn, K., Lamis, D., and Lamont, A. (2012). Initiation and persistence of alcohol use in United States Black, Hispanic, and White male and female youth. *Addictive Behaviors*, *37*(3), 299–305.

McCreanor, T. (2010). Challenging and countering anti-Maori discourse: Practices for decolonisation. *Psychology Aotearoa*, *1*(1), 16–20.

McCreanor, T., Lyons, A., Griffin, C., Goodwin, I., Moewaka Barnes, H., and Hutton, F. (2013). Youth drinking cultures, social networking and alcohol marketing: Implications for public health. *Critical Public Health*, *23*(1), 110–120.

Measham, F. (2006). The new policy mix: Alcohol, harm minimisation, and determined drunkenness in contemporary society. *International Journal of Drug Policy*, *17*, 258–268.

Measham, F., and Brain, K. (2005). 'Binge' drinking, British alcohol policy and the new culture of intoxication. *Crime, Media, Culture*, *1*(3), 262–283.

Ministry of Health. (2015). *Alcohol Use 2012/13: New Zealand Health Survey*. Wellington: Ministry of Health.

Ministry of Social Development. (2010). The Social Report 2010. Archived by WebCite® at www.webcitation.org/6Rl8aMopH. Retrieved 12 August 2014, from www.socialreport.msd.govt.nz/introduction/index.html

Moewaka Barnes, H., Borell, B., and McCreanor, T. (2014). Theorising the structural dynamics of ethnic privilege in Aotearoa: Unpacking 'this breeze at my back'. *International Journal of Critical Indigenous Studies*, *7*(1), www.isrn.qut.edu.au/publications/internationaljournal/volume7_number1_14.jsp

Moewaka Barnes, H., McCreanor, T., Goodwin, I., Lyons, A., Griffin, C., and Hutton, F. (2016). Alcohol and social media: Drinking and drunkenness while online. *Critical Public Health*, *26*(1), 62–76.

Nicholls, J. (2012). Everyday, everywhere: Alcohol marketing and social media—current trends. *Alcohol and Alcoholism, 47*(4), 486–493.

Niland, P., Lyons, A., Goodwin, I., and Hutton, F. (2013). 'Everyone can loosen up and get a bit of a buzz on': Young adults, alcohol and friendship practices. *International Journal of Drug Policy, 24*(6), 530–537.

O'Carroll, A. (2013). Māori identity construction in Social Networking Sites. *International Journal of Critical Indigenous Studies, 6*(2), 2–16.

Oetting, E., Donnermeyer, J., Trimble, J., and Beauvais, F. (1998). Primary socialization theory: Culture, ethnicity, and cultural identification. The links between culture and substance use. IV. *Substance Use and Misuse, 33*(10), 2075–2107.

Papacharissi, Z. (2009). The virtual geographies of social networks: A comparative analysis of Facebook, LinkedIn and ASmallWorld. *New Media and Society, 11*(1 and 2), 199–220.

Pascal, R., Chikritzhs, T., and Gray, D. (2009). Estimating alcohol-attributable mortality among Indigenous Australians: Towards Indigenous-specific alcohol aetiologic fractions. *Drug and Alcohol Review, 28*(2), 196–200.

Rehm, J., Mathers, C., Popova, S., Thavorncharoensap, M., Teerawattananon, Y., and Patra, J. (2009). Global burden of disease and injury and economic cost attributable to alcohol use and alcohol-use disorders. *Lancet (Series), 373*(9682), 2223–2233.

Saggers, S., and Gray, D. (1998). *Dealing With Alcohol: Indigenous Usage in Australia, New Zealand and Canada.* Cambridge: Cambridge University Press.

Smith, P., Smith, N., Sherman, K., Goodwin, I., Crothers, C., Billot, J., and Bell, A. (2010). *World Internet Project, The Internet in New Zealand 2009.* Auckland: AUT Institute of Culture, Discourse and Communication.

Spillane, N., and Smith, G. (2007). A theory of reservation-dwelling American Indian alcohol use risk. *Psychological Bulletin, 133*(3), 395–418.

Spoonley, P., Macpherson, C., and Pearson, D. (Eds.). (1996). *Nga Patai: Racism and Ethnic Relations in Aotearoa New Zealand.* Dunmore Press: Palmerston North.

Spoonley, P., Macpherson, C., and Pearson, D. (Eds.). (2004). *Tangata Tangata: The Changing Ethnic Contours of New Zealand.* Southbank, Victoria: Dunmore Press.

Statistics New Zealand. (2013a). *2013 Census QuickStats about National Highlights,* December. http://stats.govt.nz/Census/2013-census/profile-and-summary-reports/quickstats-about-national-highlights.aspx.

Statistics New Zealand. (2013b). New Zealand Period Life Tables: 2010–12. Retrieved 27 September 2013, from www.stats.govt.nz/browse_for_stats/health/life_expectancy/NZLifeTables_HOTP10–12.aspx

Szmigin, I., Griffin, C., Mistral, W., Bengry-Howell, A., Weale, L., and Hackley, C. (2008). Re-framing 'binge drinking' as calculated hedonism—Empirical evidence from the UK. *International Journal of Drug Policy, 19*(5), 359–366.

Te Puni Kokiri. (2012). *He Kai Kei Aku Ringa – The Crown-Māori Economic Growth Partnership.* Wellington. www.tpk.govt.nz/documents/download/215/He-Kai-Kei-Aku-Ringa-Strategy.pdf

Walker, R. (2004). *Ka Whawhai Tonu Matou Struggle without End.* Auckland: Penguin.

Wetherell, M., and Potter, J. (1992). *Mapping the Language of Racism: Discourse and the Legitimation of Exploitation.* New York: Harvester Wheatsheaf.

Wicki, M., Kuntsche, E., and Gmel, G. (2010). Drinking at European universities? A review of students' alcohol use. *Addictive Behavior, 35,* 913–924.

Wilson, M., Stearne, A., Gray, D., and Saggers, S. (2010). The harmful use of alcohol amongst indigenous Australians. *Australian Indigenous Health Reviews No. 4.*

Retrieved   9   June   2016,   from   www.responsiblechoice.com.au/wp-content/ uploads/2013/01/alcohol_review_june_2010.pdf

Yan, F., Beck, K., Howard, D., Shattuck, T., and Kerr, M. (2008). A structural model of alcohol use pathways among Latino youth. *American Journal of Health Behavior, 32*(2), 209–219.

Part II

Alcohol marketing and commercialisation

6   Understanding social media as commercial platforms for engaging with young adults

Nina Michaelidou

Introduction

Theorising social networking sites is crucial to understanding how they work, what their potential for health and harm may be in the alcohol domain, and additionally what the implications of their widespread embedding in drinking cultures may be in the medium and long term. In this chapter a number of issues involving social media usage currently employed by big alcohol brands will be considered. These include how alcohol companies use social media platforms such as social networking sites (e.g. Facebook and Twitter) to engage with young people, promote alcohol and generate alcohol-related conversations, through the use of multitude marketing communication tools such as advertising, sales promotions, events and broadcast sponsorships and viral marketing. The chapter will address these issues and explore theoretical understandings with significant social implications.

Why do young people drink?

Early research identified reasons that explain why young people drink alcohol, including avoidance, socialisation, sensation-seeking and enjoyment (McCarty and Kaye, 1984). Later research highlights that social and enhancement motives explain young people's situational alcohol consumption (Kuntsche et al., 2005; Szmigin et al., 2008), as young people drink moderately when socialising with friends, and heavily to enhance their mood. Additional external factors influencing alcohol consumption include low prices, promotions and advertising (Hingson et al., 2005; Szmigin et al., 2008). According to Triggle (2009), alcohol brands spend £800 million per year to promote alcoholic beverages in the UK. Previous research shows that frequent promotions and low prices are linked to higher rates of binge drinking among university students (Hingson et al., 2005). The most recent statistics show that more than nine million people in England drink above the recommended daily limit, while alcohol reflects 10% of the UK burden of death and disease, and is the third lifestyle risk factor after smoking and obesity (Alcohol Concern, 2015). Figures also indicate that about 7.5 million people are unaware of the potential risk and damage alcohol could be posing to their health, while the cost of alcohol misuse for England is about £12 billion per year in healthcare, crime and productivity cost (Alcohol Concern, 2015).

Studies focusing on traditional media have examined associations between media exposure and young people's alcohol use (Fox et al., 1998; Russell et al., 2009). Alcohol advertising is particularly appealing to young people and can influence initial development of drinking behaviour; it has also been suggested that media depicting or promoting alcohol use may encourage drinking among young viewers (Goldberg et al., 2006; Robinson et al., 1988). Further, Hastings et al. (2010) suggest that new media such as social networking sites, viral marketing and mobile marketing are used by companies as media channels for alcohol advertising, because of their ability to interact and engage audiences with alcohol brands at a young age.

Social media

Web 2.0 has created new ways of communicating, searching for information and engaging with brands or products via social media. Social media encompass a group of internet-based applications (e.g. social networking sites, blogs, video and picture sharing sites), with different ecology and functional blocks (e.g. identity, conversations, groups, sharing) (see Kietzmann et al., 2011), and which enable interactivity and allow the creation and sharing of user-generated content (Kaplan and Haenlein, 2010). Mangold and Faulds (2009) provide extensive examples of what constitutes social media, while Smith et al. (2012) suggest that different social media have different characteristics, varied natures and varied architectures. According to these authors, social media, such as Facebook, Twitter, YouTube and Instagram are also used by users for different reasons. For example, Facebook is used to share information, catch up with friends' news and keep in touch, while Twitter is used to follow friends or brands and keep abreast of news. Statistics show increasing activity on social media sites, namely Facebook, Twitter, Instagram, Pinterest and YouTube. Specifically, there are 1.28 billion, monthly active users on Facebook, 1 billion on YouTube and 255 million on Twitter (Bennett, 2014). Statistics from Nielsen suggest that social media is an integral part of the lives of consumers in the USA. Specifically, figures show that 64% of social media users access sites at least once a day via their PCs while 47% of smartphone owners access social networking sites on their devices on a daily basis (Nielsen, 2014).

Social media tools are grounded on the ideology of Web 2.0, which fosters the establishment of web-based communities, a participatory culture, and the generation of content that has the potential to go viral (Kaplan and Haenlein, 2010; Uzunoğlu and Öksüz, 2014). Currently, Facebook is the market leader with an excess of one billion registered users, followed by Twitter with 316 million active accounts (Statista, 2016). Participatory culture (Jenkins, 2006) enables users of social media to create, store and re-circulate content (Jenkins, 2006; Moraes et al., 2014) and reflects a dynamic media environment where engagement and consumption of content is achieved through co-creation and collaboration with brands (Deuze, 2007), thus shifting the traditional paradigm of passive consumption of brand content (Mangold and Faulds, 2009).

The commercial nature of social media

The use of social media by organisations has increased drastically in the last few years, highlighting their commercial nature or value. Van Dijck and Poell (2013) argue that 'the cultural and commercial dynamics determining social media blend with existing commercial and advertising practices, while also changing them. Far from being neutral platforms, social media are affecting the conditions and rules of social interaction' (p. 3). Organisations use social media to unobtrusively collect large quantities of users' data (Gleibs, 2014) that then inform strategic practices. This information is used, for example, for creating data-driven, personalised communication and targeting to promote brands (Ashworth and Free, 2006; Johnson, 2015; Kaplan and Haenlein, 2010; Palmer, 2005). Additionally, companies use social networking sites such as Facebook and Twitter as advertising tools (Smith et al., 2012). Statistics show that advertising spending on social networking sites is expected to reach $23.6 billion worldwide, an increase of 35.5% compared to 2014 (eMarketer, 2015a). This figure is expected to rise to $35.98 billion by 2017, reflecting a 20% growth in advertising spending worldwide (eMarketer, 2015a). These figures vary by geographic region. For example, in the Asia Pacific and Western Europe regions, advertising spending on social networking sites is expected to reach $11.9 and $6.85 billion respectively in 2017. Statistics also show that Facebook's global revenues from advertising are expected to reach $26.9 billion in 2017, followed by Twitter at $3.98 billion (eMarketer, 2015b).

The 'commercial nature' of social media and their subsequent use as marketing platforms has important implications where controversial products are involved, such as alcohol. Mart (2011) argues that social networking platforms such as Facebook and Twitter are nowadays 'major players in alcohol marketing campaigns' (p. 889). Such practices raise questions about the ethical and social welfare of young social media users, and, in fact, research has identified a strong link between alcohol consumption by young people and social networking sites. For example, scholars argue that, 'as commercial platforms, social network sites use sophisticated data-miners and algorithms to combine and sell data to third parties, including commercial alcohol interests. By engaging with online marketing, site users are also providing personal data to the drinks companies' (Institute for Policy Research, 2013). Despite the existing scholarly work in this domain, social media regulations were not enforced in the UK until 2011 and there is little research that examines Facebook and other social networking sites as mediums to promote alcohol brands. Most research currently focuses on content generated by social media users which enforces the normalisation of alcohol as a social agent. However, given the increasing evidence about the impact of alcohol consumption on young people's health and lives in general, and the development of a worldwide 'binge drinking culture' (Hastings and Angus, 2009; Piacentini and Banister, 2009; Szmigin et al., 2008), additional scholarly focus on how alcohol brands use social media, and specifically social networking sites, to promote alcohol brands is needed.

Social media as an intoxigenic environment

Alcohol brands have been quick to leverage social media for advertising and promotion (Smith et al., 2012) through increasing marketing spend on such platforms (Moraes et al., 2014; Nicholls, 2012), as social media are more effective in data-driven targeting than their non-digital, non-interactive and offline counterparts (Kaplan and Haenlein, 2010). In particular, recent statistics show that alcohol spending on social media rapidly increased in 2015 by as much as 50% (Johnson, 2015), while Facebook statistics indicate that global beer brands, such as Heineken and Budweiser, have in excess of ten million Facebook page fans (Socialbakers, 2015) (see Table 6.1).

A multitude of research in various disciplines points to the increasing phenomenon of social media promoting an intoxigenic culture and the proliferation of alcohol content on such platforms which seems to encourage alcohol consumption and promote drinking cultures (Lyons et al., 2015; McCreanor et al., 2013; Moewaka Barnes et al., 2016; Moraes et al., 2014). According to Griffiths and Casswell (2010) social media platforms operate as 'intoxigenic' online spaces, and positively encourage alcohol drinking by young adults (see also McCreanor et al., 2013). In their recent study, based on qualitative data, Moewaka Barnes et al. (2016) report themes pertaining to drinking practices and social media. Specifically, the authors found that young people are often intoxicated while using social networking sites, resulting in drunken postings which often lead to regret. Additionally, the authors found that participants associated pleasure and other perceived benefits of alcohol while being online and that drinking online reflects a social engagement suggesting that: 'the performance of both consumption and intoxication [in social networking sites] was a social behavior with pleasures and

Table 6.1 Facebook alcohol brands fan statistics

Alcohol Brand	Total Fans Million
Heineken	19.9
Budweiser	12.8
Skol	12.4
Johnnie Walker	11.6
Smirnoff	11.6
Corona	8.8
Bacardi	8.0
Stella Artois	7.6
Bud Light	7.4
Kingfisher	7.2

Source: Socialbakers (2015)

identity-related value, arising from the sharing of these behaviors' (Moewaka Barnes et al., 2016: 70).

Further, scholars have examined alcohol content on social media and its impact on young people, with findings suggesting that exposure is immense and that both young adults and teenagers are aware of and often engage with alcohol content on social media (Gordon et al., 2010; Hartigan and Coe, 2012; Hastings et al., 2010; Moreno et al., 2012). For example, scholars (e.g. Lyons et al., 2015; McCreanor et al., 2013; Moewaka Barnes et al., 2016) investigating Facebook pages of young people who share alcohol experiences suggest that such environments positively encourage alcohol drinking among friends. Additionally, researchers have found that young people who post content on social networking sites, such as Facebook, that display alcohol use and intoxication (e.g. pictures of themselves consuming alcohol) are more likely to be involved in risky or problematic drinking (e.g. binge drinking) (Hebden et al., 2015; Moreno et al., 2012).

Alcohol content on social media

Young people are exposed to, and/or engage with, different alcohol content on social media, including user-generated as well as marketer-generated content. The sections below discuss the different types of alcohol content on social media.

User-generated alcohol content

According to Kaplan and Haenlein (2010), user-generated content refers to content that is 'published either on a publicly accessible website or on a social networking site accessible to a selected group of people' (p. 61). It reflects some creative effort on the part of the social media user and it is created 'outside of professional routines and practices' (Kaplan and Haenlein, 2010: 61). User-generated content is grounded on the functional blocks of *sharing* and *conversations* (Kietzmann et al., 2011) that are based on different individual motives, and facilitated by the social media platform. *Sharing* reflects 'the extent to which users exchange, distribute, and receive content' (Kietzmann et al., 2011: 245); and this is based on different reasons such as to meet new people, share opinions and ideas on specific subjects (e.g. politics) or even to keep abreast of news and developments (e.g. via Twitter). In other words, user-generated content is a means through which young people express themselves on social networking sites and can take many different forms depending on the social media platform used (e.g. a Tweet, or a Facebook status update or a video shared via YouTube). Smith et al. (2012) highlight the importance of user-generated content for marketers, and argue that 'much [user-generated content] UGC across various media is brand-related and has the potential to shape consumer brand perceptions' (p. 102).

Young people are exposed to, and engage with, user-generated alcohol content shared on social networking sites by themselves, friends and others (Ali and Dwyer, 2010; Griffiths and Casswell, 2010; McCreanor et al., 2013; Moraes et al.,

2014; Mundt, 2011). Within the context of alcohol consumption, research indicates that such content involves wall posts, event replies, status updates, displays of memberships or links to drinking-related groups and communities, photographs displaying consumption or intoxication, and other social communications which involve alcohol consumption (Egan and Moreno, 2011; Griffiths and Casswell, 2010; Mart, 2011; Moraes et al., 2014). Additionally, user-generated alcohol content is linked to specific types of alcohol and brands, and thus communicates information about the product to other members of the social media user's network (Mart, 2011; Moraes et al., 2014; Moreno et al., 2010). For example, Moraes et al.'s (2014) research on Facebook and alcohol consumption shows that alcohol content shared by young people on Facebook is linked to alcohol types such as vodka or beer; while social media users tend to associate alcohol consumption and particular alcoholic drinks with specific situations, such as Friday nights, events and pre-party alcohol sessions.

Marketer-controlled content

In addition to being exposed to content produced by other social media users, young people are exposed to social media content including advertising and promotions posted by marketers of alcohol brands and clubs (e.g. Moraes et al., 2014; Nicholls, 2012; Winpenny et al., 2014). Studies have examined Facebook pages of alcohol brands and highlight the large volume of alcohol marketing which exists to promote drinking to young adults and teenagers (e.g. Carah, 2014; Moraes et al., 2014; Moreno et al., 2010; Nicholls, 2012; Winpenny et al., 2014). Exposure to alcohol marketing on social media appeals to young people and influences their attitudes towards alcohol brands (Moraes et al., 2014). This stream of research draws attention to the use of certain marketing techniques (including real-time techniques) adopted by alcohol brands such as advertising and sales promotions, viral marketing and marketer-shaped consumer engagement with alcohol brands (Carah, 2014; Mart, 2011; Montgomery and Chester, 2009; Nicholls, 2012).

Types of marketer-controlled alcohol content

Alcohol content controlled by marketers exists in various formats on social media sites such as Facebook, Twitter and YouTube, including sales promotions, event and broadcast sponsorships, as well as advertising. Such content targets users who indicate alcohol or bars as an interest (Hoffman et al., 2014; Mart et al., 2009). Limited research, however, has investigated marketer-generated content on social networking sites, focusing primarily on Facebook. For example, Winpenny et al. (2014) examined Facebook, YouTube and Twitter, Nicholls (2012) collected alcohol content from Twitter and Facebook alcohol pages, while Moraes et al. (2014) focused exclusively on Facebook pages of alcohol brands as well as clubs. Similarly, Carah (2014) conducted a content analysis of the Facebook pages of 20 alcohol brands in Australia. This line of research enquiry identifies common themes in terms of the type of content and the associated marketing communication strategies employed by alcohol brands to promote alcohol and drinking to young adults on social media.

Alcohol sales promotions

Alcohol promotions on social media are rapidly growing (Chester et al., 2010; Jernigan, 2012) and include primarily monetary, product and competition promotions. Monetary promotions include money savings (e.g. price discounts, coupons) and are said to offer utilitarian benefits. On the contrary, product promotions and competitions offer hedonic benefits, such as fun in participating, gratification and/or entertainment, as well as fulfilling intrinsic stimulation and novelty seeking needs (Chandon et al., 2000). In contrast to monetary and product promotions, competitions often require more effort or additional engagement on the part of the consumer. Within the context of social media, the use of all three types of sales promotion is widespread, and varies according to the social media platform. With regard to alcohol promotions, Winpenny et al. (2014) identify a multitude of different promotions that alcohol brands utilise in order to encourage interaction with the brands among young people, which may eventually lead to positive attitudes about alcohol and the consumption of alcohol. In particular, Winpenny et al. (2014) examined social media sites (e.g. Facebook, Twitter and YouTube) of five alcohol brands including beer, liqueur and cider brands (e.g. Fosters, Carling, Magners, Stella Artois, Tia Maria). The authors found that all Facebook brand pages studied included forms of sales promotions such as competitions. Further, Carah (2014) argues that alcohol brands such as Rekorderlig ran competitions asking their fans to post photographs as part of entering the competition. The author found that images uploaded by users 'functioned as micro-advertisements that packaged the product into the individual cultural moments and memories of fans' (p. 40). Similarly, Moraes et al. (2014) and Nicholls (2012) observed the Facebook pages of various alcohol brands of vodka and lager and equally identified the use of competitions to win music, prize draws, or tickets to sports events (e.g. beer). Specifically, Moraes et al.'s (2014) netnographic study identified five different types of alcohol promotions used by alcohol brands and clubs on Facebook, namely:

1   Competitions and prize draws for holidays/trips, shopping vouchers, tickets for sporting events, movie, festival and VIP parties, music and headphones, drink supplies, t-shirts, and glassware.
2   Free-gifts (or free giveaways) including free t-shirts, free entry to clubs and free transportation and free drinks.
3   Price discounts including price-cut-off drinks and 2 for 1.
4   Loyalty or membership benefits.
5   Auctions, such as a link to Ebay auctions for vodka bottles.

Additionally, the study identified that alcohol brands and clubs' Facebook pages encouraged competition-related posts as this type of content triggers electronic word of mouth (e-WOM) and increases traffic on the Facebook page (Moraes et al., 2014). In this case, winners post feedback on Facebook pages to highlight their winnings and the importance of winning such prizes.

Events, broadcast sponsorships and alcohol advertising

Alcohol brands associate themselves with real events and reinforce a drinking culture among social media users (e.g. 'watch football–drink beer') (Moraes et al., 2014; Nicholls, 2012). Nicholls (2012) found that alcohol brands on Twitter encouraged users to upload pictures of themselves attending real-life events using specified hashtags thus reinforcing the alcohol brand among its Twitter followers, and linking it to a valued event. Similarly, Carah (2014) found that alcohol brands (e.g. Absolut and Smirnoff) partner with popular artists or culture, music and fashion events, and sponsor charity auctions in an attempt to generate 'user-image' content that enhances the brand. Moraes et al. (2014) argue that application of events is a key Facebook feature which is used by alcohol brands to communicate with fans to advertise and promote such events.

Further, Nicholls (2012) reports that alcohol brands such as Fosters and Stella Artois undertake various marketing communication strategies on their Facebook pages including sponsoring TV programmes and live comedy, which extend their Facebook sites. Additionally, the author found that, quite commonly, brands upload links to their ads on their Facebook pages to raise awareness and elicit responses to new or existing advertising content, which often stimulate conversations with social media users who engage with the brand (Nicholls, 2012). Similarly to the work of Nicholls (2012), Winpenny et al. (2014) identified that four out of the five Facebook alcohol pages studied included video ads about their brands as well as videos that were unrelated to the brand. The authors found that alcohol brands' integrated marketing activity on YouTube and Facebook also consisted of product ads, demonstrations of how to make drinks, how ads were created and other comedy videos, and these were further discussed on Twitter (Winpenny et al., 2014). Carah (2014) also reports that many alcohol brands of whisky, vodka and liqueur (e.g. Jim Beam, Johnnie Walker, Absolut, Baileys) post advertisements on their Facebook pages, often without an accompanied responsible alcohol consumption message. Specifically, the author states that, of the advertisements on the Facebook pages studied (at the time of the research), only 14% displayed responsible consumption messages (Carah 2014).

Viral marketing and e-WoM of alcohol brands

Mart (2011) argues that the main objective of social media tactics for alcohol campaigns is to trigger positive word-of-mouth (WoM). WoM reflects 'informal communications directed at other consumers about the ownership, usage, or characteristics of particular goods and services and/or their sellers' (Westbrook,

1987: 261). Electronic word-of-mouth (e-WOM), or viral marketing, refers to marketing messages relevant to a specific company, product or brand transmitted through the use of social media applications (Kaplan and Haenlein, 2010). Within the context of alcohol consumption, research has highlighted the increasing use of viral marketing as a marketing strategy to promote alcohol brands (Casswell, 2004; Gordon et al., 2010; Mart, 2011; Montgomery and Chester, 2009; Winpenny et al., 2014). Authors agree that viral marketing's impact on exposure to alcohol content is important, however, research in this area remains limited. In a recent experiment conducted by Alhabash et al. (2015), the authors investigated viral behavioural intentions towards alcohol marketing status updates on Facebook. Their results indicated that viral intentions towards alcohol marketing status updates predict intentions to consume alcohol (Alhabash et al., 2015).

Encouraging and 'shaping' alcohol user-generated content and conversations

Kietzmann et al. (2011) state that social media sites allow or facilitate conversations among users depending on the social medium in question. Such platforms encourage engagement via participation, where creating and consuming content are intertwined. In the case of social networking sites, for example, companies share their content with their fans or followers, and allow them to engage or participate by posting comments and sharing their brand experiences with the brand. Additionally, users create conversations with other users, and control of the flow and content on social networking sites is seriously biased towards the social media user (Jenkins, 2006). As a result, marketers can no longer fully control the content about their brands generated by themselves and social media users and then circulated within social networking sites. Mangold and Faulds (2009) explain that brands attempt to 'shape' discussions or conversations on social media using various data-driven tactics (e.g. targeted message and posts) in an attempt to engage social media users with marketer-generated content and their brands. However, a fundamental issue here is the manipulation of such conversations which has ethical implications. Kietzmann et al. (2011) argue that while there maybe benefits in 'shaping' conversations (e.g. showing audiences that they care, and contributing to the discussion), companies may be accused of deliberately 'flooding conversations that were not theirs in the first place' (p. 245).

Within the context of alcohol consumption, research asserts that brands attempt to engage with young people via encouraging consumers to post images and questions about the product, popular culture or sport. Concurrently companies ask social media users to share their views following questions and images (e.g. drinks, shot glasses) posted by the brands (Carah, 2014; Moraes et al., 2014). In his content analysis of alcohol Facebook pages, Carah (2014) found that 46.7% of content posted by brands asked fans to interact. Additionally, in doing do, brands also leverage specific contexts, situations or calendar events, to encourage their followers to start conversations or engage in conversations. Nicholls (2012), Moraes et al. (2014) and Carah (2014) found that alcohol brands attempt to initiate alcohol conversations among followers using a number of themes or cues such as the weather, music and popular culture, sports, certain occasions and celebrations (e.g. national days), time and/or place. For example, Carah (2014) found that brands post most content on Fridays, while on Mondays content asks followers to recall their weekend, and on Thursdays content posted by brands aims to elicit anticipation for Friday evening. Further, the author found that content posted by brands pertained to the origin, foundations or history of alcohol brands in an attempt to highlight brand personality and authenticity (Carah, 2014). Alcohol brands found to engage fans with such content included Jameson Irish Whisky, Jim Beam and Jack Daniels as well as Jacobs Creek. Notably, Carah (2014) identified that alcohol brands also used a 'story-telling mode' to share content with fans. This tactic of encouraging or 'shaping' conversations is more engaging or involving than other forms of marketing communication (Mangold and Faulds, 2009). The author states for example: 'When brands tell stories that locate the product in particular places and ways of life, they are producing content that flows seamlessly through Facebook's news feeds. Fans are more likely to interact with an item of content that "fits" their profile rather than looks like an advertisement' (Carah, 2014: 46). Overall, by linking alcohol brands to such themes, social media users are encouraged to generate content and thus interact with the alcohol brands.

Conclusions

Scholarly research as well as anecdotal evidence indicate that alcohol brands are increasing their leverage on new media to promote alcohol (Carah, 2014; Hoffman et al., 2014; Mart, 2011; Mart et al., 2009; Moraes et al., 2014; Saffer and Dave, 2006). Relative to offline marketing, social media marketing practices seem to have a greater impact in increasing young people's engagement with alcohol brands, and this can eventually lead to normalisation of alcohol consumption (Alhabash et al., 2015; Hoffman et al., 2014; Montgomery and Chester, 2009). Such marketing techniques include the use of interactive content to increase engagement (Chester et al., 2010), viral marketing (Mart, 2011; Montgomery and Chester, 2009) as well as advertising and sales promotions (Moraes et al., 2014; Nicholls, 2012; Winpenny et al., 2014). In particular, studies (e.g. Moraes et al., 2014) show that that sales promotions involving price discounts impact on young adults' consumption of alcohol, and Facebook has proven an effective medium through which to disseminate such promotions. Facebook enables extended media exposure (Russell et al., 2009) of young adults to alcohol-related promotional content, which becomes even more engaging than offline content due to Facebook's participatory and co-creative nature. Also relevant is the evidence that nightclubs, not just alcohol brands, are playing a significant role in fostering such exposure (Moraes et al., 2014).

However, the extent to which social media is used to promote alcohol raises significant social implications. Of particular concern is the fact that online identities of social media users are in some instances impossible to ascertain (Moraes et al., 2014). This posits a major challenge to policy makers, self-regulating bodies and alcohol marketers, given that social media depicting alcohol use encourages drinking among young users (Anderson et al., 2009; Goldberg et al., 2006); while at the same time young adults' receptiveness to alcohol promotional content seems to be very high whilst on social networking sites. On this basis various authors (Hastings et al., 2010; Moraes et al., 2014; Nicholls, 2012) have suggested that alcohol promotions should be banned on social networking sites due to the harmful effects that they are likely to have on young people's drinking culture.

References

Alcohol Concern. (2015). Statistics on alcohol. Retrieved 15 April 2016, from www.alcoholconcern.org.uk/help-and-advice/statistics-on-alcohol

Alhabash, S., McAlister, A., Quilliam, E., Richards, J., and Lou, C. (2015). Alcohol's getting a bit more social: When alcohol marketing messages on Facebook increase young adults' intentions to imbibe. *Mass Communication and Society, 18*, 350–375.

Ali, M., and Dwyer, D. (2010). Social network effects in alcohol consumption among adolescents. *Addictive Behaviors, 35*(4), 337–342.

Anderson, P., de Bruijn, A., Angus, K., Gordon, R., and Hastings, G. (2009). Impact of alcohol advertising and media exposure on adolescent alcohol use: A systematic review of longitudinal studies. *Alcohol and Alcoholism, 44*(3), 229–243.

Ashworth, L., and Free, C. (2006). Marketing dataveillance and digital privacy: Using theories of justice to understand consumers' online privacy concerns. *Journal of Business Ethics, 67*(2), 107–123.

Bennett, S. (2014). Facebook, Twitter, Instagram, Pinterest, Vine, Snapchat – Social Media Stats 2014. Retrieved 27 November 2015, from www.adweek.com/socialtimes/social-media-statistics-2014/499230

Carah, N. (2014). *Like, Comment, Share: Alcohol Brand Activity on Facebook.* Brisbane: Foundation for Alcohol Research and Evaluation, University of Queensland.

Casswell, S. (2004). Alcohol brands in young peoples everyday lives: New developments in marketing. *Alcohol and Alcoholism, 39*(6), 471–476.

Chandon, P., Wansink, B., and Laurent, G. (2000). A benefit congruency framework of sales promotion effectiveness. *Journal of Marketing, 64*(4), 65–81.

Chester, J., Montgomery, K., and Dorfman, L. (2010). Alcohol marketing in the digital age. Center for Digital Democracy and Berkeley Media Studies Group, a project of the Public Health Institute. Retrieved 18 April 2016, from www.digitalads.org/documents/BMSG-CDD-Digital-Alcohol-Marketing.pdf

Deuze, M. (2007). Convergence culture in the creative industries. *International Journal of Cultural Studies, 10*, 243–263.

Egan, K., and Moreno, M. (2011). Alcohol references on undergraduate males' Facebook profiles. *American Journal of Men's Health, 5*(5), 413–420.

eMarketer. (2015a, 23 September). Social network ad revenues accelerate worldwide. Retrieved 15 April 2016, from www.emarketer.com/Article/Social-Network-Ad-Revenues-Accelerate-Worldwide/1013015

eMarketer. (2015b, 15 April). Social network ad spending to hit $23.68 billion worldwide in 2015. Retrieved 15 April 2016, from www.emarketer.com/articles/results.aspx?q=Social%20Network%20Ad%20Spending%20to%20Hit%20%2423.68%20Billion%20Worldwide

Fox, R., Krugman, D., Fletcher, J., and Fischer, P. (1998). Adolescents' attention to beer and cigarette print ads and associated product warnings. *Journal of Advertising, 27,* 57–68.

Gleibs, I. (2014). Turning virtual public spaces into laboratories: Thoughts on conducting online field studies using social network sites. *Analyses of Social Issues and Public Policy, 14*(1), 352–370.

Goldberg, M., Niedermeier, K., Bechtel, L., and Gorn, G. (2006). Heightening adolescent vigilance toward alcohol advertising to forestall alcohol use. *Journal of Public Policy and Marketing, 25,* 147–159.

Gordon, R., Hastings, G., and Moodie, C. (2010). Alcohol marketing and young people's drinking: What the evidence base suggests for policy. *Journal of Public Affairs, 10*(1–2), 88–101.

Griffiths, R., and Casswell, S. (2010). Intoxigenic digital spaces? Youth, social networking sites and alcohol marketing. *Drug and Alcohol Review, 29,* 525–530.

Hartigan, A., and Coe, N. (2012). *Internet Influences on Adolescent Attitudes to Alcohol.* London: Institute of Alcohol Studies.

Hastings, G., and Angus, K. (2009). *Under the Influence: The Damaging Effect of Alcohol Marketing on Young People.* London: British Medical Association.

Hastings, G., Brooks, O., Stead, M., Angus, K., Anker, T., and Farrell, T. (2010). Failure of self regulation of UK alcohol advertising. *British Medical Journal, 340,* 184–186.

Hebden, R., Lyons, A., Goodwin, I., and McCreanor, T. (2015). 'When you add alcohol it gets that much better': University students, alcohol consumption and online drinking cultures. *Journal of Drug Issues, 45*(2), 214–226.

Hingson, R., Heeren, T., Winter, M., and Wechsler, H. (2005). Magnitude of alcohol-related mortality and morbidity among US college students ages 18–24: Changes from 1998 to 2001. *Annual Review of Public Health, 26,* 259–279.

Hoffman, E., Pinkleton, B., Weintraub Austin, E., and Reyes-Velázquez, W. (2014). Exploring college students' use of general and alcohol-related social media and their associations with alcohol-related behaviors. *Journal of American College Health, 62,* 328–335.

Institute for Policy Research. (2013). Would you 'like' a drink? Youth drinking cultures, social media and alcohol marketing online. *University of Bath.* Retrieved 18 April 2016, from www.bath.ac.uk/ipr/our-publications/policy-briefs/youth-drinking.pdf

Jenkins, H. (2006). *Convergence Culture: Where Old and New Media Collide.* New York: New York University Press.

Jernigan, D. (2012). Who is minding the virtual alcohol store? *Archives of Paediatric and Adolescent Medicine, 166*(9), 866–868.

Johnson, L. (2015, 16 June). With better targeting, alcohol brands bet big on digital: Annual budgets increase as much as 50 percent. *Adweek.* Retrieved 15 April 2016, from www.adweek.com/news/technology/better-targeting-alcohol-brands-bet-big-digital-165357

Kaplan, A., and Haenlein, M. (2010). Users of the world, unite! The challenges and opportunities of Social Media. *Business Horizons, 53*(1), 59–68.

Kietzmann, J., Hermkens, K., McCarthy, I., and Silvestre, B. (2011). Social media? Get serious! Understanding the functional building blocks of social media. *Business Horizons, 54*(3), 241–251.

Kuntsche, E., Knibbe, R., Gmel, G., and Rutger, E. (2005). Why do young people drink? A review of drinking motives. *Clinical Psychology Review, 25,* 841–861.

Lyons, A., Goodwin, I., McCreanor, T., and Griffin, C. (2015). Social networking and young adults' drinking practices: Innovative qualitative methods for health behavior research. *Health Psychology*, *34*(4), 293–302.

Mangold, W., and Faulds, D. (2009). Social media: The new hybrid element of the promotion mix. *Business Horizons*, *52*(4), 357–365.

Mart, S. (2011). Alcohol marketing in the 21st century: New methods, old problems. *Substance Use and Misuse*, *46*(7), 889–892. www.scopus.com/inward/record. url?eid=2-s2.0–79957523498andpartnerID=40andmd5=bd9f019dad2437703f1172f3f 6bbe596

Mart, S., Mergendoller, J., and Simon, M. (2009). Alcohol promotion on facebook. *Journal of Global Drug Policy and Practice*, *3*(3). Retrieved from http://globaldrugpolicy. org/3/3/1.php

McCarty, D., and Kaye, M. (1984). Reasons for drinking: Motivational patterns and alcohol use among college students. *Addictive Behaviors*, *9*, 185–188.

McCreanor, T., Lyons, A., Griffin, C., Goodwin, I., Moewaka Barnes, H., and Hutton, F. (2013). Youth drinking cultures, social networking and alcohol marketing: Implications for public health. *Critical Public Health*, *23*(1), 110–120.

Moewaka Barnes, H., McCreanor, T., Goodwin, I., Lyons, A., Griffin, C., and Hutton, F. (2016). Alcohol and social media: Drinking and drunkenness while online. *Critical Public Health*, *26*(1), 62–76.

Montgomery, K., and Chester, J. (2009). Interactive food and beverage marketing: Targeting adolescents in the digital age. *Journal of Adolescent Health*, *45*(3), S18–S29.

Moraes, C., Michaelidou, N., and Meneses, R. (2014). The use of Facebook to promote drinking among young consumers. *Journal of Marketing Management*, *30*(13–14), 1377–1401.

Moreno, M., Briner, L., Williams, A., Brockman, L., Walker, L., and Christakis, D. (2010). A content analysis of displayed alcohol references in a social networking web site. *Journal of Adolescent Health*, *47*, 168–175.

Moreno, M., Christakis, D., Egan, K., Brockman, L., and Becker, T. (2012). Associations between displayed alcohol references on Facebook and problem drinking among college students. *Archives of Paediatric and Adolescent Medicine*, *166*(2), 157–163.

Mundt, M. (2011). The impact of peer social networks on adolescent alcohol use initiation. *Academic Pediatrics*, *11*(5), 414–421.

Nicholls, J. (2012). Everyday, everywhere: Alcohol marketing and social media—current trends. *Alcohol and Alcoholism*, *47*(4), 486–493.

Nielsen. (2014, 10 February). What's empowering the new digital consumer? Retrieved 15 April 2016, from www.nielsen.com/us/en/insights/news/2014/whats-empowering-the-new-digital-consumer.html

Palmer, D. (2005). Pop-ups, cookies, and spam: Toward a deeper analysis of the ethical significance of Internet marketing practices. *Journal of Business Ethics*, *58*(1–3), 271–280.

Piacentini, M., and Banister, E. (2009). Managing anti-consumption in an excessive drinking culture. *Journal of Business Research*, *62*(2), 279–288.

Robinson, T., Chen, H., and Killen, J. (1988). Television and music video exposure and risk of adolescent alcohol use. *Pediatrics*, *102*(5), e54.

Russell, C., Russell, D., and Grube, J. (2009). Nature and impact of alcohol messages in a youth-oriented television series. *Journal of Advertising*, *38*(3), 97–112.

Saffer, H., and Dave, D. (2006). Alcohol advertising and alcohol consumption by adolescents. *Health Economics, 15*, 617–637.

Smith, A., Fischer, E., and Yongjian, C. (2012). How does brand-related user-generated content differ across YouTube, Facebook, and Twitter? *Journal of Interactive Marketing, 26*(2), 102–113.

Socialbakers. (2015). Facebook brands stats – alcohol. Retrieved 1 November 2015, from www.socialbakers.com/statistics/facebook/pages/total/brands/alcohol/

Statista. (2016). Leading social networks worldwide as of January 2016, ranked by number of active users (in millions). Retrieved 15 April 2016, from www.statista.com/statistics/272014/global-social-networks-ranked-by-number-of-users/

Szmigin, I., Griffin, C., Mistral, W., Bengry-Howell, A., Weale, L., and Hackley, C. (2008). Re-framing 'binge drinking' as calculated hedonism—Empirical evidence from the UK. *International Journal of Drug Policy, 19*(5), 359–366.

Triggle, N. (2009, 8 September). Doctors want booze marketing ban. *BBC News*. Retrieved 9 September 2016, from http://news.bbc.co.uk/2/hi/health/8242385.stm

Uzunoğlu, E., and Öksüz, B. (2014). New opportunities in social media for ad-restricted alcohol products: The case of 'Yeni Rakı'. *Journal of Marketing Communications, 20*(4), 270–290.

van Dijck, J., and Poell, T. (2013). Understanding social media logic. *Media and Communication, 1*(1), 2–14.

Westbrook, R. (1987). Product/consumption-based affective responses and postpurchase process. *Journal of Marketing Research, 24*, 258–270.

Winpenny, E., Marteau, T., and Nolte, E. (2014). Exposure of children and adolescents to alcohol marketing on social media websites. *Alcohol and Alcoholism, 49*(2), 154–159.

7 Alcohol corporations and marketing in social media

Nicholas Carah

Introduction

This chapter offers a conceptual intervention in how we understand the role of media technologies in the marketing machinery of alcohol corporations. Policy makers, critics and activists need to develop an account of the infrastructural and computational dimensions of media in order to respond to participatory, culturally embedded and data-driven alcohol branding. A critical move here is to position analysis of the current capacities of platforms such as Facebook, Instagram or Snapchat as part of a larger trajectory of experiments in media engineering (McStay, 2013). What we variously call digital, online, social, mobile or interactive media might be more productively approached as a series of interrelated processes by which media become social and participatory, mobile and locative, entangled with our bodies, and data-driven, experimental and algorithmic. This chapter aims to map out some of the ways alcohol brands are becoming social, mobile, experimental and embodied in order to prompt productive ways to conceptualise and calibrate the harms that are intensified by alcohol marketing.

Critical examination of alcohol marketing and associated calls for policy reform have focused on the content, volume and exposure of audiences to advertising (Anderson et al., 2009; Jones, 2010, 2014; Pettigrew et al., 2012). For the most part, these studies define the harms of alcohol advertising in terms of excessive consumption, health impacts and violence (Babor et al., 2010). Studies of alcohol and social media have categorised the content produced by marketers (Mart et al., 2009; Nicholls, 2012) and the portrayal of drinking by young people (Griffiths and Casswell, 2010; Moreno et al., 2010; Ridout et al., 2012). While the description of the content that marketers produce and the quantification of harms in terms of health impacts and violence are important, I argue that we also ought to consider the impact the alcohol industry's marketing machinery has on the composition of urban spaces, the development of media infrastructure and the quality of our public and mediated lives. By this I mean that as much as we might be concerned with the economic cost to the health system of alcohol consumption or the rates of alcohol-related assault, we also need to ask questions such as 'What qualities of urban spaces such as nightlife precincts are worth cultivating and investing in?' and 'How is the industry investing in the iterative development of media platforms that enable modes of promotion that unfold beyond the purview of public scrutiny?' The marketing machinery of the alcohol industry raises questions that go to the foundation of how we understand media and manage public space and culture.

This chapter proceeds in five parts. First, I connect current perspectives on branding and digital media to argue that alcohol brands operate as open-ended computational applications on digital media platforms. This enables us to think of 'social media' as not only the currently existing or emerging platforms, but rather to turn our attention to their expanding data-processing, sensory and participatory capacities. Second, I examine how alcohol brands leverage the capacity of media platforms to collect and process data to shape user engagement. Third, I explore the role that real-world activations and material objects play in stimulating and organising brand engagement on media platforms. Fourth, I consider the expansion of 'below the line' forms of promotional labour and culture used by alcohol brands on media platforms. These sections draw attention to how cultures of alcohol consumption are integrated with the calculative and participatory nature of digital media. Throughout, I examine a range of scenarios that illustrate the complicated interplay between drinking culture, media platforms and alcohol brands. Each facet illustrates how the industry's marketing strategies are woven into everyday drinking culture. Finally, I offer regulatory interventions that might go beyond attempting to contain the content of brands and instead directly address the platform protocols, algorithms and interfaces that are the critical infrastructure of alcohol branding. Throughout the chapter I argue that we must train our attention on the infrastructure rather than the representational content of alcohol brands. Of course the symbolic still matters, but it is no longer enough to only attempt to conceptualise, account for and regulate the symbolic interventions brands make in the world. Self-regulatory systems that focus on monitoring the representational content of campaigns are not capable of apprehending the brand activity on media platforms.

The material presented in this chapter is drawn from analysis of alcohol brand content on Facebook and Instagram, observation at cultural events such as music festivals where alcohol brands create activations, and fieldwork with informants who are patrons of nightlife venues and precincts, promoters or photographers. I aim in this chapter to synthesise findings across this work into a conceptual account of how media platforms and alcohol brands are interdependent.

Media platforms and computational brands

In recent years, media scholars have developed the concept of 'media platforms' to conceptually undergird a range of terms that are often used to describe contemporary media: social, mobile, digital, participatory, locative, sensory, algorithmic, interactive and so on (Gillespie, 2014; van Dijck, 2013). Jose van Dijck (2013: 29) argues that:

> [Media] platforms are computational and architectural concepts, but can also be understood figuratively, in a sociocultural and a political sense, as political stages and performative infrastructures. A platform is a mediator rather than

an intermediary: it shapes the performance of social acts instead of merely facilitating them. Technologically speaking platforms are the providers of software, (sometimes) hardware, and services that help code social activities into a computational architecture; they process (meta)data through algorithms and formatted protocols before presenting their interpreted logic in the form of user-friendly interfaces with default settings that reflect the platform owner's strategic choices.

While this definition is conceptually dense, it usefully connects together the technical elements of media platforms that we need to place at the centre of any consideration of alcohol marketing in the digital era. Media platforms are computational architectures in the sense that they are primarily organised around collecting, storing and processing data, rather than producing content in the way that 'traditional' print or broadcast media institutions do. Van Dijck (2013: 29) defines five technical elements – data, algorithm, protocol, interface and default – that together offer a schema for investigating the interplay between media platforms and the creative capacities of users. This directs us towards the experimentation of alcohol marketers with the technical capacities of platforms, rather than just the content that flows through the user interface. Advertisers such as alcohol corporations invest in media platforms not just because of their capacity to capture audience attention, but also because of their capacity to 'engineer sociality' and experiment with market formations (van Dijck, 2013).

A media platform is a technology stack – the infrastructure necessary to run applications – upon which brands operate as computational applications. In making this claim, I connect van Dijck's (2013) account of media platforms with Lury's (2004) conceptualisation of brands as 'programming devices'. Lury (2004) takes the concept of the brand beyond the symbolic to examine how brands work to coordinate action. A brand is 'a way not of representing but of modelling markets in many dimensions'. Brands are devices for experimenting with, modulating and calibrating relationships between markets and consumers. The work of branding involves the 'soft' interpretation of cultural judgements and the 'hard' calculus of analytical experiments. Brands are computational applications in the sense that they operate in an ongoing and iterative way to calibrate action; they are open-ended processes that seek to optimise and harmonise the interplay between market imperatives and cultural life. A brand, in this sense, is a part of a larger infrastructure that coordinates market exchange. The brand is not confined to symbolic meaning-making, but rather is any aspect of the coordination of the touchpoints between marketing machinery and the open-ended nature of cultural life.

Brands that run as computational apps on media platforms comprise software, hardware and living users. Software organises, calculates and shapes flows of information. It sequences that information in an interface for specific users. Hardware is the range of input/output (I/O) devices between the calculative capacities of software and the living capacities of users. Hardware such as smartphones can be understood as having sensory capacities: collecting data such as expression and movement from users, and conveying sensory stimulus to users in the form of images, sounds and vibrations. Users generate social action and creativity that is channelled onto media platforms via hardware where software is able to make calculations about how to calibrate the ongoing action of those users and others like them. The value of understanding alcohol brands in the digital era as computational apps that run on media platforms is that it enables us to account for how the participatory aspects of branding (Arvidsson, 2005; Moor, 2003) are interdependent with their analytic capacities (Andrejevic, 2011; Turow, 2012). Media platforms are computational architecture for bringing together the creative and generative capacities of users with the analytical capacities of computational systems. In the section to follow we examine alcohol brand activities that operate on this computational media platform logic.

Platforms such as Facebook and Instagram are commercially driven media engineering projects. When Facebook was launched as a public company in 2012, the platform had a significant infrastructural problem that market analysts anticipated could undermine performance of the stock. Facebook users were rapidly moving to the mobile app, which had no advertising model. To solve the problem, Facebook had to develop a native content model that integrated paid advertiser content into the news feed along with all the other content users saw from friends and pages they followed. By 2015 about 87% of Facebook's audience used the mobile app and advertising revenue from the mobile app accounted for 73% of their total revenue.[1] Also in 2012, Facebook purchased the mobile photo-sharing app Instagram for US$1 billion.[2] Like Facebook's mobile app at the time, Instagram had no advertising or revenue model. The acquisition was arguably about acquiring Instagram's technology stack, design capabilities and the flow of images and metadata that users generated. But, Facebook have also worked to monetise Instagram's growing and highly engaged user base. In 2015 Instagram have progressively rolled out a native advertising model on the platform.[3] The integration of advertising into the Facebook and Instagram mobile apps is the first time that a native advertising model has been implemented at scale.

The emergence of these native content models is significant because, to use van Dijck's (2013) schema, the default interface is now one where advertising content uses the same protocols as all other content on a platform. Advertising material appears like any other story in the Facebook news feed, or like any other image in the Instagram home feed. These native content models are iterative and ongoing experiments. They accumulate data over time that enable them to improve their targeting, predictions and real-time customisation. Furthermore, native models stimulate more complicated interplay between advertisers and other users on the platform. Both consumers and cultural intermediaries such as celebrities, stylists, hipsters, musicians, photographers and models become producers of brand content. Brands contract intermediaries to incorporate the brand into their flow of images by sending them product or inviting them to branded events (Carah and Shaul, 2016; Marwick, 2015).

Alcohol brand activity within Facebook's native content model is extensive and growing (Carah, 2014). By the end of 2012 the top 20 alcohol brands in Australia had 2.5 million followers on their Facebook pages. During the year they posted more than 4500 items of content. Their followers interacted with that content – liking, sharing or commenting on it – over 2.3 million times. Each of those interactions increase the reach of the brand into the news feeds of users and the affinity between brands and users within the network. In 2012, Facebook's advice was that an average post reached 16% of fans. If the posts of these top 20 brands reached 16% of their fan base on average, they would have generated 90 million impressions on Facebook in Australia in 2012. Reach is increased by generating engagement and affinity within the network and by paying Facebook to promote content into the news feeds of target audiences. Alcohol brands have above-average engagement and we do not know what they spend promoting content. It is likely their reach is much higher than this 16%. The industry does not often disclose details of its partnerships with social media platforms. Occasionally information will be published in trade press or at industry conventions. For example, at the 2013 Australian Media Federation Awards, Wild Turkey won the Best Demonstration of Results award. Recognising that alcohol sponsorship of professional sport was over crowded, Wild Turkey used Facebook to engage with local sporting clubs. The brand reported that the campaign helped make it the number one bourbon brand on Facebook in Australia with a '60% increase in top of mind and a 42% increase in intention to purchase. Its sales outstripped the bourbon category's 2.5% annual growth by a factor of 8.5 times, realising 21% growth' (Media Federation of Australia, 2013). These observations are just some indications of the strategic partnerships between media platforms such as Facebook and alcohol marketers.

A follow-up study conducted of brand activity on Facebook in 2014 reveals continuing growth in fan bases. Furthermore, while brands are posting content less frequently, many are generating more engagement. This is attributable to investment in higher quality content from brands in response to changes in Facebook's architecture. Brands generate less organic reach in the news feed, but Facebook has opened up more opportunities for brands to generate paid reach by 'sponsoring' content into the feeds of targeted users. Rather than buy advertisements, brands can pay to have their content 'natively' integrated into the news feeds of select users, where it appears like any other item of content. In order to protect overall user engagement, Facebook limits the number of 'spots' available in each user's news feed for this native promoted content. Spaces are sold via auction, advertisers bid for space in specific users' feeds at specific times of day. Brands pay more for users and times for which there is more demand.

Speaking at the Australian Association of National Advertisers Connect conference in 2014, Helen Crossley, Facebook's head of measurement and insights in Australia, made a pitch to advertisers about the platform's capacity to use data to create custom and lookalike audiences (Australian Association of National Advertisers, 2014). Custom audiences are created by integrating marketers' in-house data, third-party data and Facebook's data to locate specific users on the platform. Lookalike audiences are created by using marketers' data and third-party data to locate users on the platform who are similar to a client's existing market. Crossley promoted Facebook's capacity to work with major brands to integrate data from the platform with corporations' own marketing analytics. Facebook's custom and lookalike audience features enable advertisers to leverage data to simulate potential audiences based on a range of criteria. In 2011, Diageo announced that its partnership with Facebook involved 'unprecedented levels of interaction and joint business planning', but since then no major distributor has revealed any details of their partnerships with Facebook publicly (Diageo, 2011). While the industry is highly secretive about its partnerships and investments in media platforms, it is plausible to argue that the partnerships aim to leverage user data to more seamlessly integrate brands into the lived cultural experiences of consumers. The value proposition that platforms make to advertisers is not just about selling audience attention, or even about being able to target highly customised audiences. It is also about the capacity of the platform to leverage data to simulate and experiment with potential audience configurations. For alcohol brands owned by global distributors, this experimentation with potential audiences involves the profiles and datasets of millions of Facebook users worldwide.

Alcohol branding on data-driven media platforms

Media platforms use data to shape user engagement in ongoing loops. Data (van Dijck, 2013: 30) are any type of information converted to digital form. This can include media content such as text, images or sound and other information that users enter such as demographic details, opinions or preferences. An important category of data is metadata – data about data – that adds context to a user's engagement with a platform. Metadata might, for instance, record when, where and in proximity to whom users engage with certain types of content in the platform database. For alcohol marketers, data enables time and context-specific targeting of content. A platform might be able to discern that a consumer is a fan of a rugby team because they follow the team's Facebook page, have read news stories about the team, or have posted content relating to a game in the past. During a game, an alcohol brand may be able to use that data to target content at fans of specific teams at critical moments in the game. When Team A scores a try, fans of Team A will receive a promotional post such as an image or video replaying the try. They can then share that content to their networks. In a moment when they have their smartphone in their hand and want to express their joy to their social network, the alcohol brand offers a compelling item of content that enables them to do that. While, moments later if Team B scores a try, fans of that team will receive customised content featuring the highlight from their team. Fans act as nodes or transfer points between cultural moments and brand content, switching brand content into their own social networks as part of their enjoyment of a game. Australian beer brands have used this kind of data-driven content targeting during games such as Rugby League's State of Origin. Data about cultural pastimes is also increasingly geo-spatial. If fans at a rugby game open their Facebook app while at a sporting stadium, they may register their location on the platform, enabling real-time targeting of promotional content during the game as well as registering themselves a fan of that sporting code and one of those teams for future engagement.

The data that platforms collect are leveraged by algorithms. In computer science, an algorithm is a 'finite list of well-defined instructions' for processing data (van Dijck, 2013: 30). The emergence of algorithm-driven media platforms has led cultural researchers to articulate the emergence of 'algorithmic' cultural formations and practices, where flows of cultural information and everyday cultural practices are shaped by algorithmic decisions. When we search for information on Google, when we look for a film on Netflix, when we load our Facebook news feed, algorithms sort and order content from a database for us (Hallinan and Striphas, 2014). Alcohol brands, like all content producers in an algorithmic media system, must 'address' the decision-making logic of algorithms if they want to be visible to other users. If a brand is using a platform such as Facebook, they must create content that the news feed algorithm will notice and favour in decision making. Facebook's news feed uses an expanding array of data to decide how to select and order items of content in each user's feed. One of these judgements is 'affinity' between users in a network. In simple terms, a user is more likely to see content posted by other users determined by the news feed algorithm determined as 'similar' to them. Alcohol brands must address this algorithmic logic by behaving in a similar manner to their target audience.

Brands time their posts to 'intersect' with consumers' drinking practices. This makes them more visible in news feeds because consumers incorporate the brand into their own 'real-time' expressions about drinking. In our 2012 study we found that Friday afternoon was the most common time and day for brands to post content (Carah, 2014). One way to understand this is that content posted at this time generates more engagement and therefore more visibility in users' news feeds because it coincides with their cultural practices. On average an item of content generates 530 interactions. When it is targeted at a specific event or time of day, that rises to 792. On a Friday afternoon, many users have 'knocked off' work for the week and are enjoying a drink, often with smartphone in hand, seeking to link up with their friends for the weekend. The orchestration of a drinking ritual in conjunction with a media platform generates data that the platform can harness to calibrate interplay with brands. For example, at 3pm on a Friday afternoon Bundaberg Rum posted an image of the Bundy Bear looking at his watch and saying '118 minutes till Rum O'Clock'. The post received 830 interactions, a selection of comments in the first half hour included: 'sorry, too late, couldn't hang in anymore!'; 'it's always rum o clock on my watch!'; and 'you need to get your watch checked 10am was 4 hours ago'. Likewise, on another Friday afternoon the beer brand Victoria Bitter posted 'is there anything better than your first cold VB on a Friday afternoon?' Fans' comments included: 'yeah the second cold VB cause the first 1 don't touch the sides'; 'yeah, the 18th'; and 'yep, ya first VB Saturday morning'.

We can understand this engagement between brands and consumers as a participatory mode of branding. The comments of fans are user-generated content. They perform the brand as part of their identities and self-narratives. Consumer fans deploy their position in the social world and the tone and vernacular of their expression to create a resonant performance of the brand for their peers. These two examples are broadly reflective of 'Friday afternoon' conversations that consumers have with each other about drinking. Many of these Friday afternoon conversations involve fans celebrating forms of excessive drinking that alcohol brands themselves could never explicitly endorse. In their response to the Alcohol Beverages Advertising Code regarding user-generated content of this nature, VB in fact argued that the exchanges were akin to being 'privy to a conversation say at a restaurant or pub in Glen Waverley or Subiaco or Wallsend or Kirribilli'. They argued that users on the Facebook page chose to be part of and participate in the conversations and therefore found their tone and content acceptable. In their view, because the VB page would most likely only be accessed by consumers familiar with the brand's 'tone', it should not be considered marketing but rather a conversation between like-minded peers (Brodmerkel and Carah, 2013). VB explicitly used the concept of 'affinity' – a shared drinking culture – between brand and users as an explicit defence of its activity on Facebook. They infer that the 'affinity' dimension of Facebook's algorithmic content sorting ensures that people who would find content offensive would be unlikely to see it.

What VB's argument evades, however, is that the critical issue emerging here is not the content so much as the creation of a media infrastructure for leveraging and exploiting cultural identities and performances. The protocols of the platform, which I discuss below, are the key devices that enable the brand to function. The algorithms ensure content is seen by users who share affinity with the brand. Facebook now also provide 'gating' devices, where advertisers can choose to target content directly at specific users. They can also use gating to ensure that specified users do not see content. This is most commonly used for age and region to ensure that consumers who have declared their age as under 18 do not see alcohol brand pages, or where brands wish to post region-specific content to the platform. But, it is also easy to imagine how gating could be used as a risk management strategy by brands. For instance, a brand targeting young males could ensure that no consumers who were female or over say 21 years old see certain content and the conversations around it. This means that brands could engage in forms of marketing that, while breaching a self-regulatory code such as the Australian Alcohol Beverages Advertising Code, fit well within the vernacular of a specific target market. Marketing of this kind contributes to public harms over time but is increasingly not open to any kind of public scrutiny.

We also need to consider the calculative and algorithmic dimension of branding unfolding in these interactions. By interacting with the brand as part of their drinking rituals, users initiate vectors that link their cultural world, alcohol consumption and a brand together in time and place. That enables the brand to respond in real time, by boosting posts within peer networks or lookalike networks where it is generating engagement. Preliminary research has illustrated a link between engagement with alcohol content on social media and risky drinking (Ridout, et al., 2012). This finding is logical when considered in relation to the platform infrastructure. Those whose social networks and activities on social media indicate engagement with or consumption of alcohol are more likely to be determined to share 'affinity' with alcohol brands, and therefore more likely to be exposed to their appeals. Social media platforms are different to other media technologies in that they are configured to disproportionately target heavier or riskier drinkers with alcohol-related content. For instance, imagine the likely public concern if advertising breaks in television broadcasts could target heavier drinkers with more alcohol advertising than other viewers. The protocols and algorithms of media platforms such as Facebook are weighted towards determining heavier drinkers to share a higher affinity with alcohol brands and other heavy drinkers. The array of data that might indicate this affinity is extensive. In addition to direct engagement with an alcohol brand page or content, other useful data could include: a social network with peers who follow alcohol brands, interaction with nightlife-related pages or content such as following the page of a club night, following particular cultural intermediaries such as musicians or sports clubs, geo-locational data that indicate patterns of consumption in a nightlife precinct, and so on. Platforms archive this range of associations for future analysis and action. For instance, in future Friday afternoon posts the brand will be able to more accurately predict which users are engaged in afternoon drinking rituals and what kind of content they might interact with. Bundaberg Rum produce customised content for different niche audiences on the platform. Content featuring the Bundy Bear and afternoon drinking rituals appears to be targeted at an older working-class demographic, while content featuring savvy internet memes appears to target a younger demographic. For example, Bundaberg use of the '99 Problems' meme would likely only make sense to younger users who are part of the vernacular use of these images.[4] We can assume, if Bundaberg Rum are using the technical capacities of the platform to their full extent, that they are using data to target these different streams of content at customised user groups in designated locations and at specific times of the day and week.

Media platforms are governed by protocols that open and close possible actions to users. Any action a user takes depends on a protocol. A platform such as Facebook enables activities such as adding friends, joining groups, sharing and liking content. The protocols that platforms develop in part serve the interests of investors. For instance, platform protocols only enable users to 'like' a brand; they can not 'dislike' it. While Facebook is moving towards giving users a range of 'emojis' instead of a like button to express a wider array of reactions to items in their news feeds, it seems likely that brands will be able to control the selection of 'emojis' available to users on their items of content. On an alcohol brand page, protocols ensure that any unsolicited content posted by a user is not logged on the brand's timeline unless the brand chooses to share it to their timeline. This grants the brand control over which user engagements are made visible. If a user posts content critical of a brand, it is not likely to be visible to other users. Platform protocols are set to the preferred defaults of powerful actors on the platform, like advertisers (van Dijck, 2013: 30). The platform interface – buttons, icons, boxes and devices a user can interact with – prompts and governs behaviour on the platform, enacting the 'protocolized relations' between data, software and hardware that enable the platform to function (van Dijck, 2013: 31). On a media platform, a brand is usefully understood as an interface that users interact with. A media platform's user interface is the touchpoint between the computational capacities of the brand and the creative capacities of the consumer. To think of a brand as interface, rather than a persuasive symbolic message, is to understand the production of brand value as the use of data to orchestrate, engineer, predict and shape the relationship between brand, users, cultural practices and contexts of consumption. As users engage with platforms, they register connections between their lives, social networks, patterns of movement, moods and so on that brands can leverage in real time or in the future.

Platform protocols configure a commercial productive user; one who is engaged with a platform often, integrating use of it into their everyday practices. Protocols such as share and like buttons prompt users to circulate brand images and content. Protocols such as comment boxes enable users to extend brand narratives, incorporating them into their own life narratives and social worlds. Protocols such as photo capture and upload enable users to create content that incorporates brands into rituals of alcohol consumption. The data collection and analysis components of a platform make users visible to brands. Algorithms enable that data to be leveraged to generate engagement, simulate and experiment with audience configurations, and target specific users in time and space. Alcohol brands' creation of symbolic content is one part of this larger technical infrastructure of the media platform. As I discuss in the following sections, media platforms also shape the activity of alcohol brands in real-world cultural spaces.

Real-world entanglements between brands, users and platforms

In recent years alcohol brands have installed a range of brand activations at cultural events. Yellowglen wines installed an old fairground carousel at race days. Strongbow cider placed an antique sailing ship on the grounds of the Splendour in the Grass music festival. At the same festival, Kopparberg set up a traditional Swedish village where festival-goers could play traditional games such as Kubb. XXXX leased a tropical island and changed its name to XXXX Island. These are just a few of the most spectacular real-world activations brands have implemented. Brands also send promotional staff into venues and nightlife precincts with more ad hoc or low-cost devices to generate interaction and engagement with consumers. Jim Beam took a cardboard cut-out of Jim Beam V8 Supercar drivers around pubs, getting consumers to pose with their face in the driver's racesuit. Jägermeister took an oversize cardboard cut-out bottle and passed it among patrons in venues. They posed with the bottle, danced with it and pretended to skol from it.

These activations and material objects take on a variety of utilities on media platforms. A pre-platform view of an object such as a cardboard cut-out bottle of Jägermeister would understand it as a symbolic device. The purpose of a bottle would be to increase brand awareness, make the brand present in a specific cultural setting, and perhaps capture images that can be used in word-of-mouth promotion.

For instance, in the era before social media, promotional staff would frequently enter bars and venues with various branded props. Often they would carry Polaroid cameras and get patrons to pose with the props for photos that were then given to them as a memento of the night out. A cardboard cut-out bottle still functions in this way, though when considered as a device that acts in relation to a media platform, it takes on additional properties. The bottle (or carousel, or island, or Swedish village, or supercar driver) acts as a stimulus for patrons to mediate the experience. Consumers take their smartphones out and create images that get circulated via their peer networks. The material action of the brand generates media content and data. While it creates peer-to-peer brand promotion, perhaps more importantly it registers connections in databases. If several people in a bar take images of themselves with a branded object and post it to a media platform, then the platform can link them together determining other relationships in social networks and cultural tastes of people who go to the venue, the cultural entertainment at the venue, and the brand.

Objects such as a bottle, carousel or bespoke village might also come to operate as scannable codes. Facebook's algorithms already recognise faces and landmarks to suggest user and location tags. From here, it is not difficult to see how platforms could recognise specific logos or objects in images and use them analytically. Brands format themselves to algorithmic cultural formations (Carah, 2014; Hallinan and Striphas, 2014). Part of what a brand does is undertake actions within cultural spaces that address the decision-making architecture of algorithmic media platforms. Understanding alcohol marketing in the age of social media platforms involves more than tracking the interaction that takes place on the platform itself, but further how the platform is shaping material spaces of consumption. The infrastructure of a media platform extends beyond the databases, hardware and interface to include smartphones, venues, nightlife precincts, cultural events and the bodies of consumers.

Promotional culture and below the line branding on platforms

Promoters or 'promos' are critically important labourers in the marketing of alcohol on media platforms. Promos promote venues, club nights, artists and DJs for a combination of cash and in-kind payment. Many are 'paid' in free access to venues and free drinks. A thorough understanding of alcohol marketing on social media must account for the growth of this below the line workforce, especially because as more scrutiny is applied to above the line or mainstream modes of alcohol marketing, the incentive to invest in below the line activities increases. Promos use their own bodies, sense of taste and style and social networks to generate engagement with venues and products. They most often work by circulating images of themselves at specific venues, events or parties. Many promos acquire a large following online because of their ability to put people on the 'door list' at clubs, their provocative and entertaining content, or their advice and insider knowledge on events and venues. They are a particularly valuable class of labour because they directly insert brands into their own life-casting.

They are also adept at moving across media platforms to promote brands and events. For instance, they might simultaneously use Facebook, Instagram, Snapchat and Tinder to promote a night, venue or product. In the specific case of alcohol marketing, promos operate at arm's length from the alcohol brands and venues. Hardly any are formally employed or associated with a venue or alcohol brand. This means that they can incorporate brands into narratives of excessive alcohol and drug consumption, intoxication, sexual promiscuity and so on without indicting the company.

Promos play an important role within the calculative operation of media platforms. As they generate engagement and following online, and encourage people within their peer networks to follow their venues, brands and club nights, they create associations between users, cultural spaces and practices, times of the day and week, venues and brands in the databases of media platforms. These associations can then be leveraged by both humans and algorithms. Promos might head into a venue or nightlife precinct and use their smartphone to recruit people to a particular club night, scrolling through their Facebook or Instagram feed they might see people who are headed out for the night and send a message giving them an invite or offering them a free drink at their venue. They might create a Snapchat video of wild dancing in their club and send that out to their network as evidence that their venue has a good atmosphere. Some even use Tinder to find dates and hook-ups who they invite to their venue. In this respect media platforms can be understood as live catalogues of available bodies that promos can access and guide towards their venues to consume alcohol.

Furthermore, platform algorithms become more adept at shaping flows of images and content around nightlife practices. A user might be having pre-drinks with friends in one part of the city and post an image to Facebook. They might then catch a cab into a nightlife precinct, and post an image or even just open their Facebook app. In doing so, their news feed will recognise their proximity to friends also in the precinct and to venues they have visited before and post content to their feed. The news feed reinforces drinking narratives in real time. Alcohol brands might target promotional content based on data such as people who have checked in, been in an image from, or followed, a particular venue or promoter. They effectively use the venue or promoter as a node that assembles a niche market of consumers available in a specific place and time. The important issue to consider here is the work that users and promos do in 'knitting' media platforms into their cultural and consumption practices and, in doing so, making those practices visible to platforms and the brands that run on them. This enables a range of below the line, culturally embedded and data-driven promotional practices to emerge. These practices fall well outside of any existing regulatory or policy frameworks but are key sites for incubating brand and promotional strategies.

Icon and dashboard: regulating protocol, interface and database

To conclude, I consider how policy makers, critics, activists, lobbyists and scholars might approach the question of regulating alcohol marketing on media platforms. In *The New York Times* in 2009, Saul Hansell considered a proposition by Joseph Turow, a leading figure in scholarly and public debate about interactive advertising (see Turow, 2012). Turow suggested to Hansell that online advertisements have an interactive icon: 'If you click the icon, you will go to what he calls a "privacy dashboard" that will let you understand exactly what information was used to choose that ad for you. And you'll have the opportunity to edit the information or opt out of having any targeting done at all.' Turow envisages the dashboard would display the whole range of data used to select that item of content from the marketer, media platform and third-party providers. In this configuration the icon is a transparency initiative.

By requiring platforms to disclose how data is used to tailor content, they are more accountable to their users. While the icon Turow suggests would be politically unpalatable to a powerful industry used to regulating itself, it would be technically simple and relatively low cost. Platforms would zealously resist a privacy dashboard that revealed how data are used to customise content not only because it would undermine the 'seamless' and apparently 'natural' flow of content through the user interface, but also because it would erode competitive advantages between platforms by revealing how different configurations of data are used. We ought to contend though that media platforms are now significant public institutions that societies need to place certain responsibilities upon with regard to how they construct public space, culture and discourse. Societies did this with broadcast media during the twentieth century and the time has come for a similar approach to media platforms. Despite likely political resistance from platforms and advertisers, the icon proposal is worth further consideration because it illustrates how platforms open up new possibilities for how we might understand regulation and user control.

One of the limitations of the current self-regulatory scheme for alcohol advertising in Australia is that it relies on complaints from the public. However, awareness of the scheme is low and even if a person was sufficiently motivated to make a complaint, the system is wilfully obtuse. The icon proposition builds on the already existing protocols of Facebook, Instagram and Twitter. Every item of content on these platforms contains a 'button' that enables users to report it for breaching the platform's terms of service. Turow's (2012) suggestion is that technically the button could offer users the capacity to manage their data profile: what data is kept about them, its accuracy and how it is used.

His provocation can be productively applied to the specific case of alcohol brands. Most content posted by alcohol brands to social media platforms in Australia has a 'Drink Responsibly' watermark put there by the advertiser and the item of content also has a drop-down menu within the Facebook interface that enables users to 'report' the post. We already have a symbolic commitment by the brand to regulation on the advertisement, and a button that enables users to make and report a judgement about the content in relation to a regulatory framework (the platform's terms and conditions). What if, for alcohol brands, the 'Drink Responsibly' logo was replaced with a button that users could click? This would drop down a menu that would alert users to the regulatory code under which the content is produced and enable them to report the post by clicking any guideline breached by the content. This would be 'one-click' reporting of content from within the platform interface. Of course, it is likely that very few users would use this function, but if the industry were serious about their self-regulatory code being accessible, then an innovation of this sort would be far more effective than the awareness advertising campaigns the industry has funded on television in recent years. Furthermore, following Turow's (2012) suggestion, the icon could also take users to a dashboard that indicates what information alcohol brands are leveraging to target and customise content for them. Users ought to be able to delete data as they choose. In practice, the icon would draw consumers' attention to how brands operate in a computational way. The icon explicitly makes user-experience design a critical part of the politics of regulation.

If the icon proposal intervenes in the user interface of media platforms, we ought to also consider how regulation might more productively bring public scrutiny to alcohol marketing. This means going beyond specifying what kind of content is acceptable and instead seeking to define and regulate the infrastructure, devices and databases that alcohol brands run on. This is a much larger structural reform, but at the very least we must open up the public debate about how the alcohol industry's use of media platforms can be subjected to meaningful public scrutiny. The current paradox is that at the very moment when the industry has gained the greatest real-time visibility of consumers and their engagement with brands it has ever had, its own marketing activities have become far more impervious to regulation.

In a broadcast media system it was relatively easy to quantify the volume of alcohol marketing. If you wanted to know how many advertisements the industry ran in newspapers, magazines, radio and television, you just monitored the streams of content. On social media platforms this is not possible. Customised and gated content means that only the industry and the media platforms know how much content is actually produced. But, in a broadcast media system it was relatively difficult and expensive to quantify the reach of alcohol marketing in anything other than crude terms. Ratings data would give an understanding of the size of an audience and rudimentary demographic characteristics. If researchers or policy makers wanted to know the reach of alcohol advertising to specific target markets, they would need to conduct audience research. This research is expensive and limited by the recall bias of respondents. Media platforms generate a fine-grained portrait of reach for alcohol marketers. The marketers know how many people view and engage with an item of content and can associate that engagement with detailed information about who these people are, what their interests are, where they were when they engaged with the content, and perhaps even predictions about their alcohol consumption practices. If alcohol marketing is a matter of public concern and media platforms are understood as significant institutions the public has a stake in, then we must acknowledge that it is technically possible in a way it has never been before for alcohol brands' reach and engagement with specific audiences to be opened to public scrutiny. And, that furthermore, such scrutiny would have a negligible financial cost because it is information that is already provided in dashboards by media platforms to alcohol marketers.

The icon and dashboard are each low-cost proposals that would give individual users greater control over the regulation of alcohol advertising and open up alcohol marketing to greater public scrutiny. We ought to set aside the fact that they might well be politically unpalatable, and instead seize the upside in shifting the conversation away from content and volume, and make this a critical debate about a mode of branding that uses protocols, interfaces and databases. The current self-regulatory code does not define how alcohol brands operate in the age of media platforms, so critical analysis and proposals for change need to start by engaging with the marketing machinery the industry is building. The dashboard proposal would explicitly make a platform's databases objects of public scrutiny. Databases, algorithms, interfaces and protocols are the objects in the media system that alcohol marketers deploy and these are the devices via which harm is done to individuals and the quality of our public life. The data architecture of media platforms is not just a question of individual privacy, but also much more a question of how marketers shape social life. If we enter the debate about regulation with technical proposals about the configuration of platform interfaces, protocols and algorithms we engage the industry and politicians on more productive ground. In pointing not just to the critical issues, but also to making concrete low-cost demands about what might be done, we would undertake the generative move of not seeing media platforms as a threat but instead an opportunity for more fine-grained public scrutiny and control of alcohol marketing.

Notes

1   Facebook Investor Relations, online: https://investor.fb.com/home/default.aspx
2   Instagram 'Our Story', online: https://instagram.com/press/
3   Instagram's advertising model, online: https://business.instagram.com/advertising/
4   For an etymology of the 99 Problems meme. see Know Your Meme, online: http://knowyourmeme.com/memes/i-got-99-problems-but-a-bitch-aint-one

References

Anderson, P., de Bruijn, A., Angus, K., Gordon, R., and Hastings, G. (2009). Impact of alcohol advertising and media exposure on adolescent alcohol use: A systematic review of longitudinal studies. *Alcohol and Alcoholism, 44*(3), 229–243.

Andrejevic, M. (2011). Surveillance and alienation in the online economy. *Surveillance and Society, 8*(3), 278–287.

Arvidsson, A. (2005). Brands a critical perspective. *Journal of Consumer Culture, 5*(2), 235–258.

Australian Association of National Advertisers. (2014, 20 May). AANA Connect: Helen Crossley – The Future of Online Marketing. Retrieved 9 June 2016, from https://youtu.be/ceKvWJd8ALM

Babor, T., Caetano, R., Casswell, S., Edwards, G., Giesbrecht, N., Graham, K., Grube, J., Hill, L., Holder, H., Homel, R., Livingston, M., Osterberg, E., Rehm, J., Room, R., and

Rossow, I. (2010). *Alcohol: No Ordinary Commodity Research and Public Policy* (2nd edn). Oxford: Oxford University Press.

Brodmerkel, S., and Carah, N. (2013). Alcohol brands on Facebook: The challenges of regulating brands on social media. *Journal of Public Affairs*, *13*(3), 272–281.

Carah, N. (2014). *Like, Comment, Share: Alcohol Brand Activity on Facebook*. Brisbane: Foundation for Alcohol Research and Evaluation, University of Queensland.

Carah, N., and Shaul, M. (2016). Brands and Instagram: Point, tap, swipe, glance. *Mobile Media and Communication*, *4*(1), 69–84.

Diageo. (2011, 19 September). Diageo takes multi-million dollar global partnership with Facebook to the next level. Retrieved 9 June 2016, from www.diageo.com/en-row/newsmedia/pages/resource.aspx?resourceid=1072

Gillespie, T. (2014). The relevance of algorithms. In T. Gillespie, P. Boczkowski and K. Foot (Eds.), *Media Technologies*, *Essays on Communication, Materiality and Society* (pp. 167–194). Cambridge, MA: MIT Press.

Griffiths, R., and Casswell, S. (2010). Intoxigenic digital spaces? Youth, social networking sites and alcohol marketing. *Drug and Alcohol Review*, *29*, 525–530.

Hallinan, B., and Striphas, T. (2014). Recommended for you: The Netflix Prize and the production of algorithmic culture. *New Media and Society*, *18*(1), 117–137.

Jones, S. (2010). When does alcohol sponsorship of sport become sports sponsorship of alcohol? A case study of developments in sport in Australia. *International Journal of Sports Marketing and Sponsorship*, *11*(3), 250–261.

Jones, S. (2014). Commentary on Morgenstern et al. (2014): As channels for alcohol marketing continue to increase, so will alcohol marketing receptivity and youth drinking. *Addiction*, *109*(12), 2016–2017.

Lury, C. (2004). *Brands: The Logos of the Global Economy*. London: Routledge.

Mart, S., Mergendoller, J., and Simon, M. (2009). Alcohol promotion on facebook. *Journal of Global Drug Policy and Practice*, *3*(3). Retrieved from http://globaldrugpolicy.org/3/3/1.php

Marwick, A. (2015). Instafame: Luxury selfies in the attention economy. *Public Culture*, *27*(1), 137–160.

McStay, A. (2013). *Creativity and Advertising: Affect, Events and Process*. Abingdon, Oxon: Routledge.

Media Federation of Australia. (2013). 2013 Media Federation Awards. Retrieved 9 June 2016, from www.mediafederation.org.au/uploads/award-results/2015–05/1430845200_d577793d1c3f922ed17d19f571b0ec94.pdf

Moor, E. (2003). Branded spaces: The scope of 'new marketing'. *Journal of Consumer Culture*, *3*(1), 39–60.

Moreno, M., Briner, L., Williams, A., Brockman, L., Walker, L., and Christakis, D. (2010). A content analysis of displayed alcohol references in a social networking web site. *Journal of Adolescent Health*, *47*, 168–175.

Nicholls, J. (2012). Everyday, everywhere: Alcohol marketing and social media—current trends. *Alcohol and Alcoholism*, *47*(4), 486–493.

Pettigrew, S., Roberts, M., Pescud, M., Chapman, K., Quester, P., and Miller, C. (2012). The extent and nature of alcohol advertising on Australian television. *Drug and Alcohol Review*, *31*(6), 797–802. www.scopus.com/inward/record.url?eid=2-s2.0-84858974943andpartnerID=40andmd5=da30aae50732c51c4b080b752d371d32

Ridout, B., Campbell, A., and Ellis, L. (2012). 'Off your Face(book)': Alcohol in online social identity construction and its relation to problem drinking in university students. *Drug and Alcohol Review*, *31*(1), 20–26.

Turow, J. (2012). *The Daily You: How the New Advertising Industry is Defining Your Identity and Your Worth.* New Haven, CT: Yale University Press.

van Dijck, J. (2013). *The Culture of Connectivity: A Critical History of Social Media.* New York: Oxford University Press.

8 Mobile technologies and spatially structured real-time marketing

Rebecca Monk and Derek Heim

The ubiquity of mobile phones and continuously open social media channels has fundamentally transformed how people interact with each other. This has not gone unnoticed by the alcohol industry which, faced with increased regulation in the 'real world', has sought to capitalise on the marketing possibilities – and the lack of online regulation – afforded by the mobile internet. With a particular focus on mobile social media websites and applications, this chapter examines the links between online advertising and alcohol consumption. It details marketing and subtle promotion strategies by the alcohol industry, and also considers public health and research opportunities.

We begin with a brief review of literature illustrating the efficacy of (mobile) alcohol advertising and examine how advertisers, in particular, enlist young people in their efforts to normalise alcohol behaviours. The chapter then turns to discussing links between mobile social media and alcohol consumption. We highlight that far from being exposed uncritically to direct effects of advertisers, young people actively interpret media messages and construct their own online social identity in ways that are not necessarily always compatible with the aims of the alcohol industry. With this in mind, the chapter ends by highlighting public health opportunities afforded by the increasing popularity of mobile media technologies: first, as a means to target key populations through the use of established marketing techniques to promote responsible alcohol consumption patterns, and, second, as a research tool which offers the potential to examine vast amounts of real-time data, which may help us gain a greater understanding of alcohol behaviours in both on- and offline contexts.

Mobile alcohol marketing: combining the old with the new

By now it has become clear that alcohol advertising represents an effective means of encouraging drinking, with accumulating evidence suggesting that alcohol-related advertisements increase consumption (Anderson et al., 2009; Atkinson et al., 2011; Dobson, 2012; Gordon et al., 2011; Hanewinkel et al., 2012; Parry et al., 2012; Pettigrew et al., 2012; Smith and Foxcroft, 2009). The methods used to assess the extent to which individuals are susceptible to alcohol advertising, however, often rely on indirect measures such as people's ability to name specific alcohol-related advertisements, which is a limitation in the field. Nevertheless, there is also evidence indicating that alcohol marketing is related to adolescent binge drinking at both initial assessment and longitudinally (Morgenstern et al., 2011). This association appears evident even when controlling for other contributory factors such as peer drinking and time spent watching television. Traditional advertising approaches (e.g. via television) are a well-researched driver of alcohol consumption (see Anderson et al., 2009 for a review), and they continue to be a source of concern. However, understanding the changing ways the alcohol industry advertises through 'new media' (Brooks, 2010) is highly important to the interests of both the alcohol industry and public health professionals.

Alcohol marketers are extremely knowledgeable about their target market and where alcohol consumers spend their time (Jones, 2014). It is partly for this reason, for example, that alcohol-related marketing is greater during sporting events (Lindsay et al., 2013; O'Brien and Kypri, 2008; O'Brien et al., 2015) and during prime-time television for certain audiences (e.g. visual references to alcohol during high-profile football games (Adams et al., 2014)). However, as young people have begun to spend more time using the internet, social network sites (SNS) and mobile communications, so too have alcohol advertisers begun to target these platforms (Hoffman et al., 2014; Jones, 2014).

Traditional ('buy this brand') advertisements tend to rely on persuasive communications to evoke engagement with a particular brand with the aim of stimulating purchasing behaviour. These approaches are also evident in mobile alcohol marketing. Many of the key brands which target a younger and more IT literate market (e.g. students and those in their late teens/early twenties) have, among many other social media platforms, Twitter, Facebook and Youtube accounts that are frequently used for brand promotion (Winpenny et al., 2014). As mobile alcohol marketing has become increasingly sophisticated, traditional marketing strategies have been augmented with more interactive and subtle forms of brand promotion. The rise in these amalgamated marketing strategies has been documented by a concurrent growth in 'netnographic research', the ethnographic study of online communications and interactions, and analyses of alcohol-related social media activities (Purves et al., 2014). These research efforts have revealed a number of deliberate, and perhaps more pervasive, online marketing strategies (cf. Brooks, 2010; Nicholls, 2012; Purves et al., 2014). The notion of exposure to alcohol-related marketing, for instance, differs from that used to conceptualise more traditional forms of advertising (cf. Anderson et al., 2009; Jernigan, 2006; Jernigan et al., 2005).

In contrast to these established methods, mobile strategies seek to facilitate brand promotion and product engagement by making use of the inherently interactive nature of SNS. This is evidenced by the variety and intricacy of social media marketing strategies. First, they encourage conversations about alcohol through the use of online advertisements and social media pages. Here, participants are encouraged to offer opinions on products and brands (Nicholls, 2012; Purves et al., 2014). Second, social media is used to endorse a need for celebrations that are associated with particular alcohol products (e.g. Bacardi's 'celebrate Mojito

Monday') to promote the notion that celebration with alcohol is routine (Nicholls, 2012). Third, they encourage drinking to demarcate specific events (e.g. after proposing), on specific days and over the weekend. This notion even extends to encouraging consumption when there is no specific event, for example 'Hump-day Monday' – where drinking is promoted as a means of getting through the day when there is nothing happening (Nicholls, 2012). Advertisers also sponsor and create online alcohol-related events and interactive games, all with little or no encouragement of responsible modes of consumption (Nicholls, 2012). Defining what should be classified as advertising has become somewhat blurred as a result of these evolving strategies (Nicholls, 2012) but it is evident that traditional, passive advertisements are no longer the sole or even the predominant method used. As such, there has been a shift from doing 'digital marketing' towards strategies that are seen to facilitate effective marketing in the digital age (Diageo, 2015).

Alcohol marketers have also responded to the popularity of mobile applications and adapted the marketing strategies accordingly. There has thus been a proliferation of alcohol-related mobile applications such as the 'Let's get WASTED drinking game'. A search of Apple and Android Smartphone alcohol-related applications reveals that 78% (of the 282 applications uncovered at the time the research was conducted) were concerned with overtly promoting alcohol consumption (Eagle et al., 2014).

Social network sites, identities and consumption

Even more fundamental than promoting positive representations of alcohol by seeking opinions of users, or linking its consumption to events, mobile alcohol marketing via SNS offers the potential of much more subtle and user-generated forms of advertising. Mobile technologies allow people to live 'life online and in public via these sites' (Subrahmanyam and Greenfield, 2008: 417), and are used by individuals as a means of defining their identities and interpersonal connections (Livingstone, 2008). These technologies are tools through which identities and (virtual) communities are constructed on a momentary basis (cf. Cova, 1996) and can represent amplified versions of the self and groups via visual, written or multimedia means (Senft, 2008). As public and private identity spheres have become increasingly blurred, shared practices of consumption have become an important means through which young people create and claim meaning in their lives by shaping identities and their status vis-à-vis others (McCreanor et al., 2005; Purves et al., 2014). Indeed, the facilitation of story-telling and narrative self-presentation is one of the key affordances of modern SNS (van Dijck, 2013) and the move towards these abilities (away from their use as static databases of personal information) has been a key factor in their growing popularity (Carah and Shaul, 2013). Accordingly, detailed social media content analyses and focus group data suggest that the need to belong to, and identify with, a group influences the extent to which individuals attempt to foster social connectedness through the representation of online drinking practices (Atkinson et al., 2014). Alcohol marketing strategies have sought to capitalise on this shared sense of identity and belonging in online spaces to subtly promote and help ensure continued engagement with brands. Here the appeal of SNS for alcohol marketers is clear as it facilitates a targeted and purposeful weaving together of discourses relating to pleasure, identity and culture (Senft, 2008). In the context of TV ads and prior to SNS becoming as popular as they are now, McCreanor and colleagues (2008) documented that the marketing materials ultimately aimed at promoting consumption are often valued by young people themselves, and become embedded into their social practices. As we outline below, it is likely that this has increased with the mainstreaming of SNS.

Alcohol identities on SNS help to create and maintain 'intoxigenic' environments where positive messages about alcohol are transmitted peer-to-peer among members of social networks (McCreanor et al., 2008). As well as serving to encourage drinking, such SNS may normalise heavy drinking practices in this way (Moewaka Barnes et al., 2016). The additional appeal of this type of marketing is that SNS providers are able to data mine and use detailed interaction records of users for marketing purposes. The ability to record and combine vast amounts of data from a number of sources or posts also allows for targeted and unregulated (possibly uncontrollable) alcohol marketing campaigns which aim to maintain pro-alcohol environments in both public and private spaces (McCreanor et al., 2013). Even drinking in the privacy of one's living room can, via SNS, become instantaneously integrated into both virtual and physical spaces, and incorporated into the commercial world (van Dijck, 2013).

The link between SNS, social identity and alcohol consumption is further highlighted by research which indicates that posting images depicting personal alcohol consumption (Glassman, 2012), creating alcohol-related status updates and sharing and/or 'liking' alcohol-related online content (Alhabash et al., 2015) on SNS is associated with self-reported drinking and intentions to consume alcohol. Similarly, high rates of alcohol-related posts have been linked with higher AUDIT scores (Moreno et al., 2012), and work by Ridout et al. (2012) suggests that SNS postings of pictures used to signify 'alcohol identities' are correlated with consumption. Portraying oneself as 'a drinker' therefore appears to be important to young people's online identities (Ridout, 2016). Recent research using the Alcohol-Related Facebook® Activity (ARFA) questionnaire corroborates further the link between alcohol social media postings and potentially risky patterns of consumption (Marczinski et al., 2016). Such findings highlight the extent to which users of mobile SNS may inadvertently promote alcohol and indeed celebrate intoxication by constructing identities that promote drinking.

The apparent link between advertising and alcohol consumption has been used to highlight the need for increased alcohol marketing regulation that is responsive to rapidly evolving youth cultures (Jackson et al., 2000). However, in view of the frequently blurred boundaries between SNS content that is user-generated and that which is aimed at brand-promotion and normalising alcohol behaviours (Nicholls, 2012), it is not always easy to tell whether users are more responsive to traditional or more novel and subtle methods of online brand promotion. For instance, this type of research does not typically tell us whether people are posting images because they want to portray themselves in a good light by constructing an intoxigenic social identity (Griffiths and Casswell, 2010), or whether they are responding to brand-specific encouragement to do so (or indeed whether both forces are at play). Furthermore, it is difficult to disentangle the extent to which such posts normalise and encourage alcohol consumption and the extent to which they are novel ways of documenting behaviours that previously occurred, largely undocumented, in offline settings. More longitudinal research is needed to help unpick questions of causality in this domain.

Online competition and critical media engagement: challenges for mobile alcohol marketing?

It is, however, important to consider these mobile marketing developments in the broader context of online (alcohol) consumption more generally. In addition to representing an effective subtle tool for the promotion of alcohol, it is prudent to remember that mobile technologies enable users to engage in activities that, to a greater or lesser extent, had previously been associated with alcohol-salient environments. Mobile technologies enable people to meet, talk and even to engage in sexual activities from just about any location with or without involvement of alcoholic beverages. In view of the concurrent rise in the popularity of mobile technologies, it is therefore possible to speculate that the noted international decline in alcohol consumption in recent years (De Looze et al., 2015; Pennay et al., 2015) may, in some way, be related to changes in activity patterns as a result of the mobile communications boom (Katz and Aakus, 2002). Mobile technologies, from this perspective, may have facilitated interpersonal leisure activities that do not necessarily involve alcohol consumption to the extent that had previously been the case among young people wanting to meet each other and socialise. So while SNS and mobile technologies have undoubtedly opened up manifold ways of promoting alcohol, it may be that (somewhat ironically) in the mobile marketplace of constructed identities, those identities related to alcohol may not always compete favourably with the many other identities and activities that do not include alcohol consumption. The overall significance of alcohol-related social identities for young people's interactions may therefore be less than might have been the case in offline contexts, in which much previous research documenting the significance of alcohol to young people's interactions was carried out. However, such speculation needs to be tempered by acknowledging that alcohol producers themselves are upbeat about the role that social media marketing is playing in their profitability (Diageo, 2015; Mosher, 2012), and that decreased levels of overall consumption may not be associated with concomitant reductions in alcohol-related harms across society as a whole (cf. Buck and Frosini, 2012). Changing patterns of alcohol consumption and associated harms in relation to altering leisure activities in the digital mobile age therefore require longer-term examination.

In addition to having to compete with constantly evolving possibilities of interaction and self-presentation afforded by the internet, mobile alcohol-related advertising (and the extent to which this is related unequivocally to increases in alcohol consumption) needs also to be considered in relation to how young people engage with media. Media theorists have long moved away from more simplistic notions of direct causal effects of media on its consumers. It therefore appears prudent for alcohol researchers to view the links between media content and alcohol use as a complex interplay between various influencing factors (Cherrington et al., 2006). Audience reception theory, for example, notes the potential for the media to control agendas, but moves beyond the idea that media directly causes certain behaviours (Hall, 1980, 1993). Rather, this theory outlines that the same message can lead to different outcomes (as each message can be encoded in multiple ways). In other words, whilst the media may present a preferred story (the 'preferred reading'), this does not mean that the reader will necessarily take this on board in the way intended. This perspective further notes that, dependent upon their current setting, individuals may take different interpretations from a given message (Hall, 1980). It therefore seems particularly relevant to young people's continuous online engagement, where interconnected and active participants are not passive audiences. Rather, individuals modify, negotiate and interpret messages in manifold ways that are altered by the psychological, social and environmental settings in which they are encountered.

For example, alcohol-related SNS messages will also reach media users who may be oppositional audiences and seek to counter or avoid the information provided. As such, their behaviour is unlikely to be affected. Similarly, in support of research conceptualising young people as active interpreters of media messages (Livingstone, 2013a, 2013b), the construction of alcohol-related social identities on SNS is a proactive and highly managed process (Atkinson et al., 2014). The normalisation of consumption via online identity processes, for example, represents a purposeful construction of identities and individuals who are unlikely to be passive 'sponges' that simply absorb external pressures to drink (Atkinson et al., 2014). It is equally feasible therefore that non-alcohol-related identities, or identities which emphasise moderation or even abstinence, may be constructed and become fashionable despite both industry and user-generated alcohol-related SNS content. In short, the processes that link SNS engagement, content and consumption are highly complex. Living in a constantly and instantaneously mediatised society in which people are afforded ever-increasing opportunities to engage with each other (Livingstone, 2013b) therefore presents particular challenges for research.

Mobile opportunities for public health

Mindful that the complex and socially mediated nature of mobile media use presents challenges to those with an interest in alcohol, and notwithstanding the challenges posed by the online promotion of harmful behaviours, this chapter now turns to considering opportunities for public health afforded by the ever-present use of mobile technologies. Drawing on principles promoted by social marketing advocates, and the recognition that SNS use in itself does not appear to increase alcohol consumption, SNS sites such as Facebook may therefore represent opportunities for interventions (Hoffman et al., 2014). The 'mass transformative effects' of SNS marketing, from this viewpoint, may be harnessed in the promotion of positive health (Nicholls, 2012). Indeed, a systematic review by Ross and colleagues (2006) found that commercial marketing can be used to inform and facilitate interventions aimed at reducing alcohol consumption, with some programmes showing apparent reductions in alcohol consumption up to two years later. It is near impossible to discern the degree to which online interventions causally reduce consumption in view of the complexities of the (online) world. Nevertheless, this work does highlight that health promotion campaigns, at the very least, can inform public discourses around alcohol in ways that may, to a degree, counteract the messages promoted by the alcohol lobbies. Examining how best to utilise targeted messages on specific new media channels, as an antidote to pro-alcohol messages, is therefore likely to be a significant and challenging endeavour for alcohol researchers and public health professionals in the coming years. Illustrating these complexities, Atkinson and colleagues (2014), for example, note that the careful construction of one's social identity on SNS is dependent upon the promotion of the 'right' form of drinking, with disapproval and social isolation potentially greeting those who display socially unacceptable forms of drinking behaviours. The gendered nature of alcohol consumption identities (Lyons and Willott, 2008; Simonen et al., 2014; Törrönen and Roumeliotis, 2014) needs also to be noted in this context as this, alongside the influences of social class and ethnicity (e.g. Lui et al., 2015), is likely to reinforce particular modes of consumption and associated online behaviours.

Interventions aimed at achieving behavioural change may henceforth benefit from an awareness of the importance of (online) social identities in shaping alcohol behaviours. Indeed, given the significance of alcohol-related behaviours to some young people's sense of self and their (online) identity, outlined earlier, social marketing strategies aimed at promoting responsible drinking may, if not implemented carefully, run the risk of being defied or even eliciting a backlash. In other words, messages that seek to directly discredit or admonish alcohol consumption may become a direct source of conflict to those for whom alcohol consumption is a key part of their identity and social life. This may result in opposition or purposeful disregarding of such messages, in the same way as health warnings related to smoking, for example, may be ignored for this reason (cf., e.g., Hansen et al., 2010).

Another way in which mobile technologies represent opportunities for public health lies in their possible utility for alcohol interventions; for example, for those individuals at particular risk of alcohol-related problems. Mobile technologies are already being implemented as one of the many tools in alcohol treatment approaches (cf. Quanbeck, 2015). For example, specifically designed smartphone applications that send text-messages to patients and monitor their current location in order to supply timely support when clients are in potential 'high risk' environments are becoming more widely used. Early research suggests that such mobile technologies may help reduce the number of risky drinking days following alcohol-related interventions (cf., e.g., Gustafson et al., 2014). It has long been noted that it is impossible to provide simple and scientifically defensible guidance in response to queries about the levels of alcohol that are (not) suitable for one's health (e.g. Kendell, 1987). More research in this area appears necessary. However, the use of mobile interventions in this way presents clear opportunities to deliver affordable and personalised interventions.

In addition to possibly transforming social marketing and acute interventions, in the longer term, mobile technologies are also likely to help transform alcohol policy and practice by opening up new research opportunities that will improve the evidence base and afford a more nuanced understanding of alcohol consumption. To date, many theoretical accounts of alcohol consumption have been based on questionnaires or diary studies, where participants are asked to keep a record of their daily drinking. However, the limitations of autobiographical memory and issues with retrospective recall mean that the findings from studies relying on such methods may be limited and prevent researchers from garnering a more objective perspective on alcohol consumption practices (cf. Shiffman et al., 2008). For example, a diary study which utilised covert photoreceptors found that 90% of participants responded to the study, yet, in fact, only 11% had actually complied with the task instructions (Stone and Shiffman, 2002). Such research suggests that diary-based methods of research may be prone to 'parking-lot compliance', where participants retrospectively answer questions in order to fulfil task requirement (Smyth and Stone, 2003). Asking people to directly report their consumption also creates issues relating to demand characteristics, where participants may alter their responses in an effort to meet the perceived demands of the researcher, or to avoid negative perceptions (Verster et al., 2012). Traditional research methods have also tended to be reliant on analyses of responses that are provided in environments which are far removed from the settings in which actual alcohol consumption usually occurs (Verster et al., 2012). This is problematic as it necessitates recall in the absence of any associated environmental stimuli, which may aid memory (cf. Godden and Baddeley, 1975). Finally, the difficulty of a task requiring the retrospective recall of multiple occasions may be further exacerbated by the alcohol consumption itself (cf. Walker and Hunter, 1978).

In contrast, 'Ecological Momentary Assessment' (EMA), also known as the Experience Sampling methodology (Collins et al., 1990; Collins et al., 1998), utilises portable devices to contact participants at varying time intervals. In doing so, this method has, evolved beyond the reliance on the administration of paper and pen questionnaires in contexts that are far removed from the settings in which drinking typically takes place. Rather, research can be conducted in vivo, reducing reliance on autobiographical memory. Moving beyond the use of beepers, hand-held computers and voice-response systems (cf. Collins et al., 2003; Collins et al., 1990; Collins et al., 1998) to prompt participants, research has begun to use participants' mobile phones to prompt responses and collect EMA data. Data capture has taken the form of phone calls (Courvoisier et al., 2010) and text messages (Kuntsche and Robert, 2009), an approach that appears popular amongst participants (Kuntsche and Labhart, 2013).

In addition to helping to combat research limitations relating to retrospective self-report, mobile research technologies provide a number of additional advantages over more conventional assessments. Smartphone-based EMA provides instantaneous, highly rich and useful data obtained using the user's own phone (Miller, 2012). The familiarity, proximity, social importance and frequent use of such devices means that taking part in research is easy and increases the likelihood of participation (Miller, 2012). Smartphone applications also offer various additional features to capture and record sound, pictures and movements, all of which can be useful for researchers (Kuntsche and Labhart, 2013; Santani et al., 2016). Applications also provide data which are electronically time-stamped (Miller, 2012), meaning that researchers can be sure that responses are provided close to the time of asking, rather than retrospectively. Concerns regarding alcohol-impaired cognitive functioning during participation (Weissenborn and Duka, 2002) may also be reduced by the use of smartphone technology, as it provides a familiar, straightforward method of question and response (Collins et al., 2003). Smartphone technology is also 'context-aware' (Miller, 2012) meaning that it can monitor dynamic changes across contexts. This allows researchers to identify subtleties that would not be evident in laboratory testing, which may be particularly useful for monitoring alcohol behaviours that are episodic and contextually bound. For example, earlier research that pre-dates more user-friendly EMA techniques, revealed important situational influences on round buying and drinking rates (Van de Goor et al., 1990). Indeed, the technology can even geo-locate participants – taking an instant and highly accurate measure of current location for analysis purposes.

The use of mobile alcohol research methods therefore enables researchers to better account for the long-established influences of people's current situational contexts (cf., e.g., Beck et al., 1993; Beck and Treiman, 1996) and present environment (cf., e.g., Clapp and Shillington, 2001; Clapp et al., 2006) which are important factors in shaping both the frequency and the quantity of alcohol consumed, and indeed intoxicated behaviours (cf. MacAndrew and Edgerton, 1969). Alcohol-related cognitions, for example, have been demonstrated to be environmentally variable (e.g. Monk and Heim, 2013a, 2014a; Neighbors et al., 2006; Wall et al., 2001; Wall et al., 2000). In other words, the ways people think about their own consumption, and what they expect as a result of drinking, do not appear to be static thought processes. Rather, they seem to change depending on where people are (environmental context) and who they are with (social context).

Evidence for the role of context in real-time accounts of alcohol consumption has also been furnished by smartphone-based research (Monk et al., 2015). This work compared real-time alcohol consumption reports with both daily and weekly retrospective accounts of consumption and examined the impact of drinking contexts. Findings suggest that retrospective accounts underestimate the amount of actual alcohol consumed and increased consumption appeared to exacerbate differences between real-time and retrospective accounts. Environmental and social contexts also appeared to interact with the type of alcohol consumed and the time frame given for reporting (weekly vs daily retrospective) to further impact discrepancies between real-time and retrospective reports of alcohol consumption.

For example, real-time consumption in a bar/pub was associated with increases in the discrepancy observed between real-time and weekly retrospective accounts of consumption (Monk et al., 2015). Similarly, smartphone-based assessments of student drinking every Thursday, Friday and Saturday evenings for five weekends revealed that drinking as part of larger friendship groups appears to be associated with increases in the frequency of drinking (Thrul and Kuntsche, 2015). The amount of alcohol consumed on Saturday night also seems to be exacerbated by the presence of same-sex friends (Kuntsche et al., 2015). Mobile technology may therefore offer researchers important insights into the dynamic nature of consumption and associated beliefs. Continued use of such technologies in this area is also recommended to inform the development of interventions that should ideally be able to respond to contextually varying demands if they are to be successful in reducing consumption (Davies, 1997).

Conclusion

The popularity and widespread use of mobile technologies and associated applications has, in a relatively brief period of time, begun to have a transformative impact on the way in which alcohol is marketed. It is not only alcohol advertisers who take advantage of the interactive nature of the (mobile) internet and social network sites. Evidence indicates that users themselves frequently further the aims of the alcohol industry by generating and normalising alcohol-related content and behaviours. At the same time, the complex and uncontrollable nature of the mobile internet means that the alcohol industry has to compete with numerous other messages and opportunities. This may inadvertently dilute the effectiveness of alcohol promotions and be related to falling levels of alcohol consumption in some way. Persuasive communications on the internet are (re)interpreted and (re) negotiated by media-literate consumers who are in no way passive recipients of alcohol advertising. With this in mind, there are a number of potential ways in which the mobile internet may help promote identities and behaviours which emphasise more responsible forms of consumption. Researchers certainly have a challenging agenda mapped out when seeking to understand complex mobile online alcohol interactions. At the same time, the very technologies which have created this task are likely to contribute towards a better understanding of the behaviour in question, and also enable researchers to better understand offline alcohol behaviours.

Acknowledgement

The authors would like to thank to Dr James Nicholls of Alcohol Research UK for fruitful discussions around this topic.

References

Adams, J., Coleman, J., and White, M. (2014). Alcohol marketing in televised international football: Frequency analysis. *BMC Public Health, 14*, 473–479.

Alhabash, S., McAlister, A., Quilliam, E., Richards, J., and Lou, C. (2015). Alcohol's getting a bit more social: When alcohol marketing messages on Facebook increase young adults' intentions to imbibe. *Mass Communication and Society, 18*, 350–375.

Anderson, P., de Bruijn, A., Angus, K., Gordon, R., and Hastings, G. (2009). Impact of alcohol advertising and media exposure on adolescent alcohol use: A systematic review of longitudinal studies. *Alcohol and Alcoholism, 44*(3), 229–243.

Atkinson, A., Elliot, G., Ellis, M., and Sumnall, H. (2011). *Young People, Alcohol and the Media*. York: Joseph Rowntree Foundation.

Atkinson, A., Ross, K., Begley, E., and Sumnall, H. (2014). *Constructing Alcohol Identities: The Role of Social Network Sites (SNS) in Young People's Drinking Cultures*. London: Alcohol Research UK. http://alcoholresearchuk.org/downloads/finalReports/Final Report_0119.pdf

Beck, K., Thombs, D., and Summons, T. (1993). The social context of drinking scales: Construct validation and relationship to indicants of abuse in an adolescent population. *Addictive Behaviors, 18*, 159–169.

Beck, K., and Treiman, K. (1996). The relationship of social context of drinking, perceived social norms, and parental influence to various drinking patterns of adolescents. *Addictive Behaviors, 21*, 633–644.

Brooks, O. (2010). *Routes to Magic: The Alcoholic Beverage Industry's Use of New Media in Alcohol Marketing*. Edinburgh: Scottish Health Action on Alcohol Problems.

Buck, D., and Frosini, F. (2012). Clustering of unhealthy behaviours over time: Implications for policy and practice. *The King's Fund*. Retrieved November, 2015, from www.kingsfund.org.uk/sites/files/kf/field/field_publication_file/clustering-of-unhealthy-behaviours-over-time-aug-2012.pdf

Carah, N., and Shaul, M. (2013). Leveraging social media. *Prevention Research, June*, 1–25.

Cherrington, J., Chamberlain, K., and Grixti, J. (2006). Relocating alcohol advertising research: Examining socially mediated relationships with alcohol. *Journal of Health Psychology, 11*, 209–222.

Clapp, D., and Shillington, A. (2001). Environmental predictors of heavy episodic drinking. *American Journal of Drug and Alcohol Abuse, 27*(2), 301–313.

Clapp, J., Reed, M., Holmes, M., Lange, J., and Voas, R. (2006). Drunk in public, drunk in private: The relationship between college students, drinking environments and alcohol consumption. *American Journal of Drug and Alcohol Abuse, 32*, 275–285.

Collins, L., Kashdan, T., and Gollnisch, G. (2003). The feasibility of using cellular phones to collect ecological momentary assessment data: Application to alcohol consumption. *Experimental and Clinical Psychopharmacology, 11*, 73–78.

Collins, R., Lapp, W., Emmons, K., and Isaac, L. (1990). Endorsement and strength of alcohol expectancies. *Journal of Studies on Alcohol, 51*, 336–342.

Collins, R., Morsheimer, E., Shiffman, S., Paty, J., Gnys, M., and Papandonatos, G. (1998). Ecological momentary assessment in a behavioral drinking moderation training program. *Experimental and Clinical Psychopharmacology, 6*(3), 306–315.

Courvoisier, D., Eid, M., Lischetzke, T., and Schreiber, W. (2010). Psychometric properties of a computerized mobile phone method for assessing mood in daily life. *Emotion, 10*, 115–124.

Cova, B. (1996). The postmodern explained to managers: Implications for marketing. *Business Horizons, 39*, 15–23.

Davies, J. B. (1997). *The Myth of Addiction* (2nd edn). Amsterdam: Harwood Academic Publishers.

De Looze, M., Raaijmakers, Q., Bogt, T., Bendtsen, P., Farhat, T., Ferreira, M. E. G., Kuntsche, E., Molcho, M., Pförtner, T.-K., Simons-Morton, B., Vieno, A., Vollebergh, W., and Pickett, W. (2015). Decreases in weekly adolescent alcohol use in Europe and North America: Evidence from 28 countries from 2002 to 2010. *European Journal of Public Health*, 25(Supplement 2), 69–72.

Diageo. (2015). Full year results 2015 (Year ended 30 June 2015). Retrieved January 2016, from www.diageo.com/Lists/Resources/Attachments/2800/Final%20Fast%20Facts%20-%20F15[1].pdf

Dobson, C. (2012). *Alcohol Marketing and Young People: Time for a New Policy Agenda*. Kingston, ACT: Australian Medical Association.

Eagle, L., Dahl, S., Low, D., and Mahoney, T. (2014). Alcohol promotion via mobile phone apps: Gaps in impact evaluation and regulatory coverage. Paper presented at the Proceedings ANZMAC Annual Conference 2014: Agents of Change, 1–3 December 2014, Brisbane, QLD, Australia.

Glassman, T. (2012). Implications for college students posting pictures of themselves drinking alcohol on facebook. *Journal of Alcohol and Drug Education*, 56, 38–58.

Godden, D., and Baddeley, A. (1975). Context-dependent memory in two natural environments: On land and underwater. *British Journal of Psychology*, 66, 325–331.

Gordon, R., Harris, F., Marie MacKintosh, A., and Moodie, C. (2011). Assessing the cumulative impact of alcohol marketing on young people's drinking: Cross-sectional data findings. *Addiction Research and Theory*, 19(1), 66–75.

Griffiths, R., and Casswell, S. (2010). Intoxigenic digital spaces? Youth, social networking sites and alcohol marketing. *Drug and Alcohol Review*, 29, 525–530.

Gustafson, D., McTavish, F., Chih, M., Atwood, A., Johnson, R., Boyle, M., Levy, M., Driscoll, H., Chisholm, S., Dillenburg, L., Isham, A., and Shah, D. (2014). A smartphone application to support recovery from alcoholism: A randomized clinical trial. *JAMA Psychiatry*, 71(5), 566–572.

Hall, S. (1980). Encoding/decoding. In D. Hall, A. Hobson, A. Lowe et al. (Eds.), *Culture, Media, Language: Working Papers in Cultural Studies, 1972–79* (pp. 128–138). London: Hutchinson.

Hall, S. (1993). Encoding, decoding. *The Cultural Studies Reader*, 4, 90–103.

Hanewinkel, R., Sargent, J., Poelen, E., Scholte, R., Florek, E., Sweeting, H., Hunt, K., Karlsdottir, S., Jonsson, S., Mathis, F., Faggiano, F., and Morgenstern, M. (2012). Alcohol consumption in movies and adolescent binge drinking in 6 European countries. *Pediatrics*, 129(4), 709–720.

Hansen, J., Winzeler, S., and Topolinski, S. (2010). When death makes you smoke: A terror management perspective on the effectiveness of cigarette on-pack warnings. *Journal of Experimental Social Psychology*, 46(1), 226–228.

Hoffman, E., Pinkleton, B., Weintraub Austin, E., and Reyes-Velázquez, W. (2014). Exploring college students' use of general and alcohol-related social media and their associations with alcohol-related behaviors. *Journal of American College Health*, 62, 328–335.

Jackson, M., Hastings, G., Wheeler, C., Eadie, D., and MacKintosh, A. (2000). Marketing alcohol to young people: Implications for industry regulation and research policy. *Addiction*, 95(Supplement 4), S597–S608.

Jernigan, D. (2006). Importance of reducing youth exposure to alcohol advertising. *Archives of Paediatric and Adolescent Medicine*, 160, 100–102.

Jernigan, D., Ostroff, J., and Ross, C. (2005). Alcohol advertising and youth: A measured approach. *Journal of Public Health Policy*, 26, 312–325.

Jones, S. (2014). Commentary on Morgenstern et al. (2014): As channels for alcohol marketing continue to increase, so will alcohol marketing receptivity and youth drinking. *Addiction, 109*(12), 2016–2017.

Katz, J., and Aakus, M. (2002). Framing the issues. In J. Katz and M. Aakus (Eds.), *Perpetual Contact: Mobile Communication, Private Talk, Public Performance* (pp. 170-192). Cambridge: Cambridge University Press.

Kendell, B. (1987). Drinking sensibly. *British Journal of Addiction, 82*, 1279–1288.

Kuntsche, E., and Labhart, F. (2013). ICAT: Development of an Internet-based data collection method for ecological momentary assessment using personal cell phones. *European Journal of Psychological Assessment, 29*, 140–148.

Kuntsche, E., and Robert, B. (2009). Short message service (SMS) technology in alcohol research–a feasibility study. *Alcohol and Alcoholism, 44*, 423–428.

Kuntsche, E., Otten, R., & Labhart, F. (2015). Identifying risky drinking patterns over the course of Saturday evenings: An event-level study. *Psychology of addictive behaviors, 29*(3), 744–752.

Lindsay, S., Thomas, S., Lewis, S., Westberg, K., Moodie, R., and Jones, S. (2013). Eat, drink and gamble: Marketing messages about 'risky' products in an Australian major sporting series. *BMC Public Health, 13*(1), 719–730.

Livingstone, S. (2008). Taking risky opportunities in youthful content creation: Teenagers' use of SNSs for intimacy, privacy and self-expression. *New Media and Society, 10*(3), 393–411.

Livingstone, S. (2013a). *Making Sense of Television: The Psychology of Audience Interpretation*. London: Routledge.

Livingstone, S. (2013b). The participation paradigm in audience research. *Communication Review, 16*, 21–30.

Lui, C., Chung, P., Ford, C., Grella, C., and Mulia, N. (2015). Drinking behaviors and life course socioeconomic status during the transition from adolescence to adulthood among Whites and Blacks. *Journal of Studies on Alcohol and Drugs, 76*, 68–79.

Lyons, A., and Willott, S. (2008). Alcohol consumption, gender identities and women's changing social positions. *Sex Roles, 59*, 694–712.

MacAndrew, C., and Edgerton, R. (1969). *Drunken Comportment: A Social Explanation*. Chicago: Aldine Publishing.

Marczinski, C., Hertzenberg, H., Goddard, P., Maloney, S., Stamates, A., and O'Connor, K. (2016). Alcohol-related Facebook® activity predicts alcohol use patterns in college students. *Addiction Research and Theory*, published online 29 February, doi.10.3109/1 6066359.16062016.11146709.

McCreanor, T., Lyons, A., Griffin, C., Goodwin, I., Moewaka Barnes, H., and Hutton, F. (2013). Youth drinking cultures, social networking and alcohol marketing: Implications for public health. *Critical Public Health, 23*(1), 110–120.

McCreanor, T., Moewaka Barnes, H., Gregory, A., Kaiwai, H., and Borell, S. (2005). Consuming identities: Alcohol marketing and the comodification of youth. *Addiction Research and Theory, 13*(6), 579–590.

McCreanor, T., Moewaka Barnes, H., Kaiwai, H., Borell, S., and Gregory, A. (2008). Creating intoxigenic environments: Marketing alcohol to young people in Aotearoa New Zealand. *Social Science and Medicine, 67*(6), 938–946.

Miller, G. (2012). The smartphone psychology manifesto. *Perspectives on Psychological Science, 7*, 221–237.

Moewaka Barnes, H., McCreanor, T., Goodwin, I., Lyons, A., Griffin, C., and Hutton, F. (2016). Alcohol and social media: Drinking and drunkenness while online. *Critical Public Health, 26*(1), 62–76.

Monk, R., and Heim, D. (2013a). Environmental context effects on alcohol-related outcome expectancies, efficacy and norms: A field study. *Psychology of Addictive Behaviors, 27*, 814–818.

Monk, R., and Heim, D. (2014a). A real-time examination of context effects on alcohol cognitions. *Alcoholism: Clinical and Experimental Research, 38*, 2452–2459.

Monk, R., Heim, D., Qureshi, A., and Price, A. (2015). 'I have no clue what I drunk last night': Using Smartphone technology to compare in-vivo and retrospective self-reports of alcohol consumption. *PLoS ONE, 10*(5), e0126209.

Moreno, M., Christakis, D., Egan, K., Brockman, L., and Becker, T. (2012). Associations between displayed alcohol references on Facebook and problem drinking among college students. *Archives of Paediatric and Adolescent Medicine, 166*(2), 157–163.

Morgenstern, M., Isensee, B., Sargent, J. D., and Hanewinkel, R. (2011). Attitudes as mediators of the longitudinal association between alcohol advertising and youth drinking. *Archives of Pediatrics and Adolescent Medicine, 165*(7), 610–616. www.scopus.com/inward/record.url?eid=2-s2.0–79953276639andpartnerID=40andmd5=52 3f17e5d67711fcbdeb314ec098ab17

Mosher, J. (2012). Joe Camel in a bottle: Diageo, the Smirnoff brand, and the transformation of the youth alcohol market. *American Journal of Public Health, 102*(1), 56–63.

Neighbors, C., Oster-Aaland, L., Bergstrom, R., and Lewis, M. (2006). Event-and context-specific normative misperceptions and high-risk drinking: 21st birthday celebrations and football tailgating. *Journal of Studies on Alcohol, 67*, 282–289.

Nicholls, J. (2012). Everyday, everywhere: Alcohol marketing and social media—current trends. *Alcohol and Alcoholism, 47*(4), 486–493.

O'Brien, K., and Kypri, K. (2008). Alcohol industry sponsorship and hazardous drinking among sportspeople. *Addiction, 103*(12), 1961–1966.

O'Brien, K., Carr, S., Ferris, J., Room, R., Miller, P., Livingston, M., Kypri, K., and Lynott, D. (2015). Alcohol advertising in sport and non-sport TV in Australia, during children's viewing times. *PLoS ONE, 10*(8), e0134889.

Parry, C., Burnhams, N., and London, L. (2012). A total ban on alcohol advertising: Presenting the public health case. *SAMJ: South African Medical Journal, 102*(7), 602–604.

Pennay, A., Livingston, M., and Maclean, S. (2015). Young people are drinking less: It's time we found out why. *Drug and Alcohol Review, 34*, 115–118.

Pettigrew, S., Roberts, M., Pescud, M., Chapman, K., Quester, P., and Miller, C. (2012). The extent and nature of alcohol advertising on Australian television. *Drug and Alcohol Review, 31*(6), 797–802. www.scopus.com/inward/record.url?eid=2-s2.0–84858974943 andpartnerID=40andmd5=da30aae50732c51c4b080b752d371d32

Purves, R., Stead, M., and Eadie, D. (2014). *'What Are You Meant to Do When you See It Everywhere?': Young People, Alcohol Packaging and Digital Media.* December. London: Alcohol Research UK. http://alcoholresearchuk.org/downloads/finalReports/FinalReport_0120.pdf.

Quanbeck, A. (2015). Mobile delivery of alcohol treatment: A systematic review of the literature. *Addiction Science and Clinical Practice, 10*(Supplement 1), a50.

Ridout, B. (2016). Facebook, social media and its application to problem drinking among college students. *Current Opinion in Psychology, 9*, 83–87.

Ridout, B., Campbell, A., and Ellis, L. (2012). 'Off your Face(book)': Alcohol in online social identity construction and its relation to problem drinking in university students. *Drug and Alcohol Review, 31*(1), 20–26.

Ross, G., McDermott, L., Stead, M., and Angus, K. (2006). The effectiveness of social marketing interventions for health improvement: What's the evidence? *Public Health, 120*, 1133–1139.

Santani, D., Biel, J. I., Labhart, F., Truong, J., Landolt, S., Kuntsche, E., & Gatica-Perez, D. (2016, September). The night is young: urban crowdsourcing of nightlife patterns. In *Proceedings of the 2016 ACM International Joint Conference on Pervasive and Ubiquitous Computing* (pp. 427–438). ACM.

Senft, T. (2008). *Camgirls: Celebrity and Community in the Age of Social Networks*. New York: Peter Lang.

Shiffman, S., Stone, A., and Hufford, M. (2008). Ecological momentary assessment. *Annual Review of Clinical Psychology, 4*, 1–32.

Simonen, J., Törrönen, J., and Tigerstedt, C. (2014). Femininities of drinking among Finnish and Swedish women of different ages. *Addiction Research and Theory, 22*, 98–108.

Smith, L., and Foxcroft, D. (2009). The effect of alcohol advertising, marketing and portrayal on drinking behaviour in young people: Systematic review of prospective cohort studies. *BMC Public Health, 9*(51), 1–11. Retrieved 9 September 2016, from http://bmcpublichealth.biomedcentral.com/articles/10.1186/1471-2458-9-51

Smyth, J., and Stone, A. (2003). Ecological momentary assessment research in behavioural medicine. *Journal of Happiness Studies, 4*, 35–52.

Stone, A., and Shiffman, S. (2002). Capturing momentary self-report data: A proposal for reporting guidelines. *Annals of Behavioral Medicine, 24*, 236–243.

Subrahmanyam, K., and Greenfield, P. (2008). Virtual worlds in development: Implications of social networking sites. *Journal of Applied Developmental Psychology, 29*, 417–419.

Thrul, J., and Kuntsche, E. (2015). The impact of friends on young adults' drinking over the course of the evening—an event-level analysis. *Addiction, 110*, 619–626.

Törrönen, J., and Roumeliotis, F. (2014). Masculinities of drinking as described by Swedish and Finnish age-based focus groups. *Addiction Research and Theory, 22*, 126–136.

Van de Goor, L., Knibbe, R., and Drop, M. (1990). Adolescent drinking behavior: an observational study of the influence of situational factors on adolescent drinking rates. *Journal of Studies on Alcohol, 51*, 548–555.

van Dijck, J. (2013). *The Culture of Connectivity: A Critical History of Social Media*. New York: Oxford University Press.

Verster, J., Tiplady, B., and McKinney, A. (2012). Mobile technology and naturalistic study designs in addiction research [Editorial]. *Current Drug Abuse Reviews, 5*, 169–171.

Walker, D., and Hunter, B. (1978). Short-term memory impairment following chronic alcohol consumption in rats. *Neuropsychologia, 16*, 545–553.

Wall, A., Hinson, R., McKee, S., and Goldstein, A. (2001). Examining alcohol outcome expectancies in laboratory and naturalistic bar settings: A within-subjects experimental analysis. *Psychology of Addictive Behaviors, 15*, 219–226.

Wall, A., McKee, S., and Hinson, R. (2000). Assessing variation in alcohol outcome expectancies across environmental context: An examination of the situational-specificity hypothesis. *Psychology of Addictive Behaviors, 14*, 367–375.

Weissenborn, R., and Duka, T. (2002). Acute alcohol effects on cognitive function in social drinkers: Their relationship to drinking habits. *Psychopharmacology, 165*, 306–312.

Winpenny, E., Marteau, T., and Nolte, E. (2014). Exposure of children and adolescents to alcohol marketing on social media websites. *Alcohol and Alcoholism, 49*(2), 154–159.

9 Creating powerful brands

Richard Purves

Introduction

The consumption of alcohol plays an important part in the way young people create desired identities and live their social lives. Alcohol marketing is an important focus for investigation by alcohol researchers because of its potential to influence drinking behaviour, particularly amongst young people. There is a wealth of evidence that exposure to alcohol advertising increases the likelihood that young people will start to consume alcohol and will drink more if they already do so (Anderson et al., 2009; Smith and Foxcroft, 2009). Through marketing practices, alcohol brands have become embedded in everyday life and this is amplified by the increase in new technologies that facilitate the transfer of marketing messages. The emergence of online technologies such as social networking sites (SNS) has raised questions regarding the nature and content of marketing and the implications this has for policy and regulation. This chapter discusses how alcohol brands use SNS as part of their repertoire of marketing activities to create and reinforce powerful brands, and how consumers respond to and engage with these activities.

In order to understand alcohol marketing and its significance to young people, we need to not only examine evidence of direct effects – increased sales or consumption – but also to explore how marketing works; how marketing activities contribute to the creation and reinforcement of desired brand values. Although part of the function of marketing communications is to convey information about a product, a much more important function is to appeal to consumers' emotions and to create an emotional connection between the consumer and the product by building a brand.

Building a brand

Branding can be seen as a process whereby intangible emotional benefits and attributes such as 'luxury', 'coolness' or 'popularity' come to be associated in consumers' minds with particular products. In categories such as alcohol where there are very few differences between products in terms of their tangible characteristics, branding is a key strategy for differentiation and adding value.

Every time a customer is in contact with a brand, there is a potential opportunity to say something about that brand and reinforce its positioning (Elliott and Leonard, 2004). These points of contact are provided not only through advertising, but also through every aspect of marketing: how products are designed, how they are priced, how they are sold and displayed in shops, how they are packaged, where and how they are consumed in public and private places, and how they are talked about in conversations and popular culture (Babor et al., 2010). For example, a trade press content analysis by Stead et al. (2014) demonstrates how even something as simple as the glass can be used as a means of communicating brand values and enhancing the drinking experience, recruiting new segments to a particular drink category, reviving interest in a brand, complementing the launch of new products and building market share.

All these points of contact are used to shape consumers' thoughts and feelings about a brand in such a way that they want to purchase, consume, display and associate themselves with it. Marketing tools are used to communicate the brand's attributes, both its tangible benefits (e.g. taste, affordable price) and its intangible emotional benefits – the emotions, images and values it evokes (Gigerenzer, 2007). Marketing seeks to confer personalities on brands and to associate them with values and experiences which will resonate with their target groups (Stead et al., 2011). The most effective marketing actions and messages are those which consistently reinforce the brand's desired personality and set of associations. Advertising often appeals to emotion and imagination rather than rational thought, and most effective influence occurs when the person does not realise they are being influenced (Binde, 2007). Advertising messages attract because of appealing images of people consuming the products and their implied lifestyles, such that 'the brand becomes symbolically invested with the positive attributes of the lifestyle itself' (Casswell, 1995).

Branding and identity in youth culture

Youth culture attaches great value to brand labels and symbols (Casswell, 2004). Adolescence can be a period of transition in which young people seek to establish their personal identity and young people use brands to help create and present their desired identity (Hill, 2001). Within the context of peer group culture, young people must learn how to present themselves as the same or as different from others, and to manage the tensions between conformity and individuality (Wills, 2005). Valentine (2000) refers to this process as 'social competence' and describes it as being acknowledged and accepted by a peer group, rather than being anonymous among the crowd, while at the same time being careful not to single one's self out and be stigmatised or excluded as an outsider. Young people's identities are entrenched in complex networks of relations where the power to include or exclude others is central to how they relate to each other (Stead et al., 2011). Therefore, the act of consumption takes on new significance in adolescence. The products a person consumes lead others to make judgements about their personality and it is important for young people that they be seen to be consuming what their peer groups would consider 'the right brands' (Belk et al., 1984; Wooten, 2006).

Branding plays an important role in young people's consumer behaviour since they encapsulate the perceived value and attributes of products. Branding can also communicate social status and aspirations and is important to personal identity and peer acceptance (Jackson et al., 2000). Brands can market themselves as adventurous, fun-loving or sophisticated, reinforcing this identity through affiliations with popular culture, sports or music (Stead et al., 2011). As discussed, marketers build intangible emotional benefits into their brands in a bid to evoke certain feelings when consumers use their product. In essence, the brand becomes an extension of the consumers' self-identity through a process known as 'symbolic self-completion' whereby the meanings and values of the brand transfer to the individual who is seen to be consuming it (Belk, 1988; Elliott and Wattanasuwan, 1998). Therefore, the consumption of brands serves two important functions for adolescents – it helps them create and present a desired identity, and it helps them fit in with their desired peer group (Elliott and Wattanasuwan, 1998; Patterson and O'Malley, 2006).

Alcohol marketing strategies and young people

In many cultures, the act of consuming alcohol in adolescence can act as a sign of rebellion or independence, coupled with a desire to emulate the lifestyle of young adults (Babor et al., 2010). For young people, consuming alcohol with their peers can also play an important role in group identity formation, with drinking to excess normalised and accepted as essential to fitting in (Griffin, 2008). There is evidence that links young people's alcohol consumption with their expectations of social success. A review by Kuntsche et al. (2005) found that most young people reported drinking for social motives. A further review of empirical research by Kuntsche et al. (2006) found that social and enhancement motives were very important reasons adolescents drank, particularly for boys. This review also highlighted social coping motivations amongst young girls as a motivation for alcohol use. Much of the alcohol marketing that targets young people is driven by this concept of friendship and socialising (Babor et al., 2010; Griffin, 2008; Hastings et al., 2010). Marketing codes prevent advertisers from suggesting that alcohol can enhance the social success of either an individual or an event. However, an analysis of UK alcohol industry documents found examples of brands doing both of these things (Hastings et al., 2010). Marketing strategy documents for Carling beer made reference to positioning the brand as a 'social glue' which should 'own sociability', as this was the way to 'dominate the booze market'. In internal documents for Lambrini (a sparkling perry), the brand was described as a 'social lubricant' in a creative brief for a summer campaign, and brand positioning strategy documents referred to it as 'the perfect start to the night', with its 'essence' being to 'make the night sparkle' and 'the best way to make your night light, bubbly and full of flavour'. Similarly, for the Ready to Drink (RTD) brand WKD, campaign documents stated that the single most important message to convey to consumers was that the brand 'is all about having a laugh with your mates' (Hastings et al., 2010).

There is strong evidence that having positive emotional responses to alcohol marketing, usually measured in terms of liking advertising, is linked to increased levels of alcohol consumption in young people. Younger adolescents appear to be particularly susceptible to the persuasive messages contained in alcohol commercials broadcast on TV. There is evidence from a range of systematic reviews and primary studies to demonstrate that awareness/recall of or exposure to marketing is associated with increased likelihood of alcohol consumption (Anderson et al., 2009; Booth et al., 2008; Smith and Foxcroft, 2009). Alcohol marketing appeals to extraversion, impulsivity and sensation-seeking (Kuntsche et al., 2006). A key strategy for alcohol marketers is to generate excitement about a brand, activity or brand-sponsored event. A content analysis of alcohol adverts in the USA gave examples of how alcohol advertising subtly implied positive outcomes associated with drinking such as having fun, excitement and pleasure (Zwarun and Farrar, 2005). This is evident in WARC (World Advertising Research Centre) industry documents such as that describing the Smirnoff 'Nightlife Exchange Project' (McGregor and Martinez, 2012). This campaign report described how the campaign sought to communicate 'in the moment' experiences, generate buzz and excitement for the brand and encourage consumers to 'Be There'. Qualitative research conducted to inform the campaign 'revealed the motivating force of FOMO – the Fear Of Missing Out'. This involved hosting events and generating excitement to such a degree that consumers were worried they would miss out on an exciting, once in a lifetime opportunity to be part of something special.

Branding has been found to have an effect on young people's awareness and appreciation of alcohol marketing, as well as their likelihood to consume alcohol. Research has shown that children as young as ten are familiar with and can identify alcohol company brands and logos (Alcohol Concern, 2015). A study examining the relationship between measures of awareness of marketing and drinking among a sample of young people in New Zealand aged between 13 and 14 found that brand allegiance (respondents were asked if they had a favourite brand of alcohol) increased the odds of being a drinker by 356%. Brand allegiance was also associated with more frequent alcohol consumption (1.65 times more drinking occasions per year) and 86% more alcohol consumed on a typical occasion (Lin et al., 2012). Other studies have found a link between liking of alcohol advertising and brand allegiance at age 18 and the volume of beer consumed at age 21 (Casswell and Zhang, 1998). A cross-sectional study with 15–20 year olds in the USA found that having a favourite brand to drink was significantly associated with binge drinking (McClure et al., 2013), providing evidence of a link between alcohol marketing and heavy drinking. Owning and using branded items can be seen as an indicator of an emotional attachment to the brand; consumers choose and use branded items because they like the brand itself and feel that it conveys a desirable identity. There is evidence that owning branded merchandise is associated with higher levels of alcohol consumption among young people (Fisher et al., 2007; Gordon et al., 2011; Gordon et al., 2010).

Branding creates and evokes particular attributes and emotional responses through minimal cues such as brand names and logos, and producers invest tremendous effort in building loyalty to particular brands. Loyalty is achieved through creating identification with the brand and associating the brand with other phenomena to which the consumer is loyal, such as music and sport. One such way marketers will attempt to create these associations is through sponsorship. Sponsorship acts as a way of raising brand awareness, creating positive brand attitudes and building emotional connections with consumers. Its power comes not from direct advertising messages but through associating the brand with an already engaging event or celebrity, and gaining power and credibility in the process. Sponsorship works by creating indirect associations in consumers' minds and often uses themes which are designed to appeal to young people. For example, a content analysis by Kelly et al. (2015) of sponsorship-linked marketing communications in Australia found frequent use of themes likely to appeal emotionally to youth, including humour, success and pop music. Internal industry documents indicate that producers seek to associate their brands with sports or music events in order to benefit from the existing strong emotional connections which sports and music fans have with particular teams or bands (Hastings et al., 2010). An analysis of internal UK alcohol industry documents described various sponsorship activities involving the Carling brand. Self-regulatory codes in the UK prohibit any link between alcohol and youth culture or sporting achievement. However, industry documents examined by the researchers were found to discuss in detail sponsorship deals with football clubs and tournaments, and 'lad magazines' aimed at young men and music festivals. Carling's sponsorship of the Carling Cup Final (football) was described specifically in internal documents as a way to 'recruit young male (LDA-21) drinkers into the brand'.

Alcohol industry documents refer to the need to build credibility with consumers and one way of doing this is through the use of sponsorship. Carling's football sponsorship strategy was underpinned by concepts describing the brand 'earning the right to play'; in other words, to be perceived by consumers as an authentic fan and genuine source of authority on sport. Carling's music sponsorship deals included free branded tents for 'festival virgins', free cans of beer, free t-shirts and comfort kits, and a free laundry service. One campaign brief for a festival sponsorship deal described the aim in these terms: 'Ultimately, the band are the heroes at the venue and Carling should use them to "piggy back" and engage customers' emotions' (Carling campaign brief, cited in Hastings et al., 2010). Alcohol marketing, and in particular alcohol sponsorship, is clearly making an impression on young people. Research has shown that alcohol sponsorship can have an effect on alcohol consumption, attitudes and expectations (Babor et al., 2010). For example, a recent study found that half of 837 children surveyed in England and Scotland associated beer brands with their favourite football teams and tournaments (Alcohol Concern, 2015). In addition, a study of awareness of alcohol sponsorship of sport in Ireland (Houghton et al., 2014) found high awareness among 7–13 year olds, indicating that sponsorship reached those well below the legal age of purchase for alcohol.

A fundamental point about alcohol marketing is that these strategies work in combination; they interact with one another to produce cumulative effects (Babor et al., 2010). The effect of one particular marketing channel or tool such as alcohol advertising or sponsorship is incredibly difficult to isolate and to measure; furthermore, to measure one channel or tool in isolation is to examine only a fraction of marketing's influence. Individual encounters with a brand combine to produce a cumulative effect which cements the brand identity in consumers' minds (Gordon and Harris, 2009).

The increasing presence of alcohol brands on SNS

A particularly noteworthy trend in alcohol marketing has been a dramatic increase in the use of social media alongside more traditional forms of marketing communications. Online advertising became the largest channel in the UK in 2011, overtaking television for the first time (Winpenny et al., 2012). Alcohol brand websites can be accessed by anyone with internet access or a smartphone, with age verification procedures being in most cases weak and easily circumvented (Hastings et al., 2010). Brand activity on social media comprises considerably more than brand websites and paid advertising, however, and includes the production of content for pages on SNS, conversation and interaction with users, and the accumulation of 'likes' and 'followers' who will spread and discuss content through their own networks (Carah, 2014; Purves et al., 2014). As such, the internet is an area where exposure of young people to alcohol marketing is potentially high (Winpenny et al., 2014). An analysis of commercial data on internet usage found that Facebook and YouTube each had an average monthly reach of around 90% of young people aged 15–24, indicating that this is a channel with huge potential to create marketing awareness among young people (Winpenny et al., 2014). Alcohol producers have a major presence on social media – a global partnership between beer producer Heineken and Google in 2011 enabled an increase in the brand's YouTube activity, estimated to result in exposure of at least 103 million minors around the world to alcohol advertising on a monthly basis (EUCAM 2011, cited in de Bruijn, 2013). Another partnership deal in the same year between global alcohol producer Diageo and Facebook had the explicit aim to 'drive unprecedented levels of interaction and joint business planning and experimentation between the two companies' (Carah, 2014). Diageo claims that the deal boosted its sales by 20% (Alcohol Focus Scotland et al., 2011). Exposure to online alcohol marketing has been found to have an effect on young people's alcohol consumption. A four-country study of over 9000 young people in Germany, Italy, the Netherlands and Poland found that higher exposure to online alcohol marketing increased the odds of binge drinking in the previous 30 days in all four countries (de Bruijn, 2013). Research by Critchlow et al. (2016) found that digital marketing was more successful than traditional marketing in reaching young adults, and had a stronger association with increased frequency of heavy episodic drinking. As described above, the effects of marketing exposure have been found to be aggregative: greater awareness of marketing across multiple channels increases the strength of the association (Booth et al., 2008).

The large volume of alcohol-related content identified on SNS such as Facebook and Twitter has been highlighted as an area of growing concern regarding the inadequacies of current regulations to protect young people from exposure to alcohol marketing (Moreno et al., 2010; Nicholls, 2012). Although many adults use SNS, research has found that that online social networking is an important part of youth culture, which facilitates participation in a peer network and the development of social identity (Moraes et al., 2014). Recent studies have demonstrated the power and ubiquity of social media in young people's lives (Chou and Edge, 2012; Paradise and Sullivan, 2012). Access to online technologies, particularly SNS, has fundamentally altered traditional conditions of identity construction (Wood and Smith, 2001). Sites such as Facebook and Twitter provide a platform for users to establish and explore self-identity through interaction with others by providing users with feedback on their own behaviour and allowing them to monitor the behaviour of their peers and how others react to this behaviour (Chou and Edge, 2012). SNS also offer new avenues for young people to create 'consumer identities' by engaging directly with brands and also help in the creation and maintenance of certain social norms and behaviours (McCreanor et al., 2005). This is particularly important when it comes to alcohol use because research has identified alcohol expectancies and perceptions of peer consumption habits as predictors of alcohol use (Moreno et al., 2009).

Alcohol brand practices on SNS

It has been argued that alcohol brands use a number of distinct marketing methods on SNS which undermine policies aimed at normative beliefs and normalise daily alcohol consumption (Nicholls, 2012). Alcohol brands perform a number of actions on SNS: they use SNS as an advertising platform, for product and distribution information; they use SNS to solicit feedback from users and open up a conversation; they use SNS to encourage users to act (e.g., by 'liking', or posting comments, or entering competitions, or re-tweeting brand-authored content); and they use and co-opt user-generated content to support their own branding (Purves et al., 2014). These types of brand actions, however simple they may appear, could all be seen as having been carefully designed to reinforce the values and identity of the brand. For example, when brands post content or 'talk' to users, the tone of voice, the selection of images and wording, the cultural references and so on all appear to have been carefully selected to evoke particular associations and emotional responses in users' minds which are consistent with what the brands are trying to achieve. A key aspect of brand identity is the persona or personality which the brand chooses to project. Brand personality is an expression of the brand's core values and characteristics with an emphasis on human traits such as, for example, trustworthiness, excitement, stylishness or warmth and SNS offer a unique opportunity for alcohol brands to communicate directly with users on a day-to-day basis. Brand personality can be seen to be constructed through the language a brand uses when 'talking' to users, through cultural references which say something about the brand's values, through use of imagery and language designed to appeal to a particular gender or age group, and so on. For example, a content analysis of alcohol brands' social networking pages found that some brands used masculine and feminine values to project their desired identity and appeal to specific target markets (Purves et al., 2014). Another content analysis of Australian alcohol brands' Facebook posts (Carah, 2014) found that many beer and spirits brands appealed directly to men by asking them about the rules of male rituals. These activities associated the brand with Australian masculine identities. They make the brand authentic and credible by providing resources for men to convey how 'Aussie' and 'blokey' they are. By contrast, brands such as Baileys, Midori and Rekorderlig were found to target women. For example, they posed questions directly to women such as when Baileys asked 'There's nothing better than a good Girls' Night Out. When was your last one?' Responses from fans define what a 'girls' night out' is to them.

Digital marketing strategies include competitions, interactive games and association with real-world events. Brands can also co-opt user-generated material alongside brand-authored images (McCreanor et al., 2013). Digital alcohol marketing aims to promote interaction between brands and SNS users, as well as user-to-user conversations among potential consumers (Nicholls, 2012). These interactions and conversations may not always revolve around alcohol consumption, but will often reflect brand values, revealing the subtlety and complexity of branding. This creates social and emotional bonds between users which are beneficial in creating a feeling of belonging and acceptance. As individuals 'like' brands and comment on them or share their content, brand messages are passed on to the news feeds of their friends, normalising alcohol advertising in the everyday lives of SNS users (McCreanor et al., 2013; Nicholls, 2012). Branded posts on social media invoke pleasure, relaxation, socialising, drinking after work and at the weekend, drinking in the sun outdoors or on holiday in a bid to promote interaction between users (Purves et al., 2014). Alcohol brands use SNS to associate themselves with particular cultural references and events or with particular organisations. Brands seek to create desirable brand associations because they contribute to brand identity and values, and also because they will be of intrinsic interest to users, who will in turn be happy to be associated with such references and share them with their social networks. Different types of associations have been identified: associations with popular culture and music, association with sporting events, and association with other brands, retailers and producers (Carah, 2014; Purves et al., 2014). Similarly, a market research conference paper discusses how alcohol brands can be used to 'activate', 'fuel' and be part of online conversations with consumers (Verhaeghe et al., 2011). This paper notes that conversations about alcohol often involved people bonding with each other, and suggests that 'Diageo could facilitate this' by bringing together people with similar interests. The research was conducted by 'friending' key consumers online and using their conversations as a source of consumer insight, allowing the marketers to further hone their brand and marketing messages.

Marketers measure a brand's success in digital conversations by analysing the tone of conversations, the extent to which the brand is mentioned and the likelihood that the user will purchase the brand's products (Verhaeghe et al., 2011).

Research suggests that some of the brands' uses of SNS could be seen not just to encourage and drive feelings about the particular brand but also to promote the idea of habitual consumption. Messages and images on social media often encourage consumption of alcohol on particular days of the week (McCreanor et al., 2013). For example, Purves et al. (2014), in an analysis of alcohol brand content on social media websites, found instances of images and messages being regularly used to link alcohol use to particular times of the week, implying a habitual routine. Examples cited in the study urge social media users to 'grab a Bud tonight' and to settle down 'for a chilled mid-week Bulmers'. Another analysis of alcohol brands' posts on Facebook found that the most common time for brands to post content was a Friday afternoon, to coincide with the end of the working week when users would be planning to go out to pubs, bars and restaurants (Carah, 2014). However, brands would also post on Monday asking fans to reminisce about the weekend, on Wednesday lamenting the middle of the week, and on Thursday anticipating Friday, in this way implying that alcohol consumption was an integral part of the week and providing constant reminders (Carah, 2014). Similarly, Nicholls' (2012) content analysis of alcohol marketing on social media noted the frequent occurrence of posts encouraging users to drink which were day-specific, linking consumption to the weekend, but also linking brands to early and mid-week consumption. For example, one Smirnoff tweet read 'Sunday's fun day. Not that any day isn't fun day with #smirnoff'. Bacardi was found to make regular references to 'Mojito Monday' (e.g. 'waiting for the weekend for a mojito? We had one Monday! #mojitomonday'). Bacardi also used the phrase 'hump day' (relating to middle of the week Wednesday) in tweets such as 'Reward yourself for cresting hump day with a Bacardi cocktail!' and 'Happy hump day!' As with weekend drinking, these messages were promoted in real time, appearing on the day to which they referred (Nicholls, 2012).

As well as shaping perceptions that certain consumption behaviours are normal and widespread, marketing also helps to convey the message that they are socially desirable and approved. Marketing can influence levels of perceived peer approval by promoting drinking as a social activity and by creating brand associations which are viewed as acceptable by certain peer groups. As noted earlier, young people may be particularly susceptible to marketing because they have a heightened sensitivity to image and reputation at a time when they are struggling to develop their own identities, and actively search for cues in advertising which conforms the right way to look and behave (Hill, 2001; Wills, 2005). Drinking for some becomes an action which resolves social pressures and demands in terms of identity and role. This message is reinforced by marketing messages which convey the impression that drinking is desirable, socially acceptable and prevalent among their peers. Digital media such as SNS are a strong potential influence on social norms regarding alcohol use (Hastings et al., 2010; Purves et al., 2014). A content analysis of alcohol images on SNS found that alcohol consumption was presented primarily in a positive light, potentially skewing social norms and leading young people to the belief that the majority of people their age regularly drink alcohol (Purves et al., 2014).

Co-creating alcohol marketing messages

A particular strategic benefit of SNS for brands is that they can work with SNS users to co-create social media content. In effect, brand-authored content and user-generated content work together to create and distribute marketing messages. Brand messages are passed on, commented on and transformed by users who become part of the marketing, co-creating the branding and working in synergy to spread marketing messages. Research by Purves et al. (2014) identified three ways users engage with alcohol brand-related content on SNS. The first category of engagement, direct responses to the brand, included responses to advertising, new flavours and promotions, and direct questions or answers in response to brand content. A second type of engagement was labelled 'self-presentation' and referred to the ways in which users co-opted alcohol brand-related content to say something about themselves, their tastes, personality and lifestyle on SNS. The third type of engagement, labelled a 'space for conversation', referred to the ways in which users conversed and shared with one another content which did not directly refer to the brands or even to alcohol. While this content did not at first appear directly relevant, it was important because it took place on platforms linked to the alcohol brands. Brands are cultural signifiers which users can reference on social media, just as they do in real life when choosing to wear a particular brand of sports shoe or buy a particular model of mobile phone, to signal something about the sort of person they wish to be perceived as. More subtly, brands become conversational resources which become 'part of consumer experiences, pastimes and memories' and part of the stories which consumers tell about their everyday lives (Carah, 2014). In this way, the connections between brands and consumers' lives and identities are deepened. SNS allow the user to create and share content which is meaningful to them and brands become part of this. By discussing and creating alcohol-related content on SNS, users are able to construct their desired identity in a space which is not constrained by existing social and structural barriers (boyd and Ellison, 2007). Consumers also derive benefits from interacting with alcohol brands on SNS. An analysis of user-generated content on SNS found that users were able to respond directly to the brand, expressing opinions on new products, advertising campaigns and promotions. They appeared to respond voluntarily and with enthusiasm to brand content, spreading it to their wider social network and further increasing its reach. More subtly, users were also able to engage with alcohol brands in order to portray something about themselves to others (Purves et al., 2014).

A qualitative study by Griffiths and Casswell (2010) found that some teenagers openly presented themselves as excessive drinkers on SNS. Many participants utilised a variety of photographic and textual material to present alcohol as a major part of their identity on Facebook, with over half of participants selecting an alcohol-related profile picture. When interacting with alcohol brands online by 'liking', 'commenting' or 'sharing' content from an alcohol brand, users are openly endorsing products to an audience comprising their peers (Griffiths and Casswell, 2010). Qualitative work by Purves et al. (2014) found that young people spoke about regularly seeing examples of friends 'liking' or 'following' alcohol brands, spreading the marketing messages to their social group. Recent studies looking at alcohol use on Facebook found that pictures on users' profiles showing alcohol consumption and images featuring an alcohol brand logo were positively received by other Facebook users, receiving significantly more 'likes' than other non-drinking images (Beullens and Schepers, 2013). These images are often carefully selected by users to show alcohol consumption in a positive light and present an image of their desired identity. Research by Niland et al. (2014) found that displaying drinking photos on Facebook reinforced friendship group relationships, but time and effort was required to limit drunken photo displays in order to maintain an overall attractive online identity. Further research with young adults found that 32% uploaded pictures of themselves consuming alcohol to social media (Morgan et al., 2010) and 56% posted pictures of their peers drinking (Glassman, 2012). Some studies have also found that exposure to user-created alcohol promotion is associated with increased consumption, including daily drinking, indications of at-risk consumption, alcohol cravings and willingness to drink (Glassman, 2012; Litt and Stock, 2011; Moreno et al., 2012; Ridout et al., 2012; Stoddard et al., 2012; Westgate et al., 2014). The recent 'Neknomination' trend, where users posted online videos of themselves drinking alcohol and then nominated other online friends to take up the challenge, exemplified the level of interest that images of excessive alcohol consumption could generate. Indeed it was noteworthy that this phenomenon was responsible for images of excessive consumption and risky behaviour escalating, for example, from drinking a can of beer in one go to more extreme levels of consumption involving 'protein shakes', 'bleach' and 'petrol' (Purves et al., 2014). Not only did the Neknominate game generate content from individual users, but it also generated public 'fan pages' (Facebook, 2014) and viral video compilations (You Tube, 2014).

New media platforms allow alcohol producers to co-opt and benefit from user-generated images of branded alcohol products. Analysis of alcohol brand activity on social media in the UK by Purves et al. (2014) found that users would post images of themselves consuming a branded alcohol product onto the Facebook or Twitter pages of those brands; these images could then be seen by their 'friends' and those who 'followed' the particular brand on SNS. Messages from alcohol marketers on social media appear alongside comments and images from friends, which potentially lends them greater credibility, authenticity and persuasiveness. The distinction between brand-authored and user-generated content is not always clear, and this confusion potentially adds to the impression of social approval from multiple sources (McCreanor et al., 2013). Content analysis of Smirnoff's social media marketing material for the brand's Nightlife Exchange Project found that user-generated material such as fan photos were mixed with brand promotion such as official images and videos (Nicholls, 2012). Analyses of internal industry documents suggest that producers are aware of this and seek to take advantage of it; for example, a marketing strategy document for Carling described how online brand-authored marketing communications 'should look like it's come from your mate, but it is in fact Carling branded' (Hastings et al., 2010). By appealing to certain values and creating desirable brand associations, alcohol brands are able to craft a personality and convey to users the impression that their online content is not from faceless corporations but from friends with similar interests and a familiar outlook on life, making it easier for users to pass on the brand messages to other friends within their social network and thereby to extend the reach of the brand's marketing and lend it authenticity. On SNS, marketing content becomes entangled with the exchange of user-generated messages and information between friends, and as a consequence, many brand messages appear to come from or be endorsed by a trusted friend. In turn, brands co-opt user generated content – for example, particularly amusing tweets or attractive images – which supports their brand values. Thus, marketing and branding can be seen to be co-created on SNS.

Conclusion

All of an alcohol brand's marketing actions are designed to reinforce the values and identity of the brand. Brands adopt a particular tone of voice, appeal to certain values, use humour and associate themselves with cultural references points such as sport or music which is of intrinsic interest to consumers and encourages them to feel comfortable in the brand's presence. Alcohol marketing is a part of young people's everyday life and their dependence on SNS as a means of everyday social interaction has vast implications for marketers. The advent of SNS means that corporations can have direct access to, and form part of, a young person's social reality. If the ideal relationship between the consumer and the brand is a close one, the omnipresence of SNS means that brands are able to constantly reinforce their values, cementing the brand identity in consumers' minds. Messages from alcohol marketers on SNS appear alongside comments and images from friends, lending them greater credibility, authenticity and persuasiveness. Alcohol marketing on SNS only shows alcohol consumption in a positive light, skewing social norms. Drinking and images of excess are a central feature of the self-generated content that is widely accessed and shared on SNS. These practices not only provide a platform for endorsing specific alcohol brands, but also serve to normalise excessive consumption and potentially risky drinking behaviours. The online spaces created by alcohol brands can be seen to function as 'glue', bringing together users who share similar interests or views. This creates social and emotional bonds between users which are beneficial in creating a feeling of belonging and acceptance. Alcohol brands also use SNS to position the brand as part of everyday activities, framing alcohol consumption as a positive, everyday activity.

Current marketing regulations aimed at protecting vulnerable groups such as young people can be seen as ineffective because they seek to apply existing codes to the online environment, rather than addressing the unique challenges posed by social media (Nicholls, 2012). This chapter highlights the dynamic nature of marketing communications and the need for further research to fully understand young people's experience with digital marketing. Understanding the role that alcohol brands play in adolescent identity formation is an important first step to reforming alcohol marketing regulations.

References

Alcohol Concern. (2015). *Children's Recognition of Alcohol Marketing*. London: Alcohol Concern.

Alcohol Focus Scotland, SHAAP, Balance, and Our Life. (2011). *The Four Steps to Alcohol Misuse. How the Industry Uses Price, Place, Promotion and Product Design to Persuade Us That Too Much Alcohol is Not Enough*. Edinburgh: Alcohol Focus Scotland. www.alcohol-focus-scotland.org.uk/media/85193/The-four-steps-to-alcohol-misuse.pdf

Anderson, P., de Bruijn, A., Angus, K., Gordon, R., and Hastings, G. (2009). Impact of alcohol advertising and media exposure on adolescent alcohol use: A systematic review of longitudinal studies. *Alcohol and Alcoholism, 44*(3), 229–243.

Babor, T., Caetano, R., Casswell, S., Edwards, G., Giesbrecht, N., Graham, K., Grube, J., Hill, L., Holder, H., Homel, R., Livingston, M., Osterberg, E., Rehm, J., Room, R., and Rossow, I. (2010). *Alcohol: No Ordinary Commodity Research and Public Policy* (2nd edn). Oxford: Oxford University Press.

Belk, R. (1988). Possessions and the extended self. *Journal of Consumer Research, 15*, 139–168.

Belk, R., Mayer, R., and Driscoll, A. (1984). Children's recognition of consumption symbolism in children's products. *Journal of Consumer Research, 9*(1), 4–17.

Beullens, K., and Schepers, A. (2013). Display of alcohol use on Facebook: A content analysis. *Cyberpsychology, Behaviour and Social Networking, 16*(7), 497–503.

Binde, P. (2007). Selling dreams – causing nightmares? *Journal of Gambling Issues, 20*, 167–192.

Booth, A., Meier, T., Stockwell, T., Sutton, A., Wilkinson, A., and Wong, R. (2008). Review 1: The effect of pricing and taxation on alcohol consumption (pp. 30–79). Review 2: The effect of promotion on alcohol consumption (pp. 80–218). *Independent Review of the Effects of Alcohol Pricing and Promotion. Part A: Systematic Reviews. Project Report for the Department of Health*. Retrieved May 2016, from http://webarchive.nationalarchives.gov.uk/20130107105354/www.dh.gov.uk/prod_consum_dh/groups/dh_digitalassets/documents/digitalasset/dh_091366.pdf

boyd, d., and Ellison, N. (2007). Social network sites: Definition, history, and scholarship. *Journal of Computer-Mediated Communication, 13*(1), 210–230.

Carah, N. (2014). *Like, Comment, Share: Alcohol Brand Activity on Facebook*. Brisbane: Foundation for Alcohol Research and Evaluation, University of Queensland.

Casswell, S. (1995). Does alcohol advertising have an impact on the public health? *Drug and Alcohol Review, 14*(4), 395–403.

Casswell, S. (2004). Alcohol brands in young peoples everyday lives: New developments in marketing. *Alcohol and Alcoholism, 39*(6), 471–476.

Casswell, S., and Zhang, J. (1998). Impact of liking for advertising and brand allegiance on drinking and alcohol-related aggression: A longitudinal study. *Addiction, 93*(8), 1209–1217.

Chou, H., and Edge, N. (2012). 'They are happier and having better lives than I am': The impact of using Facebook on perceptions of others' lives. *Cyberpsychology, Behaviour and Social Networking, 15*, 117–121.

Critchlow, N., Moodie, C., Bauld, L., Bonner, A., and Hastings, G. (2016). Awareness of, and participation with, digital alcohol marketing, and the association with frequency of high episodic drinking among young adults. *Drugs: Education, Prevention and Policy*, published online 26 January, doi: 10.3109/09687637.09682015.01119247.

de Bruijn, A. (2013). Exposure to online alcohol marketing and adolescents' binge drinking: A cross-sectional study in four European countries. In P. Anderson, F. Braddick, J. Reynolds et al. (Eds.), *Alcohol Policy in Europe: Evidence from AMPHORA. The AMPHORA Project* (2nd edn). http://amphoraproject.net/w2box/data/e-book/Chapter%208%20-%20AM_E-BOOK_2nd%20edition%20-%20June%202013.pdf

Elliott, R., and Leonard, C. (2004). Peer pressure and poverty: Exploring fashion brands and consumption symbolism among children of the 'British poor'. *Journal of Consumer Behaviour, 4*(4), 347–359.

Elliott, R., and Wattanasuwan, K. (1998). Brands as symbolic resources for the construction of identity. *International Journal of Advertising, 17*, 131–144.

Facebook. (no date). Neknominate Community. Retrieved November 2015, from www.facebook.com/neknominate2014/?fref=ts

Fisher, L., Miles, I., Austin, S., Camargo, C., and Colditz, G. (2007). Predictors of initiation of alcohol use among US adolescents: Findings from a prospective cohort study. *Archives of Pediatrics and Adolescent Medicine, 161*(10), 959–966.

Gigerenzer, G. (2007). *Gut Feelings: The Intelligence of the Unconscious*. New York: Viking.

Glassman, T. (2012). Implications for college students posting pictures of themselves drinking alcohol on facebook. *Journal of Alcohol and Drug Education, 56*, 38–58.

Gordon, R., and Harris, F. (2009). Assessing the cumulative impact of alcohol marketing on young people's drinking: Cross sectional data findings. *Addiction Research and Theory, 19*(1), 66–75.

Gordon, R., Harris, F., Marie MacKintosh, A., and Moodie, C. (2011). Assessing the cumulative impact of alcohol marketing on young people's drinking: Cross-sectional data findings. *Addiction Research and Theory, 19*(1), 66–75.

Gordon, R., Hastings, G., and Moodie, C. (2010). Alcohol marketing and young people's drinking: What the evidence base suggests for policy. *Journal of Public Affairs, 10*(1–2), 88–101.

Griffin, C. (2008). Understanding youth: Perspectives, identities and practices. *Health and Social Care in the Community, 16*(1), 108–109.

Griffiths, R., and Casswell, S. (2010). Intoxigenic digital spaces? Youth, social networking sites and alcohol marketing. *Drug and Alcohol Review, 29*, 525–530.

Hastings, G., Brooks, O., Stead, M., Angus, K., Anker, T., and Farrell, T. (2010). *'They'll Drink Bucketloads of the Stuff': An Analysis of Internal Alcohol Industry Documents* (Memorandum by Professor Gerard Hastings, Institute for Social Marketing, University of Stirling and the Open University), January. London: Alcohol Education and Research Council. http://alcoholresearchuk.org/downloads/finalReports/AERC_Final Report_0071.pdf

Hill, A. (2001). Nutrition and behaviour group symposium on 'evolving attitudes to food and nutrition': Developmental issues in attitudes to food and diet. *Proceedings of the Nutrition Society, 61*, 259–266.

Houghton, F., Scott, L., Houghton, S., and Lewis, C. (2014). Children's awareness of alcohol sponsorship of sport in Ireland: Munster Rugby and the 2008 European Rugby Cup. *International Journal of Public Health, 59*(5), 829–832.

Jackson, M., Hastings, G., Wheeler, C., Eadie, D., and MacKintosh, A. (2000). Marketing alcohol to young people: Implications for industry regulation and research policy. *Addiction, 95*(Supplement 4), S597–S608.

Kelly, S., Ireland, M., Alpert, F., and Mangan, J. (2015). Young consumers' exposure to alcohol sponsorship in sport. *International Journal of Sports Marketing and Sponsorship, 16*(2), 83–102.

Kuntsche, E., Knibbe, R., Gmel, G., and Engels, R. (2006). Who drinks and why? A review of socio-demographic, personality, and contextual issues behind the drinking motives in young people. *Addictive Behaviors, 31*(10), 1844–1857.

Kuntsche, E., Knibbe, R., Gmel, G., and Rutger, E. (2005). Why do young people drink? A review of drinking motives. *Clinical Psychology Review, 25*, 841–861.

Lin, E.-Y., Casswell, S., You, R. Q., and Huckle, T. (2012). Engagement with alcohol marketing and early brand allegiance in relation to early years of drinking. *Addiction Research and Theory, 20*(4), 329–338.

Litt, D., and Stock, M. (2011). Adolescent alcohol-related risk cognitions: The roles of social norms and social networking sites. *Psychology of Addictive Behaviours, 25*(4), 708–713.

McClure, A., Stoolmiller, M., Tanski, S., Engels, R., and Sargent, J. (2013). Alcohol marketing receptivity, marketing-specific cognitions, and underage binge drinking. *Alcoholism: Clinical and Experimental Research, 37*(Supplement 1), e404–e413.

McCreanor, T., Greenaway, A., Moewaka Barnes, H., Borell, S., and Gregory, A. (2005). Youth identity formation and contemporary alcohol marketing. *Critical Public Health, 15*(3), 251–262.

McCreanor, T., Lyons, A., Griffin, C., Goodwin, I., Moewaka Barnes, H., and Hutton, F. (2013). Youth drinking cultures, social networking and alcohol marketing: Implications for public health. *Critical Public Health, 23*(1), 110–120.

McGregor, L., and Martinez, O. (2012). Were you there? The research behind the innovative and award-winning Smirnoff campaign. Paper presented at the Congress 2012, Accelerating Excellence – Celebrating 65 Years and Beyond, Amsterdam, September. www.warc.com/ (Paywall)

Moraes, C., Michaelidou, N., and Meneses, R. (2014). The use of Facebook to promote drinking among young consumers. *Journal of Marketing Management, 30*(13–14), 1377–1401.

Moreno, M., Briner, L., Williams, A., Brockman, L., Walker, L., and Christakis, D. (2010). A content analysis of displayed alcohol references in a social networking web site. *Journal of Adolescent Health, 47*, 168–175.

Moreno, M., Christakis, D., Egan, K., Brockman, L., and Becker, T. (2012). Associations between displayed alcohol references on Facebook and problem drinking among college students. *Archives of Paediatric and Adolescent Medicine, 166*(2), 157–163.

Moreno, M., Parks, M., Zimmerman, F., Brito, T., and Christakis, D. (2009). Display of health risk behaviours on MySpace by adolescents. Prevalence and associations. *Archives of Pediatrics and Adolescent Medicine, 163*, 27–34.

Morgan, E., Snelson, C., and Elison-Bowers, P. (2010). Image and video disclosure of substance use on social media websites. *Computers in Human Behavior, 26*(6), 1405–1411.

Nicholls, J. (2012). Everyday, everywhere: Alcohol marketing and social media—current trends. *Alcohol and Alcoholism, 47*(4), 486–493.

Niland, P., Lyons, A., Goodwin, I., and Hutton, F. (2014). 'See it doesn't look pretty does it?' Young adults' airbrushed drinking practices on Facebook. *Psychology and Health, 29*(8), 877–895.

Paradise, A., and Sullivan, M. (2012). (In)visible threats? The third-person effect in perceptions of the influence of Facebook. *Cyberpsychology, Behaviour and Social Networking, 15*, 55–60.

Patterson, M., and O'Malley, L. (2006). Brands, consumers and relationships: A review. *Irish Marketing Review, 18*, 10–20.

Purves, R., Stead, M., and Eadie, D. (2014). *'What Are You Meant to Do When You See It Everywhere?': Young People, Alcohol Packaging and Digital Media.* December. London: Alcohol Research UK. http://alcoholresearchuk.org/downloads/finalReports/FinalReport_0120.pdf.

Ridout, B., Campbell, A., and Ellis, L. (2012). 'Off your Face(book)': Alcohol in online social identity construction and its relation to problem drinking in university students. *Drug and Alcohol Review, 31*(1), 20–26.

Smith, L., and Foxcroft, D. (2009). The effect of alcohol advertising, marketing and portrayal on drinking behaviour in young people: Systematic review of prospective cohort studies. *BMC Public Health, 9*(51), 1–11. www.biomedcentral.com/1471–2458/1479/1451

Stead, M., Angus, K., Macdonald, L., and Bauld, L. (2014). Looking into the glass: Glassware as an alcohol marketing tool, and the implications for policy. *Alcohol and Alcoholism, 49*(3), 317–320.

Stead, M., McDermott, L., Mackintosh, A., and Adamson, A. (2011). Why healthy eating is bad for young people's health: Identity, belonging and food. *Social Science and Medicine, 72*(7), 1131–1139.

Stoddard, S., Bauermeister, J., Gordon-Messer, D., Johns, M., and Zimmerman, M. (2012). Permissive norms and young adults' alcohol and marijuana use: The role of online communities. *Journal of Studies on Alcohol and Drugs, 73*(6), 968–975.

Valentine, G. (2000). Exploring children and young people's narratives of identity. *Geoforum, 31*(2), 257–267.

Verhaeghe, A., Van Belleghem, S., and Price, D. (2011). Let's go on an online safari. Levering the power of conversations in the alcohol beverages industry. Paper presented at the Market Research Society, Annual Conference. www.warc.com/ (Paywall)

Westgate, E., Neighbors, C., Heppner, H., Jahn, S., and Lindgrem, K. (2014). 'I will take a shot for every "like" I get on this status': Posting alcohol-related Facebook content is linked to drinking outcomes. *Journal of Studies on Alcohol and Drugs, 75*(3), 390–398.

Wills, W. (2005). Food and eating practices during the transition from secondary school to new social contexts. *Journal of Youth Studies, 8*(1), 97–110.

Winpenny, E., Marteau, T., and Nolte, E. (2014). Exposure of children and adolescents to alcohol marketing on social media websites. *Alcohol and Alcoholism, 49*(2), 154–159.

Winpenny, E., Patil, S., Elliott, M., Villalba van Dijk, L., Hinrichs, S., Marteau, T., and Nolte, E. (2012). *Assessment of Young People's Exposure to Alcohol Marketing in Audiovisual and Online Media.* Cambridge: Rand Europe. http://ec.europa.eu/health/alcohol/docs/alcohol_rand_youth_exposure_marketing_en.pdf

Wood, A., and Smith, M. (2001). *Online Communication: Linking Technology, Identity, and Culture.* Mahwah, NJ: Lawrence Erlbaum Associates.

Wooten, D. (2006). From labelling possessions to possessing labels: Ridicule and socialization among adolescents. *Journal of Consumer Research*, *33*, 188–198.

YouTube. (2014, 16 January). Neknomination Neknominate Compilation #1 – January 2014 – Latest Social Media Trend. [YouTube video file] Retrieved May 2016, from https://youtu.be/6ZmQlR03J1g

Zwarun, L., and Farrar, K. (2005). Doing what they say, saying what they mean: Self-regulatory compliance and depictions of drinking in alcohol commercials in televised sports. *Mass Communication and Society*, *8*(4), 347–371.

Part III

Public health and regulating alcohol promotion

10 Social media affordances for curbing alcohol consumption

Insights from Hello Sunday Morning blog posts

Hélène Cherrier, Nicholas Carah and Carla Meurk

Introduction

In this study, we introduce the concept of 'affordances' and articulate how a particular type of social media – weblogs (hereafter, 'blogs') used in health promotion – affords unknown users opportunities to curb their alcohol consumption behaviours. Specifically, we examine how the Hello Sunday Morning (HSM) blogging site is being used, as well as users' motivations for using blogs, during a period of alcohol abstinence. Our findings show that HSM blogging sites are not perceived or used because of their qualities or properties as such, but rather as functionally meaningful entities – the 'official' HSM blogging site affords accessibility, anonymity and interactivity tied to self-understanding, self-talk and self-commitment. Our concluding remarks inform guidelines that help maximise the affordances of blogs in the context of online health promotion, in terms of the relations that arise from the interaction of HSM participants, taking into account their attitudes, preferences, intentions, motivations, experiences and desires, and HSM blogging site qualities and properties.

Alcohol interventions using social media

Social media are important platforms for the performance and promotion of alcohol consumption (Brown and Gregg, 2012; McCreanor et al., 2013). While alcohol and nightlife industries were early innovators in the use of social media to promote alcohol consumption, the health sector has taken a cautious approach to using social media for promoting behavioural change strategies.

The iterative experiments of health communicators with social media indicate at least three ways they impact and transform health interventions. These can be understood as sitting across a spectrum of knowledge production and practice, spanning the uses of social media to: 1) reproduce a hierarchy of knowledge, where expert knowledge is disseminated to a lay public; 2) facilitate knowledge exchange, where expert and lay knowledges are actively engaged in public dialogue; and, finally, 3) construct new forms of expertise through social engagement around a shared purpose. While the first presumes a linear trajectory in which expertise is assumed to inform practice, the latter two modes of engagement reconfigure the relationship between expertise and practice.

First, at the most basic level, social media have become part of the communication mix. Already existing health interventions begin to distribute content such as information, interactive resources or advertisements via social media. In these cases, social media principally act as a means for the one-way distribution of more or less 'traditional' health information to a target audience. Second, health communicators use social media to foster new modes of participation from target audiences, including modes of interactivity which allow lay publics to reformulate and transmit messages via the creation and circulation of content. Within the parameters of established interventions, this mode of practice opens up opportunities for target audiences to ask questions, create content or share ideas in more impactful ways. Third, health interventions are beginning to emerge from social media platforms which are 'natively' or 'endogenously' social. In some cases, this latter type of 'intervention' does not follow the established clinical or evaluative protocols of typical health interventions. These campaigns often mix together audience participation, lifestyle branding strategies and health intervention tactics in novel ways. Endogenous social media interventions place the active contribution of participants at the centre of the intervention. Campaigns such as Hello Sunday Morning (www.hellosundaymorning.org), Dry July and Febfast to some extent require participants to take action in their everyday lives and document that action on a social media platform. The activity of participants generates the content (and, thus, expertise) and engagement around the intervention. As social media platforms become more data-driven and calculative, health interventions can respond to participants in more structured and customised ways. Thus, there is an emerging overlap between the participatory protocols of social media and the data-driven self-quantification enabled by apps and wearables such as Fitbit. This overlap is evident where social media interventions include elements of self-monitoring and customised data visualisation. Health intervention sector apps such as My Quit Buddy, for instance, encourage users to track the health and financial progress made from quitting smoking and to share their progress on social media platforms. Nevertheless, these technologies depart from other forms of health communication inasmuch as they enable the social production of expertise through practice.

Locating online alcohol consumption interventions

Robin Room (1988) uses the term 'action models' to discuss different strategies that have been used – across space and time – to address substance use problems. In this section, we identity the different 'action' models that have been used vis-à-vis alcohol consumption: 1) the temperance model, whereby the government implements alcohol regulations; 2) the responsible decision-making model, aimed at educating the consumer; 3) the lifestyle risk-reduction model, which blames the product for alcohol-related problems; and 4) the community-level alcohol intervention model, which situates social change at the local/communal level. We first provide an overview of each of these possible intervention models before arguing that the use of social media in alcohol intervention is generating a new form of action model based on the unique, evolving affordances of social media.

The temperance model focuses on convincing people that alcohol is dangerous and destructive. The model was prominent in the nineteenth century leading to a series of governmental controls on the manufacturing, selling, distribution and consumption of alcohol (Levine and Reinarman, 1991; Room, 1988). Evidence suggests that these initiatives resulted in a rise in crime, disability, violence, unwanted sex, pregnancies and death, leading the government to loosen alcohol regulations (Blocker, 2006; Hall, 2011; Huckle et al., 2012; Slack et al., 2009; Williams, 2001).

The responsible decision-making model focuses on educating consumers about what is individually and socially best for them (Wolburg, 2005). Through a variety of political, health and social marketing prescriptions about what is considered to be healthy, good and acceptable alcohol consumption, this approach aims to make individuals responsible for their personal alcohol consumption choices. This action model uses educational interventions, including advertising campaigns on responsible drinking and healthy lifestyle promotions. Focusing on information, this model assumes that alcohol consumption is a rational, cognitive decision linked to information processing, awareness and choice and thus positions the consumer as having the capacity to engage in self-regulation and risk-management behaviours (Wolburg, 2005). Such an approach nests comfortably within a neoliberal framework that responsibilises and moralises the drinking self, while remaining uncritical of the power and persuasiveness of corporate interests that drive alcohol consumption through the marketing and sale of alcohol products (Babor et al., 2010).

In contrast to the responsible decision-making model, the lifestyle risk-reduction model problematises alcohol and accounts for the social consequences of commercial marketing activities in promoting the societal perception that alcohol is a mundane, accessible, convenient, affordable and meaningful product. This model calls for the development of alcohol intervention programmes that consider 'the role the liquor industry plays in fostering drinking' (Goldberg, 1995: 365). Studies in this domain point to the encouraging effects of contemporary alcohol marketing on drinking behaviour (Hastings, 2007; Hastings et al., 2006; McCreanor et al., 2005; Smith and Foxcroft, 2009) and note the influence of the commercialisation of events such as Spring Break in the United States or Schoolies in Australia on heavy alcohol use (Grekin et al., 2007; Weitzman et al., 2003). The aim of the lifestyle risk reduction model is to refine the way individuals perceive alcohol consumption and influence alcohol-marketing techniques (Goldberg, 1995; Gordon et al., 2011).

Another approach to alcohol intervention, known as the community-level alcohol intervention model, examines the peer and social influences that constitute the community in which alcohol consumption practices are learned and perpetuated (Holder, 2003; Perkins and Berkowitz, 1986). Several studies inform the notion that alcohol consumption reinforces communal bonding and collective identity

(Griffin et al., 2009a; Griffin et al., 2009b; Holder, 2003; Lyons and Willott, 2008; Montemurro and McClure, 2005; Perkins and Berkowitz, 1986; Rolfe et al., 2009; Smith and Foxcroft, 2009). In these studies, alcohol consumption is a visible practice that differentiates between in-group drinkers versus out-group non-drinkers. Studies of non-drinkers support that young people who resist drinking face stigmatisation and exclusion from alcohol drinkers (Cherrier and Gurrieri, 2013, 2014). By considering the importance of community in shaping drinking behaviour, the community-level alcohol intervention model encourages local-level actions (Mistral et al., 2006). These actions can range from offering non-alcoholic beverages during communal gatherings to discouraging public events at which alcohol is a prominent activity (Casswell and Gilmore, 1989; Holder, 2003).

These approaches (Perkins and Berkowitz, 1986) focus either on the individual or on the environment. In the temperance model, the focus is on consumer choice perceived as problematic and needing to be controlled and sanctioned. Likewise, the responsible decision-making model aims at responsibilising the consumer. By contrast, the lifestyle-risk reduction and the community-level intervention models both focus on the environment – one targeting the alcohol industry and the other aimed at changing aspects of our social and cultural environment that foster alcohol consumption. Consequently, these models do not explicitly account for the individual and the environment that, in interaction, can facilitate or hinder changes in alcohol consumption. Redressing this, we use the relational theory of affordance to consider the ongoing interactions between a subject and their environment in the context of changes in alcohol consumption.

Affordance theory draws on an ecological perspective whereby the subject and their environment are viewed as mutually constitutive elements. Thus, affordance theory challenges the dualism of subject and world implicit in the other models we have discussed (Bloomfield et al., 2010; Costall, 1995).

Theoretical lens: social media affordances

'Affordance' is a relational concept that grasps the actionable possibilities between two complementary systems: the environment (including artificial ones) and an organism (whether a human or an animal) situated in it (Gibson, 1977, 1979). In contrast to representation, product symbolism and cognitive evaluation of abstract data guiding actions, affordances are what individuals notice an object can offer to them. Gibson (1977) explains that a graspable rigid object of moderate size and weight affords throwing whilst a large object needs a handle to afford grasping. Crucially, 'an affordance points both ways, to the environment, and to the observer' (Gibson, 1979: 129). This means that the same object can afford different actions to different subjects – a chair affords an adult to sit and not a young child who may not have the ability to sit. In this manner, objects have an invitation character embedded in and shaped by what the object is, the subject, and the situation the subject and the object are in (Sanders, 1997; Shaw and Turvey, 1981; Shaw et al., 1982).

Given the relational nature of affordances, the theory has had obvious attractions to several fields of social science. Work on design has shown that affordances of ordinary objects are linked to cultural conventions, learned behaviours, and physical, logical and cultural behavioural constraints; a cursor that is shaped like an arrow affords clicking but it is impossible to move a cursor outside of the screen area and all users understand that by dragging the scroll bar downward they will see the rest of the page that is 'off screen' (Norman, 1988). This perspective leans on the user's experiences and goals in interaction with the object that affords possibilities for actions.

The theory has also migrated to social media research to consider the action possibilities called forth by the use of specific technology to a perceiving subject (Brzozowski et al., 2009; Hutchby, 2001; Leonardi, 2011; Majchrzak et al., 2013; Treem and Leonardi, 2012). In this field, social media technology is understood as an artefact that makes certain types of behaviour possible, and not others. Treem and Leonardi (2012) have identified four basic affordances of social media to social organisation: behaviour visibility, persistent conversation, editability and associations enabling community building/access to expertise. They argue that collaborative software or teleconferencing offer limited visibility and associations, email affords persistence and editability, but only social media portrays all four affordances. Other researchers focusing on employees' engagement in knowledge-sharing conversations note that social media affords metavoicing (potential to provide collective feedback through commenting, voting, rating of content), triggered attending (automatic notifications of changes within content to guide participation), network-informed associating (linking to others to enhance participation and engagement) and generative role-taking (emergent role to facilitate dialogue) (Majchrzak et al., 2013). Concerned with the current optimistic approach to social media and the 'ideology of openness' in organisational knowledge sharing, Gibbs et al. (2013) identify opposing affordances: visibility/invisibility (enables remote co-workers to be visible but also to hide or avoid being disturbed), engagement/disengagement (enables quick interactions but can be distracting) and sharing/control (enables knowledge sharing but is subject to leaks). Their research emphasises that using social media may be challenging and requires particular strategic thinking (Kaplan and Haenlein, 2010).

The use of the theory of affordances within social media has two main shortcomings: first, studies on social media affordances rarely distinguish among types of social media. Yet, social media differ from Web 2.0 and User Generated Content, and includes various types such as collaborative projects (i.e. Wikipedia or Wiki), blogs, social networking (i.e. Facebook or MySpace), virtual game worlds and virtual social worlds (Kaplan and Haenlein, 2010). Social media are heterogeneous, enabling a range of specific actions and thus differing in their types of affordances (Hutchby, 2001). A second shortcoming is the focus on social media affordances within social organisation, which deals with the coordination of actions of groups of people internal to an entity (Strong et al., 2014). Yet, social media are increasingly used within the public domain to foster behavioural change where external interaction amongst unknown users is prevalent.

Understanding alcohol consumption interventions and the affordances of social media: the case of Hello Sunday Morning

Hello Sunday Morning (HSM) is an online health intervention that has developed in iterative stages since 2009. The project began when a young advertising creative, Chris Raine, founded an individual blog to document a year not drinking. The blog was an observational account of drinking culture from the view of a young Australian male. Raine attracted a large readership and towards the end of the year moved into a second iteration when he invited peers to join him in a similar self-experiment. This iteration gained momentum predominantly via word of mouth as Raine personally invited a small group of peers to 'do' a HSM and these individuals, in turn, invited others. During this period, a community of bloggers bonded, and HSM crystalised as a social movement, around the practice of reading and commenting on each other's blogs regularly. This involved frequent deliberation with each other about the protocols for 'doing a HSM' such as whether a participant had to be abstinent from alcohol, for how long, whether they must blog, whether they should set goals, and whether a 'slip up' by consuming alcohol meant they had to start the period of abstinence again. Thus, HSM emerged from online peer-to-peer deliberation, as an endogenously social activity, defined by a set of socially negotiated online and offline practices that simultaneously defined the community.

The practices that solidified HSM as a social movement in its second iteration were operationalised in its third, as HSM developed a bespoke social media platform organised around user profiles and blogs. During this phase, Hello Sunday Morning was organised around inviting participants to undertake a three or six month period of abstinence from alcohol, set some personal goals and reflect on their efforts to change on a personal blog. HSM gradually became more structured as it transitioned in scale from a largely peer-to-peer exchange, to a platform hosted on generically available blogging software, to an organisation manifest as a tailored platform based on a number of unique protocols that prescribed participation in specific ways. These included: a menu of set goals for participants to choose from, direction for participants in nominating a set period for a HSM (three, six or twelve months), and automatic invitations for participants to 'check in' each week to log their progress, well-being and record any 'slip ups'. HSM also iteratively developed tools aimed at boosting engagement on the site such as customising feeds of blog content so that participants saw posts by users who were similar to them (Carah et al., 2015a).

At the same time as HSM was beginning its transformation into an organisation and lifestyle brand, it began to focus on evaluating its intervention on the basis of the qualitative expressions of participants. It purposefully resisted calls to specifically evaluate quantitative change in alcohol consumption. This decision was driven by several interrelated factors. Most significant was HSM's emergence from a non-clinical setting and its emphasis on wanting to inspire 'cultural change' rather than seeing itself as a clinical intervention. It was not so much interested in how much people drank but whether or not people understood and reflected on why they drank. Over time, a number of factors have led HSM towards evaluating the alcohol consumption of participants. Some of these include: increasing engagement with the alcohol behaviour change sector that viewed its legitimacy through the lens of consumption change, demands from funding agencies that expected evaluation to document consumption change, and the emergence of self-quantification as a routine practice on social media platforms. By 2015 HSM invited participants to complete alcohol consumption and well-being questionnaires at sign-up and via monthly check-ins. It launched a purpose-built mobile app in 2015 that prompts weekly check-ins and offers participants a customised visualisation of change in alcohol consumption and well-being.

To date, studies have examined the blog posts of HSM participants as a rich record of their reflections on alcohol consumption, cultural and behaviour change (Carah, et al., 2015a; Fry, 2014). These studies each illustrate a progressive change on participants' blogs as they establish new cultural practices and identities related to alcohol consumption. Carah et al. (2015b) profiled the demographics and quantitative alcohol consumption of participants in Hello Sunday Morning and illustrated that HSM attracts participants who are more likely to be female, younger and riskier drinkers than treatment-seeking populations. The HSM platform enables a mode of enacting identity which de-centres alcohol by virtue of the process of collective blogging on a non-alcohol named website. Participants set out to change their relationship with alcohol, but that does not mean the content they produce is only or even primarily a reflection on alcohol consumption. By setting non-alcohol-related goals, much of their content enacts an alternative identity. This enactment is activist because of the way in which it is publically performed via blogs and social media platforms (Carah et al., 2015a).

The study

To better understand the possible benefits of using social media to enact behavioural change in alcohol consumption, we consider blog affordances in the context of an alcohol intervention programme orchestrated by Hello Sunday Morning.

Blogs are types of websites that display dated entries in reverse chronological order (Kaplan and Haenlein, 2010). One particular feature of blogs is that they are usually managed by one person but provide opportunities for interaction through added comments by others. This aspect enables us to capture blog affordances by considering what and how users communicate through HSM blogs. For this study, we selected 1254 posts from the ten most active bloggers from 2011 to 2013 (see Table 11.1). The posts were selected from a spreadsheet of all posts to the website provided by HSM. The spreadsheet linked each blog post to categorical data such as a user ID, demographic data and date of post. This enabled researchers to rank participants by number of posts. For the purposes of this analysis we excluded the blog posts by the HSM founder Chris Raine.

HSM blogs provide both visual (icon, colour scheme, tiles, images, typeface or videos) and textual data. For the purposes of this study, we focused on how and why participants' communicated using HSM. Thus, we selected and solely

Table 11.1 Informants

Bloggers' Pseudonyms	# blogs	Gender
Lorraine	245	Female
Cory	222	Male
Patrick	137	Male
Danny	116	not provided
Kelly	108	Female
Mary	107	Female
Patricia	87	Female
Clara	79	Female
Karl	78	Male
Aris	75	not provided

analysed textual expression using guidelines provided by Miles and Huberman (1994). Given the large amount of data, the blog posts were first read, and summarised for topic covered and the way issues around alcohol were framed. Next, the blog posts were reread along with their summaries, and inductively coded to identify and label emerging blog affordances. Subsequent readings entailed selective coding, to identify and label the major emerging blog affordances and their actualisation. While we did not constrain ourselves to an a priori coding scheme, the emergent affordances identified included those properties articulated by Hopkins (2013) including anonymity, disembodiment and interactivity.

Findings: social media affordances in the context of HSM blog participation

For the most part, the blog posts were a reflection of everyday happenings and events that accompanied the process of discovering and experiencing what it means to be sober. Catchphrases (such as one's changing relationship with alcohol) and the use of specific language (including 'sober,' 'sobriety', 'free', 'constructive' that were explicitly contrasted with 'self-sabotage', 'poison', 'binge drinking', 'alcoholism' or 'drunk') shows a high degree of reflexivity around alcohol use and abstinence, scattered among mundane everyday descriptions of life.

The apparent development of bloggers' reflexivity on their alcohol consumption, through a dialectic reformulation of the self as transitioning from 'alcoholic/ drunk' to 'clean/sober', indicated the dynamic engagement between blog user and blog technology, and thus pointed to the existence of blog affordances guiding reflexivity. Below we discuss the main blog affordances we identified – accessibility, anonymity and interactivity – and how these were constantly modulated in unique ways in relation to each individual's particular goals and abilities. Consequently, we identified further types of blog affordances which we labelled: self-understanding, self-talk and self-commitment. This highlights that blog affordances for behaviour change are not given by the blog's technological properties per se but are co-dependent on the blog users and blog technologies.

Accessibility and self-understanding

In our data, bloggers mentioned typing late at night or during the early hours of the morning. Their physical location ranged from typing at home to blogging in a bar or even using their mobile phone to type whilst being outside on the street or in a park. For example, Cory below describes a scene on the dance floor:

> Cory: I'm currently at a dance club, making a few observations. Firstly, looking at how people are talking with each other, there seems to be this invisible boundary when you have a drink in your hand. I guess we feel safe as long as there's glass between us. I look upon the dance floor at people who are only half drunk. They look timid and their facial expressions tell me they need to be drunk to enjoy themselves. They are dancing like they were put on the dance floor by someone who has a giant mouse and they have clicked and dragged them on there in a SIMS game.

As portrayed here, and in many other similar posts created outside of the home, blogs afford the possibility to write and share information at anytime and anywhere. Cory writes whilst being at a dance club at night, and shares his experience of being sober and observing practices of drinking, dancing and people's interactions. By enabling instant (textual) recording of alcohol-related events, a prevalent blog affordance is its accessibility, that is, the invitation to write at any time and virtually anywhere (Hopkins, 2013). Blogs are characterised by instant text publishing for one single author, a reverse chronological ordered archiving system, and a feedback mechanism where readers can comment on particular posts. However, our data adds that blogs' accessibility, in the context of changes in alcohol consumption, affords the possibility for consciousness-raising and self-understanding. Striking to Cory's experience of blogging at a nightclub is his acute observation and deep reflection on the surroundings. He focuses on details of the situation, such as physical mannerisms and facial expressions, which make up the common drinking patterns and social interactions in a dance club. The process of blogging about the activities and occurrences in the dance club triggers acute attentiveness and information processing about the objects such as glasses, people and their lived experience of alcohol consumption, leading Cory to construct analogies between being drunk on the dance floor and being clicked and dragged in a SIMS game. When we consider Cory's particular circumstances, motivations and experiences, what becomes apparent is the blog's accessibility affordance is actualised alongside an affordance for *self-understanding*. Researchers have discussed that individuals are most likely to notice others' behaviour and judge others on dimensions that are relevant to them (Markus et al., 1985). In effect, we see that in the act of writing about others, Cory mainly provides an internal dialogue about his feelings in response to what he sees. In this manner, Cory is experiencing himself via blogging about others' experiences. This becomes evident when we consider the flow of Cory's posts towards deeper inquiries around individuals' interactions and how he, himself, has been behaving in social settings, and most particularly with women, as illustrated in the post below:

> I was thinking about how incredible it was to just bounce from group to group, throwing a bit of chitchats interaction then cruise onto the next one. The real problem is we have actually only learned how to communicate in these situations WITH alcohol. Even on a chemical level it's like our brains have been programed to function to only socialise with new people WITH alcohol. [...] How it impacts on my life is that I end up 'tuning' more [women] than I get to know women for who they are. And secondly, it has sometimes put my level of attention on a pretty girl over friends and family. [...] I need to practice letting go of perceived opportunities rather than snatching at them as though it will be my last.

Through repeated visits to the dance club, Cory continued to reflect on clubbing, alcohol consumption and social interactions. The accessibility of blogging enabled Cory's active reflection on himself in relation to his surroundings. Subsequent posts culminated in 'personal revelation' (Cory) as his acute attentiveness to social interactions in a club led to the realisation that alcohol consumption impinges on a process of self-understanding and he started to question how normalised alcohol consumption practices had an 'impact on my life'. This turn to the self through immediate writing has been noted in psychological studies (Wright, 2009).

Self-understanding affordances further entangled with blog *accessibility* affordances for Clara, whose night-time blogging practices led to numerous self-discoveries as when she explains: 'in the last three months I have gotten even better at identifying my strengths and weaknesses'. Clara's and other bloggers' posts show that emergent self-understanding is integrated in writing using HSM blogs at anytime and anywhere. This actualisation of the accessibility creates an opportunity to further self-understanding, such as being sensitive to alcogenic environments, thus creating the possibility to develop new skills and identities in relation to alcohol consumption.

Anonymity and self-talk

Our bloggers used weblog names, thus limiting their online exposure by remaining anonymous and relatively unidentifiable. Moreover, they often opted to conceal their physical location when describing an outside event or occurrence. This was most evident when we considered Patrick's 137 posts, representing 25,187 words, during which he never disclosed his profession, place of employment, friends' names and any other personal details that could reveal his identity. Writing text on a computer, too, permits anonymity because of the impossibility of identifying someone by their handwriting. Crucially, anonymity is not to be associated with privacy as blogs, once posted, are available to the public and cannot be deleted (at least not easily).

Further consideration of anonymity led us to view anonymous blogging as not solely an affordance picked up from the properties of blog technologies. Rather, anonymous blogging served as a means to achieve what we name here as *self-talk*. In our context, self-talk represents the bloggers' internal dialogue of the self to the self or internal monologue actualised during their acts of writing on the HSM blogging site. Self-talk is made explicit by Patrick who explains: 'I wake up this morning I start the negative self talk, telling me I am useless and pathetic.' Active bloggers on the HSM site disclosed some of their innermost stories of depression, uncertainties and fears, and struggles with alcohol.

With self-talk, we capture bloggers offering both personal details and opinions as well as evaluations on what they do, feel and think in their lives, revealing their doubts and anxieties, and also accomplishments and self-realisations. These self-talk posts are akin to an inner voice, at times positive and at others negative, something exemplified in Patrick's post below:

> I am becoming more aware of my anxiety, I'm better able to look at myself and see that I am at fault and not everyone around me, which is my usual reaction. It's them, not me. I'm still struggling with everything, friends, moods, work, etc. I think it's going to be a long time by societies standards for me to be capable of working properly, socialising easily, and being able to not over react over small things. But that's good news, I can at least see that I can get a decent life.

In this post, Patrick exposes a socially unacceptable aspect of his self, as incapable of working and socialising according to normative standards. On the one hand, we see how anonymity enables Patrick to have a voice of his own and freely give and take account for his subjectivity, thus revealing his vulnerable side, an aspect of the self that may otherwise be hidden. This behaviour is consistent with previous studies that discuss how anonymity and distance from sources of comment are thought to facilitate self-talk (Morin, 1993). On the other hand, Patrick describes a gradual process of becoming aware of his anxiety emerging through practices of blog writing. At the same time, he becomes aware of an alternative and preferred life-course, that is, the possibilities to 'get a decent life'. Yet, this blog affordance is not, in itself, sufficient to cascade into self-talk affordance. As Bloomfield et al. (2010) emphasise in their study of the affordances of technical objects, affordances emerge as situated, ongoing accomplishments. For Patrick, it is the personal accomplishment of becoming more reflexive and aware of his anxiety entangled with practices of anonymous self-talk made possible by the HSM blogging website. In this respect, the anonymity affordance is not solely linked to the property of blog technology but emerges in interaction with our bloggers' goals and capacities for self-talk, which, for example, helped Patrick 'become more aware of my anxiety'.

Our data also reveals the limitations of blog affordances. To continue Patrick's example, we note that blog affordances do not impel activity:

> I've had writers block lately. Again, I am experiencing motivational issues. So I've not been blogging how I've been feeling, because I can't be bothered and don't have the desire.

Patrick's post above highlights that actualising the blog self-talk affordance is not an immutable property determined by blogging technology, but rather emerges through human activity requiring motivations and desires. In this respect, blog affordances are clearly situated and emerge in relation to our bloggers' motivations, capacities and practices to write on the HSM blogging website.

Interactivity and self-commitment

Studies note the influence of blogging on users' social interactions and discuss how blogs enable their visitors to interact with others via the comments and blog visitor traces in server logs (Hopkins, 2013). Our analysis supports that groups of bloggers use this affordance to relate with one another, often leaving comments on blogs and referring to other bloggers' discussions in their posts. Comments on others' blogs appeared frequently, with sentences such as 'this is an interesting point', 'I learnt a lot from this post' and descriptions such as 'valuable' and 'great reading' often used. For example, Lorraine who 'always read the new Feed each morning and evening and get really chuffed when I see how well you are going', posted:

> HSM is full of people sharing love and encouragement. I wrote about headaches yesterday and received so many lovely helpful comments.

She later reinforces:

> I was thinking yesterday how much I love all you HSMers. It is funny how I can feel love for people I have only virtually met.

Kelly, too, is one blogger who often tuned to others' posts:

> [blogger name] had an interesting post last week, It's got me thinking that I want to know what I used to tell myself to justify why it was okay to drink like I did. [...] [Blogger name] posted a great poem today; It's got me thinking ... it's time to get back outside my comfort zone and become the successful person I was. Thanks team. This HSM journey sure is a bizarre ride. I appreciate you giving me a wake up call!

Kelly's blog points to the affordance for interactivity. Reading others' poems, for example, could trigger sensations, feelings and emotions that catalyse thinking about the self. In this exchange, the blogs' interactivity is modulated by Kelly's capacity for committing to improving the self. In taking into account others' poems posted on the HSM site, she pledges to learn about herself both from her participation with the HSM community and from temporal alcohol abstinence. This is explicit when we consider that Kelly not only thanks the poet but also thanks the entire HSM team for a 'wake up call' to improve the self, which, through the practice of blog-writing, actualises a self-commitment 'to get back outside my comfort zone and become the successful person I was'. By self-commitment, we understand our bloggers' discussions around their accountability, answerability and active involvement in improving the self and its relationship with alcohol consumption.

Blogging's affordance for interactivity and its potential to cascade into the affordance for self-commitment is explicit in Lorraine's post:

> I have to make time to make contact with the HSM website. That is non negotiable because I feel that putting my thoughts and actions down in writing enables me to make healthy choices regarding myself and my strategies for when I feel the urge to have a drink.

By blogging and connecting with others in the virtual space, Lorraine finds the strength to change habits and lifestyle. Clear to her post is that blogging is vital to self-commitment and even when she is unsure as to what to post, she nevertheless sits, writes and posts as she explains below:

> Sometimes I sit at my computer and wonder what I am going to blog about. That is what I am doing now. So I will just say it from my experience and thoughts. Had a good sleep last night. It is very hot and humid in [location] at the moment so my air con is getting well used.

Throughout her posts, Lorraine often discusses her day-to-day activities, her relationships with her two daughters and her granddaughter, or even the weather as described in her post above. Even though writing about the weather or mundane activities seems entirely unrelated to alcohol consumption, her posts still have a function in keeping someone 'in contact' with the community and thus prompting reflection and reinforcement of alcohol-related goals and commitment to curb her consumption. That is, placing the self in dialogue with others via the interactivity of blogging – reading and commenting on others' posts – enlarges the scope of commitment to improving the self and actively tackling personal issues around alcohol consumption, something explicit in Cory's blog below:

> Before I get into this post, I just want to say that writing these next three blogs has been one of the hardest, soul baring things I have ever had to do. Especially because I know so many people are going to read it. This really puts the spotlight on my psychological dysfunctionality (both past and present) but it is something that I need to get out. I am doing this as a commitment to the process of this year and also as a commitment to myself. I have set the intention to not have any psychological conditioning holding me back by the end of this year, so I guess now is as good a time as any to purge that which is holding me back.

Cory's post above is clearly about opening up, digging deep into personal issues and making himself vulnerable. Blogging's affordance for interactivity plays a big role in this process. In effect, Cory is directly addressing the others. Knowing that many will read his post, he warns them on his current state. The interaction with others in the virtual space nourishes a commitment to the self to open up and be vulnerable, to improve life and self-concept, and to ultimately establish a desirable relation with alcohol.

Conclusion

In this study, we sought to contribute to the understanding of the use of blogs in behavioural change interventions in the context of alcohol consumption. We used the theoretical lens of affordances. Previous studies have discussed basic blog affordances including storage, reduplication, asynchronous communication, multimedia, modularity and hyperlinking (Hopkins, 2013). These affordances capture the components of the blog medium itself, its capacity to hyperlink and to connect to other websites, webpages and the blog database. To these intrinsic affordances, Hopkins (2013) adds emerging blog affordances that arise from the interaction of the components of the blog: anonymity, disembodiment, accessibility, personalisation and interactivity.

Our analysis of 1254 posts from ten active HSM bloggers from 2011 to 2013 highlights that the interaction between blog users and blog technologies create a particular experience that unfolds into reflexivity of self on self around alcohol consumption and its abstinence. All our bloggers' posts gradually evolved to a more reflexive self, including growing a clearer perception of strengths, weaknesses, beliefs, motivations and emotions, tied with a reflection on other people's behaviour and societal norms, values and rituals around alcohol consumption (Carah et al., 2015a; Cherrier and Gurrieri, 2014). This meant drawing oneself out of a problematic relationship with alcohol consumption, breaking with unwanted alcohol habits and rituals, and getting into contact with one's feelings, thinking and daily practices. Through the platform of collective blogging, HSM provided an opportunity for participants to disengage from an alcohol-laden lifestyle-identity, and engage with a new kind community – one that afforded an opportunity to reproduce one's identity such that alcohol was less important (see Carah et al., 2015a).

Analysing how bloggers' posts changed overtime highlighted how blog affordances for accessibility, anonymity and interactivity were tied up with subsequent blog affordances for self-understanding, self-talk and self-commitment, fostering reflexivity around alcohol consumption. We thus propose a framing of blog affordances for reflexivity around alcohol consumption as cascades of affordances (Michael, 2000) that emerge from the interaction with HSM users and blog technology in the context of experiencing temporal alcohol abstinence.

First, we saw that self-understanding, self-talking and self-commitment were paramount to a process of becoming reflexive on one's alcohol consumption practices and social circumstances. These qualities were not pre-given and absolute. Rather, they existed in constant reformation, emerging in relation to blog affordances for accessibility, anonymity and interactivity. The implications of this for using blogs in the context of alcohol interventions is that they can facilitate beneficial forms of reflexivity around alcohol consumption but only in the presence of other blog affordances; in this case, accessibility, anonymity and interactivity tied to self-understanding, self-talk and self-commitment.

Our findings have important implications for developing strategies aimed at enacting behaviour change around alcohol consumption. As noted previously, alcohol interventions are multiple, ranging from the temperance model, the responsible decision-making model, the lifestyle risk-reduction model and the community-level alcohol intervention model. Common to these models is that they reproduce a dualism between human and non-human actions. Seeking to overcome the dichotomy inherent in these models, we propose a conceptual framework for behavioural change based on understanding how people make use of social media and how social media technology facilitates usage through the theory of affordances. Hello Sunday Morning is one organisation that has made use of social media to reconfigure alcohol consumption in Australia. Yet, paramount to the success of blogs in alcohol intervention are the users' interaction with technology and how this interaction actualises blogs affordances for accessibility, anonymity and interactivity, and cascades into blogs affordances for self-understanding, self-talk and self-commitment. We suggest organisations wishing to use blogging as a means to enact behaviour change facilitate such a cascade of blog affordances. On the one hand, the possibilities for blogging sites to afford accessibility, anonymity and interactivity to users should be reinforced. On the other hand, practices of self-understanding, self-talk and self-commitment should be encouraged. This may be achieved by organising weekly small group virtual discussions that facilitate interactivity, through pre-defined bloggers' names that guarantee anonymity, and/or through easy smartphone or tablet applications that foster accessibility.

One limitation of the approach taken here is that it does not analyse non-textual elements of blog affordances; for example, how website architecture, aesthetics and functionality facilitates communication. These facets of blog affordances are an important area for future research.

References

Babor, T., Caetano, R., Casswell, S., Edwards, G., Giesbrecht, N., Graham, K., Grube, J., Hill, L., Holder, H., Homel, R., Livingston, M., Osterberg, E., Rehm, J., Room, R., and Rossow, I. (2010). *Alcohol: No Ordinary Commodity Research and Public Policy* (2nd edn). Oxford: Oxford University Press.

Blocker, J. (2006). Did prohibition really work? Alcohol prohibition as a public health innovation. *American Journal of Public Health*, 96(2), 233–243.

Bloomfield, B., Latham, Y., and Vurdubakis, T. (2010). Bodies, technologies and action possibilities: When is an affordance? *Sociology*, 44(3), 415–433.

Brown, R., and Gregg, M. (2012). The pedagogy of regret: Facebook, binge drinking and young women. *Continuum: Journal of Media and Cultural Studies*, 26(3), 357–369.

Brzozowski, M., Sandholm, T., and Hogg, T. (2009). *Effects of Feedback and Peer Pressure on Contributions to Enterprise Social Media.* Palo Alto, CA: Hewlett-Packard Laboratories.

Carah, N., Meurk, C., and Angus, D. (2015a). Online self-expression and experimentation as 'reflectivism': Using text analytics to examine the participatory forum Hello Sunday Morning. *Health,* published online before print 27 July, doi: 10.1177/1363459315596799.

Carah, N., Meurk, C., and Hall, W. (2015b). Profiling Hello Sunday Morning: Who are the participants? *International Journal of Drug Policy, 26*(2), 214–216.

Casswell, S., and Gilmore, L. (1989). An evaluated community action project on alcohol. *Journal of Studies on Alcohol, 50*(4), 339–346.

Cherrier, H., and Gurrieri, L. (2013). Anti-consumption choices performed in a drinking culture: Normative struggles and repairs. *Journal of Macromarketing, 33*(3), 232–244.

Cherrier, H., and Gurrieri, L. (2014). Framing social marketing as a system of interaction: A neo-institutional approach to alcohol abstinence. *Journal of Marketing Management, 30*(7–8), 607–633.

Costall, A. (1995). Socializing affordances. *Theory and Psychology, 5*(4), 467–481.

Fry, M. (2014). Rethinking social marketing: Towards a sociality of consumption. *Journal of Social Marketing, 4*(3), 210–222.

Gibbs, J., Rozaidi, N., and Eisenberg, J. (2013). Overcoming the 'ideology of openness': Probing the affordances of social media for organizational knowledge sharing. *Journal of Computer-Mediated Communication, 19*(1), 102–120.

Gibson, J. (1977). The theory of affordances. In R. Shaw and J. Bransford (Eds.), *Perceiving, Acting, and Knowing. Toward an Ecological Psychology* (pp. 67–82). Hillsdale: NJ: Lawrence Erlbaum Associates.

Gibson, J. (1979). *The Ecological Approach to Visual Perception.* Boston: Houghton Mifflin.

Goldberg, M. (1995). Social marketing: Are we fiddling while Rome burns? *Journal of Consumer Psychology, 4*(1), 347–370.

Gordon, R., Harris, F., Marie MacKintosh, A., and Moodie, C. (2011). Assessing the cumulative impact of alcohol marketing on young people's drinking: Cross-sectional data findings. *Addiction Research and Theory, 19*(1), 66–75.

Grekin, E., Sher, K., and Krull, J. (2007). College spring break and alcohol use: Effects of spring break activity. *Journal of Studies on Alcohol and Drugs, 68*(5), 681–688.

Griffin, C., Bengry-Howell, A., Hackley, C., Mistral, W., and Szmigin, I. (2009a). 'Every time I do it I absolutely annihilate myself': Loss of (self-)consciousness and loss of memory in young people's drinking narratives. *Sociology, 43*(3), 457–476.

Griffin, C., Szmigin, I., Hackley, C., Mistral, W., and Bengry-Howell, A. (2009b). The allure of belonging: Young people's drinking practices and collective identification. In M. Wetherell (Ed.), *Identity in the 21st Century: New Trends in Changing Times* (pp. 213–230). London: Palgrave.

Hall, S. (2011). The neo-liberal revolution. *Cultural Studies, 25*(6), 705–728.

Hastings, G. (2007). *Social Marketing: Why Should the Devil Have All the Best Tunes?* Oxford: Elsevier.

Hastings, G., Anderson, S., Cooke, E., and Gordon, R. (2006). Alcohol marketing and young people's drinking: A review of the research. *Journal of Public Health Policy, 26*(3), 296–311.

Holder, H. (2003). *Alcohol and the Community: A Systems Approach to Prevention.* Cambridge: Cambridge University Press.

Hopkins, J. (2013). Assembling affordances: Towards a theory of relational affordances. *Selected Papers of Internet Research 14*. Denver, USA. http://spir.aoir.org/index.php/spir/article/view/783

Huckle, T., Pledger, M., and Casswell, S. (2012). Increases in typical quantities consumed and alcohol-related problems during a decade of liberalising alcohol policy. *Journal of Studies on Alcohol and Drugs, 73*(1), 53–62.

Hutchby, I. (2001). Technologies, texts and affordances. *Sociology, 35*(2), 441–456.

Kaplan, A., and Haenlein, M. (2010). Users of the world, unite! The challenges and opportunities of Social Media. *Business Horizons, 53*(1), 59–68.

Leonardi, P. (2011). When flexible routines meet flexible technologies: Affordance, constraint, and imbrication of human and material agencies. *Management Information Systems Quarterly, 35*(1), 147–167.

Levine, H., and Reinarman, C. (1991). From prohibition to regulation: Lessons from alcohol policy for drug policy. *The Milbank Quarterly, 69*(3, Part 1), 461–494.

Lyons, A., and Willott, S. (2008). Alcohol consumption, gender identities and women's changing social positions. *Sex Roles, 59*, 694–712.

Majchrzak, A., Faraj, S., Kane, G., and Azad, B. (2013). The contradictory influence of social media affordances on online communal knowledge sharing. *Journal of Computer Mediated Communication, 19*(1), 38–55.

Markus, H., Smith, J., and Moreland, R. (1985). Role of the self-concept in the perception of others. *Journal of Personality and Social Psychology, 49*(6), 1494.

McCreanor, T., Lyons, A., Griffin, C., Goodwin, I., Moewaka Barnes, H., and Hutton, F. (2013). Youth drinking cultures, social networking and alcohol marketing: Implications for public health. *Critical Public Health, 23*(1), 110–120.

McCreanor, T., Moewaka Barnes, H., Gregory, A., Kaiwai, H., and Borell, S. (2005). Consuming identities: Alcohol marketing and the comodification of youth. *Addiction Research and Theory, 13*(6), 579–590.

Michael, M. (2000). These boots are made for walking...: Mundane technology, the body and human-environment relations. *Body and Society, 6*(3–4), 107–126.

Miles, M., and Huberman, A. (1994). *Qualitative Data Analysis* (2nd edn). London: Sage.

Mistral, W., Velleman, L., Templeton, L., and Mastache, C. (2006). Local action to prevent alcohol problems: Is the UK Community Alcohol Prevention Programme the best solution? *International Journal of Drug Policy, 17*, 278–284.

Montemurro, B., and McClure, B. (2005). Changing gender norms for alcohol consumption: Social drinking and lowered inhibitions at bachelorette parties. *Sex Roles, 52*(5–6), 279–288.

Morin, A. (1993). Self-talk and self-awareness: On the nature of the relation. *Journal of Mind and Behavior, 14*, 223–234.

Norman, D. (1988). *The Psychology of Everyday Things*. New York: Basic Books.

Perkins, W., and Berkowitz, A. (1986). Perceiving the community norms of alcohol use among students: Some research implications for campus alcohol education programming. *International Journal of the Addictions, 21*(9–10), 961–976.

Rolfe, A., Orford, J., and Dalton, S. (2009). Women, alcohol and femininity: A discourse analysis of women heavy drinkers' accounts. *Journal of Health Psychology, 14*(2), 326–335.

Room, R. (1988). The dialectic of drinking in Australian life: From the Rum Corps to the wine column. *Drug and Alcohol Review, 7*(4), 413–421.

Sanders, J. (1997). An ontology of affordances. *Ecological Psychology, 9*(1), 97–112.

Shaw, R., and Turvey, M. (1981). Coalitions as models for ecosystems: A realist perspective on perceptual organization. In M. Kubovy and J. Pomerantz (Eds.), *Perceptual Organization* (pp. 343–415). Hillsdale, NJ: Lawrence Erlbaum Associates.

Shaw, R., Turvey, M., and Mace, W. (1982). Ecology psychology: The consequence of a commitment to realism. In W. Weimer and D. Palermo (Eds.), *Cognition and the Symbolic Processes II* (pp. 159–226). Hillsdale, NJ: Lawrence Erlbaum Associates.

Slack, A., Nana, G., Webster, M., Stokes, F., and Wu, J. (2009). *Costs of Harmful Alcohol and Other Drug Use* (Report to: Ministry of Health and ACC), July. Wellington, NZ: Business and Economic Research Limited (BERL).

Smith, L., and Foxcroft, D. (2009). The effect of alcohol advertising, marketing and portrayal on drinking behaviour in young people: Systematic review of prospective cohort studies. *BMC Public Health*, 9(51), 1–11. www.biomedcentral.com/1471–2458/1479/1451

Strong, D., Volkoff, O., Johnson, S., Pelletier, L., Tulu, B., Bar-On, I., Trudel, J., and Garber, L. (2014). A theory of organization-EHR affordance actualization. *Journal of the Association for Information Systems*, 15(2), 53–85.

Treem, J., and Leonardi, P. (2012). Social media use in organizations – exploring the affordances of visibility, editability, persistence, and association. *Communication Yearbook*, 36, 143–189.

Weitzman, E., Nelson, T., and Wechsler, H. (2003). Taking up binge drinking in college: The influences of person, social group, and environmment. *Journal of Adolescent Health*, 32(1), 26–35.

Williams, P. (Ed.). (2001). *Alcohol, Young Persons and Violence*. Australian Institute of Criminology Research and Public Policy Series No. 35. Canberra: Australian Institute of Criminology.

Wolburg, J. (2005). Misplaced marketing: How responsible are 'responsible' drinking campaigns for preventing alcohol abuse? *Journal of Consumer Marketing*, 22(4), 176–177.

Wright, J. (2009). Dialogical journal writing as 'self-therapy':'I matter'. *Counselling and Psychotherapy Research*, 9(4), 234–240.

11 Regulating social media

Reasons not to ask the audience

Andy Ruddock

Introduction

It is tempting to think that social media have unleashed a panoply of unimaginable risks into society. Extremism, violence and all manner of cybercrime threats fill the headlines. As for alcohol, the already complex business of addressing marketing power is further complicated by consumer-generated social media content, linking alcohol with fun and tradition (Alhabash et al., 2015; Carah et al., 2014; Nicholls, 2012; Ruddock, 2012, 2013; Uzunoğlu and Öksüz, 2014). As other contributions to this anthology establish, the identities and well-being of young people are frequently integral to discussions of these dynamics; brewers, distillers and retail outlets adeptly create seductive social fantasies, blending drinking, pleasure and identity. This chapter extends this focus to the policy realm: does alcohol marketing influence how people participate in the regulation of their media environment, and how does 'youth' figure here?

These questions access a historical narrative about media influence and consumer culture. To ask how the cocktail of social media and alcohol affect youth identity is to interrogate the basic dynamics of common, global symbolic environments, driven by commercial logics that infiltrate social thought. Discussions about the popularisation of drinking through social media channel earlier observations on how media advanced consumer culture. In the 1950s, Hungarian American scholar George Gerbner founded the 'Cultural Indicators Project' (CIP) to address this process. Over six decades, Gerbner demonstrated that however much technology and times changed, global media relied on a simple 'story' about consumption and happiness. The grand effect of this trend was to inculcate audiences into accepting consumer ideology as common sense. Much of his thinking, in this regard, focused on alcohol and young people.

Gerbner remains relevant for two reasons: first, present-day research has returned to the idea of cultural indicators as a method to make sense of intoxicating cultures; and second, Gerbner's ideas relate questions of youth, social media and alcohol to broader rhythms in the political consequences of media systems. This is important because analysing how people complain about alcohol marketing offers insights on bigger issues of access and participation in media culture.

When making sense of youth, social media and drinking, it pays to understand how new questions reflect established concerns. Gerbner's CIP presents a lucid framework for doing so. This chapter makes this argument through the following steps. First, it explores how social media have complicated the already difficult matter of conceiving the relationship between commercial messages and alcohol abuse. Second, it explains the value of a CIP perspective, by showing how Gerbner's late twentieth-century work on alcohol and drugs contextualised 'risk' in the political climate of global commercial media culture, predicting many of the issues that young people now face when it comes to making sense of alcohol messages.

This review leads to the hypothesis that the main 'effect' of online marketing is to naturalise the language of consumer culture as the 'normal' argot of identity and pleasure. As a test, I examine public involvement in UK advertising regulation. The objective of this section is to use CIP methods to find evidence of restrictions that advertising, marketing and regulatory frameworks build around public debate on media and well-being. Gerbner and researchers on social media and alcohol share the view that consumerism has purloined expression. Griffiths and Casswell (2010) observe that alcohol companies have adeptly used social media to get young people to share their drinking experiences in words and pictures. This has built an 'intoxigenic' culture that helps normalise heavy drinking. Their work reflects the central CIP theme: media industries encourage people to accept the basic structures and logic of consumer culture as the common sense upon which society operates. This study asks if the same effect is apparent in policy-related activism. If so, questions about alcohol marketing and social media reflect critical perspectives on the nature of democracy in commercial media cultures. That is, as well as asking how people create identities in the sharing of drinking content, it is possible to ask how they act as citizens when complaining about the same thing.

Youth and social media in intoxigenic culture

As well as investigating media's power to instigate drinking, it is also important to ask how the drinks and media industries affect social communication practices. Gunter et al. (2010) pointed out that alcohol promotion involves complicated patterns of social communication, characterised by a marketing mix where simple strategies such as supermarket placement may have far more impact than slick advertising campaigns. Their review characterised alcohol marketing as a symptom of consumer culture. It is part of a larger tale, where the cumulative power of media storytelling has made it near impossible to imagine that the path to happiness runs through anything other than consumption (Lewis, 2013). The existence of consumption as the 'common sense' language of pleasure makes regulation harder still, because audiences, as native speakers, can easily fill in the gap of the nuanced implied claims (Leiss et al., 1997). This state of affairs gestures towards how alcohol manufacturers profit from architectures of communication blending media use and social life.

Some researchers have approached the new cultural terrain by documenting the symbolic environment of drinking cultures where social media play a role in defining pleasure. In Australia, Carah et al. (2014) quantitatively analysed the Facebook communication techniques used by 11 leading alcohol brands. Thematic categorisation outlined a number of strategies those brands used to insinuate themselves into the online social networks of young consumers (e.g. asking questions about drinking cultures, or suggesting new ways to drink the product). The goal was not so much to show the effects of marketing, as to note how alcohol companies synchronise their appeal with the everyday online language – the likes and the shares – of young social media users.

Nicholls (2012) also applied thematic content analysis to 701 brand-authored Facebook posts and Tweets in the UK. His study noted the promotion of brand-sponsored live events ('real-world' tie-ins) as a distinctive feature of this genre. Like Carah et al. (2014), Nicholls read these trends as indicative of social media's ability to occupy the 'common sense' of young drinkers, making drinking appear as a natural part of youth leisure.

Notably, these studies echoed strategies used at a key point in media research to change the way that 'effects' were conceived. Like Nicholls (2012) and Carah et al. (2014), Gerbner created the 'Cultural Indicators Project' (CIP) to map the contours of commercial media messages (Gerbner, 1958, 1969, 1973). He also developed a method for connecting these structures to the formation of social attitudes. Hence, his work is worth considering as a means of explaining how to complement work on social media messages with studies of policy adjudications.

Gerbner on alcohol

The CIP mapped the social effects of living in pervasive media environments where privately owned media industries monopolise the ideas, images and stories that people have always used to make sense of the world, converting audience attention into revenue and corporate sponsorship (Gerbner, 1973). It was, at base, a reaction to the arrival of television as an unprecedented teller of popular stories, paid for by burgeoning consumer goods industries.

The CIP had three aspects. From the 1950s through to his death in 2005, Gerbner set about analysing how market pressures affected the production of media content (Gerbner, 1958), created common symbolic patterns across a variety of media genres (Gerbner, 1969) and impacted the development of social attitudes (Gerbner, 1960, 1984; Gerbner et al., 1982a). Overall, the project identified consistent symbolic patterns in media content, explained how those patterns reflected economically motivated production values, and demonstrated how exposure to these patterns correlated with (or 'cultivated') social attitudes (Gerbner, 1998; Morgan, 2012; Morgan et al., 2012; Shanahan and Morgan, 1999).

Gerbner's best-known work was on television violence. Together with colleagues at the University of Pennsylvania, Gerbner argued that commercial demand for simple stories produced a plethora of action content where violence featured prominently. Survey evidence suggested that this left people who watched a great deal of television feeling afraid and alienated (Gerbner et al., 1980a, 1980b). However, this theme was but the headline of broader interest in how media manufactured social reality. Violence became a way to discuss dominant representations of gender that victimised women. Other studies examined how limited representations of mental illness (Gerbner, 1959a, 1980), education (Gerbner, 1959b), healthcare (Gerbner et al., 1982b) and ageing (Gerbner et al., 1980c), to name but a few, 'cultivated' the perception that little could be done to address the inequalities of capitalism, other than consume and hope for protection.

Yet for all the attention that the violence argument attracted, Gerbner's work on drinking was a better reflection of his overall thesis about media, markets and democracy. For one thing, Gerbner believed that advertising was the most important media genre, marking the point of articulation between media, capitalist governance and the public:

> Advertising is (capitalism's) cultural cutting edge. To critique it as merely superficial ... fails to do it justice in several respects. Advertising has the virtues and flaws of our society and it can be changed ... only as we change the institutions that feed and depend on it.
>
> (Gerbner, 1982: 68)

Moreover, alcohol was especially significant as an intoxicant that connected advertising, fiction and entertainment. Drinking was an especially vivid example of how media could harm populations through naturalising consumption as the most accessible and effective path to happiness (Gerbner, 1978). Efforts to understand the relationship between media and alcohol use had to start with the basic symbolic power of the media. Whether talking about violence, heroes, education, religion, news or representations of intoxicants, media's 'merger of technology and culture' had transformed it into 'the chief cultural nexus of modern governance' (Gerbner, 1978: 13). Along the same lines, the selling of alcohol mattered as an integral part of the general media effect, of turning culture into consumer culture by creating 'populist commercialism' that taught audiences to equate democracy with 'instant individual gratification' (Gerbner, 1978: 17).

As the twentieth century progressed, changing media environments appeared to be accentuating the trends, and pointing them at young people (Gerbner and Ozyegin, 1996). The advent of MTV opened a new front beyond the purview of advertising and its would-be regulators.

> Music videos present alcohol more than movies or television, and illicit drugs three times more often than movies or television. ... A viewer of MTV sees alcohol use every 14 minutes compared to 17 in the movies and 22 on prime time television.
>
> (Gerbner and Ozyegin, 1996: 2).

Given these developments, it was likely that increasingly intrusive systems of media representation would naturalise the use of intoxicants, and this naturalisation would cause widespread suffering. Although cultivation cut its teeth on television, it was designed to explain how consumer culture and media can create preconditions for social harm. As such, it predicted several issues that inform contemporary concerns about social media, drinking and youth.

In fact, alcohol was the one topic where Gerbner stepped beyond the conventional interests of the CIP to address what Nicholls (2012) was later to term 'real word tie-ins'. Gerbner thought that alcohol showed how commercial interests operated as both media inputs and cultural outputs. Unlike television violence, Gerbner saw a much more direct relationship between the creation and results of consumer messages about drinking. This was because alcohol companies funded commercial messages and created places where audiences could 'act out' their desire for consumer satisfaction:

> Tobacco, alcohol, and pharmaceutical conglomerates now own television stations and other media, popular soft drinks and food products, theme parks, and many other enterprises. They sponsor sports events, art exhibits, concerts, and youth magazines.
>
> (Gerbner, 1990: 62)

To that end, Gerbner's work on alcohol showed how media create places for enacting desires (Gerbner, 1990). Again, there was a distinct youth angle in this development: the targeting of college campuses as lucrative drinking places demonstrated how marketing became a health risk, especially around gender (Gerbner and Ozyegin, 1996).

The classic cultivation formula holds that the over-representation of a particular version of media reality 'cultivates' powerful ideas about what is normal in the real world (Morgan et al., 2009). In this regard, the occurrence of alcohol on prime time television was another index of the cultivation effect. The basic idea in these works is that media stories disconnect alcohol from harm. On the rare occasion where alcoholism featured, it was easily resolved. The difference, however, is that when it came to alcohol, the damage caused by the misrepresentation of reality was exacerbated by the growing reluctance to develop policy to act against it. For example, public protest against the growing influence of corporate alcohol sponsorship in collegiate sport in the 1990s was ignored. For Gerbner, alcohol also uniquely demonstrated how the trend towards media deregulation in the late twentieth century amplified the process through which consumption and culture blended through media, even when the public protested against such moves (Gerbner, 1990).

Towards the end of his career, Gerbner was quite clear that media messages about alcohol consumption posed the same sort of risk to public health as violence. As a public health issue, publics should band together to lobby for a media environment free from monopolies of unfettered commercial speech. The ubiquity of positive alcohol images across a variety of media narratives reflected the general bias towards stories that focused, one way or another, on pleasure. Significantly, he called for a debate that went far beyond the topic of regulation: 'Citizens own the airways. We should demand that it be healthy, free and fair, and not just "rated"' (Gerbner, no date: 6).

In total, Gerbner's work shows that current concerns about social media, youth and alcohol continue a trend in the conceptualisation of media influence harking back to the days of television. The work of people such as Carah and Nicholls demonstrate how right Gerbner was to identify the mediated normalisation of alcohol abuse as a case study in how stories about consumption had a particular effect, because retailers connected media messages with real-world outlets; the phenomenon of collegiate drinking being a case in point. Gerbner saw little prospect for change until the public gained an effective voice in media policy.

This turns the spotlight onto organisations such as the UK's Advertising Standards Authority, which does provide a mechanism for complaint, and a commitment to act on every query that citizens raise. For the sake of clarity, let's restate the argument so far: Gerbner believed that the monopolisation of public discourse by privately owned, commercially dependent media industries had established consumption as the common-sense substratum of cultural participation. Effectively, it was incredibly difficult for most people to critique a consumer society when consumption was the bottom line of almost every story they saw about how the world worked. Alcohol was a vivid example of how consumer-friendly media stories crossed over into social life. This critique is highly relevant to the analysis of the ASA, and the historical milieu in which it exists. Scrutinising a decade in which the UK Labour Party's 1997 rise to power had seen significant increases in alcohol consumption and health problems, and a dramatic drop in the real price of alcoholic beverages, Anderson (2007) pointed to a key contradiction in government policy action on these problems. Labour sought to work in partnership with the drinks industry, reversing its earlier stance that one could hardly act against alcohol consumption with the help of business interests who depended on its sale. Media policy was part of the problem. Although some attention had been paid to the content of alcohol advertising, nothing had been done about its volume, with evidence from peak bodies suggesting connections between cumulative exposure and harmful drinking patterns. The idea that commercial media's power to bombard the public with the same message over and over again helps to normalise consumption was directly relevant to British discussions on twenty-first-century alcohol and media policy.

It follows that efforts to counter the effects of alcohol promotion that rest on partnerships between government, the media and the alcohol industry are vulnerable to similar criticisms. One could argue, in fact, that efforts to 'hear' what individual consumers have to say about commercial messages is little more than a smart way of keeping business as usual (Anderson, 2007). Parry et al. (2012) point out that WHO data supports the case for total advertising bans as an effective means of combating normalisation, whereas European evidence shows that voluntary advertising codes made through bodies such as the ASA do not reduce youth exposure to drinks advertising.

Parry et al. (2012) also suggest that the problem with audience-driven alcohol regulation is that, bluntly, it does not really matter what ordinary people think about what is safe in terms of alcohol consumption or advertising; overindulgence in both is harmful for a significant number of people and has a real social cost. In this sense, while the ASA's commitment to listen to each public complaint about drinks promotion might seem laudable, it can also be seen as playing to the very sentiments of individuality and choice that are the hub of the problem. This is a variant on Gerbner's theme: that media inhibit public life by limiting its terms of reference to consumption's articles of faith. From a cultivation perspective, we might ask the following questions: how do these complaints serve as 'cultural indicators'; do they 'indicate' a popular will and skill to get involved in the regulation business, or do they lend yet more evidence to Gerbner's idea that commercial media limit the public imagination?

The present study

The present study examines 86 adjudications made by the UK's Advertising Standards Authority on complaints about alcohol advertising and marketing made between 2010 and 2015. We have seen that quantitative thematic analysis has become an important device in making sense of new marketing strategies. We have also seen how these strategies reflect the logic of the cultural indicators project. Finally, we have seen how towards the end of Gerbner's career, the CIP founder turned his attention to getting audiences involved in media regulation, in a context where 'real world tie-ins' connecting media meanings with social opportunities were becoming common in drinking cultures. All of this, of course, was framed within the thesis that the main media effect in the post-war world was that audiences had been inducted into the values of consumption. Commercial media placed limits around the social imagination. Hence, the ASA complaints provide data to ask if public involvement in UK alcohol regulation is 'unimaginative'.

The UK's Advertising Standards Authority is an independent organisation tasked with enacting code compliance. The organisation is funded by a levy paid on the selling of advertising space (Advertising Standards Authority, no date-b). This funding pays for three kinds of activities. Television and radio ads are 'pre-cleared' for broadcast. 'Non-broadcast' advertising cannot be pre-cleared because of its sheer volume, and so the ASA offers advice services for these media. In the last instance, the ASA is empowered to sanction advertising which is deemed to be in breach of the Code of Advertising Practice (CAP) (Advertising Standards Authority, no date-a). An obvious observation, then, is that social media occupies the space that the ASA has the most trouble in managing.

The ASA invites complaints about any ad that consumers or public bodies deem to be 'misleading, harmful or offensive' (Advertising Standards Authority, no date-a), and stresses that they are bound to act on single complaints. The upshot of this commitment means that they average over 30,000 complaints every year (Advertising Standards Authority, no date-a). At the same time, the ASA's commitment to listen to the public as it manages a vastly expanded realm of commercial communication makes it an ideal test case to examine how loud the public voice is in public discussions on drinks marketing.

Data came from the ASA website, which archives adjudications made on advertising. The period since 2010 was chosen, since this is when the ASA began including online marketing in its considerations. Searching this archive, the study found 86 cases where the ASA has been asked to make a formal decision on commercial activities related to the promotion of alcohol in that period. This dataset provides a means of being very precise about 'changes' in the conversation that cultures have about alcohol. Nicholls (2012) reported that the post-2010 period saw a seismic shift in online marketing practices, with some major brands shifting almost all of their digital marketing to Facebook in particular, and alcohol quickly rising to the third most engaged-with consumer good on that platform. The ASA complaints data is thus significant in that it has reigistered the effects of these changes.

Method

Recall that the CIP put evidence about content together with evidence about audience response. In the same vein, this project connects what we know about how social media portray drinking, with evidence of how audiences interpret these campaigns, in relation to alcohol's larger marketing mix. The data are 'cultural indicators' of how media regulators, advertisers and the public have discussed the post-2010 marketing world. As with the content of social media itself, there is value in quantitatively and qualitatively assessing the thematic structure of this conversation. What discussions emerged? Was there a pattern of especially prevalent themes?

The method applies Clive Seale's insights on the relationship between quantitative and qualitative research approaches to the adoption of a 'cultural indicators' position on policy documents. The approach is based on the growing recognition that 'culture' is, in some regards, a quantitative notion given that it relies on patterned, replicable behaviours and themes that can be counted (Lewis, 2000; Ruddock, 2001; Seale, 2003). The idea is to develop a method that raises sensitising questions in an age where changing marketing practices create uncertainty about potential harm. Under such circumstances, Seale advocates a mixed methods approach to data that allows for the qualitative, grounded exploration of new situations while using numbers to defend against charges of 'anecdotalism' in reporting data.

To that end, the method employed here used the QDA software program Nvivo 10 in a connected quantitative and qualitative approach to outline the nature of ASA complaints documents as 'cultural indicators' of the limits placed around the debate on alcohol promotion. The cultural indicators project invited researchers to combine qualitative and quantitative approaches to analysis (Ruddock, 1995, 2001), and Seale's method applies the same idea to health messages. Seale suggested using Nvivo as a means of overcoming the false dichotomy crudely drawn between quantitative and qualitative methods, showing how the combination of approaches was especially suited to conditions where it is important to develop new questions about new cultural phenomena.

The method in this project is modelled on this idea. The challenge is to manage an enormous problem in relation to an appropriate dataset; a body of evidence that shows how a range of tendencies in mediatised alcohol cultures come to take on a specific shape in the context of a particular activity based around the alcohol and media industries. In order to answer these questions, the 86 complaints adjudicated by the ASA were loaded as pdfs into the Nvivo program. Each was then coded to assess basic patterns of complaint. The coding operation asked:

- Who lodged the complaint (private consumer or public body)?
- What kind of 'risk' did they complain about (encouraging 'bingeing', linking alcohol with success, exposure of minors or appeal to minors, offensiveness, misleading claims)?
- What medium was involved (television, social media, below the line promotion, radio, press and cinema ads)?
- What kind of organisation prompted the offence (alcohol manufacturer, media company or retail outlet)?
- What was the outcome of the complaint?
- How did the defendant respond (did they apologise or mount defences based on disputed readings of ethical practices)?

These coding procedures achieved two goals. First, they established basic patterns in complaints in the 2010–2015 period; who complained about what and for what reason. Second, it provided a systematic way to find case studies of especially complex cases, as such indicating how the changes in marketing practices introduced by social media have made discussing and regulating promotion more difficult. The coding scheme identified patterns across all cases – the overall picture of the kinds of media that attracted attention, the source of the complaint, the reason for the complaint etc. However, because it was possible for complaints to come from more than one source, be directed at more than one medium and comprise multiple perceived code violations, the coding scheme also allowed for the identification of 'rich' cases. These were complaints that raised multiple objections about multimedia campaigns, reflecting how the post-2010 era had complicated the adjudication business.

Results

One way to make sense of the data is to report the 'modal' trend – the most frequent kind of complaint dealt with by the ASA panel. In that regard, the most common scenario the panel faced was a grievance from a private individual (50) directed at an alcohol company (48) about a television ad (37) where the most frequent concern was that the message in question was likely to reach and/or be especially appealing to under 18s (46). Such complaints were most likely to be upheld (47). Defendants were unlikely to offer apologies (only 17 of the 86), and in the case of age appeals usually maintained that they had followed appropriate age protocols (38), thus underlining the difficulties of interpreting and implementing regulations.

At this very early stage, the numbers suggest a few interesting aspects of the difficulties of constructing a complaints mechanism that gives the public a meaningful range of expression. To begin, the total number of complaints, in relation to the volume of commercial messages, is low. Second, a significant number of complaints come from public bodies, local councils, alcohol awareness groups, and even the ASA itself (43 complaints). Third, the youth exposure angle suggests that the question of distribution is more concerning than content. The most common thing to complain about is the notion that young people might be exposed to promotional content – whatever that content might be. This is a first indication of the limits placed on public debate through a policy framework; for the most part, the public seem to think that the alcohol industry can say whatever it wants, as long as it is not in front of the children. Remembering that we are in an exploratory research phase, this raises the question of whether this is evidence that the connection of drinking and pleasure in commercial discourse is generally seen as acceptable, as long as the audience are adults. It also indicates a lack of attention to the issue of how promotion naturalises drinking across populations.

The spirit of the mixed methods approach essentially holds that numbers are a useful raw material in telling a research story through the identification of patterns that stimulate questions, rather than simple conclusions. In that respect, drilling down into the numbers demonstrates some of the complications in determining how regulatory frameworks give the public a forum to speak about commercial culture, and the extent to which social media has impacted structures that are, according to the ASA itself, best suited to handle broadcast material. Taking on board the likelihood that we are currently in a period of intense change brought about by new marketing practices instigated by social media, it is worth noting that while TV continues to dominate, social media has assumed a relatively high profile (Figure 11.1).

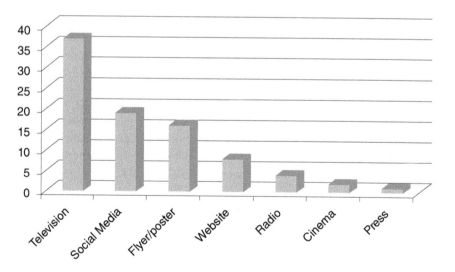

Figure 11.1 Medium complained about

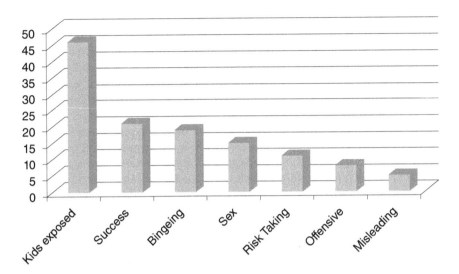

Figure 11.2 Issue complained about

One lesson that Gerbner valuably taught us was that quantitative thematic analysis can reveal surprising patterns. In that regard, it is interesting that, after age, the most frequent reason for complaining about alcohol promotions was their articulation of drinking, popularity and success (Figure 11.2). The relative frequency of this item suggests sensitivity to the idea that promotional culture is a discourse on lifestyle. Hence, the ASA has established a medium for such reservations to be articulated. However, the overall numbers suggest that critical consumer language is a bit like Welsh: people appreciate its existence, but hardly anyone speaks it.

Qualitative analysis: processes in action

One challenge here is to make sense of the relationship between what is and how that 'is' picture speaks to change and cultural tension; that is, it is important to address how this snapshot of the 2010–2015 period addresses what went before, and what is to come, in making sense of the role of media promotion in drinking cultures. The method adopted here is to use the coding exercise to identify a smaller number of dense cases – instances where multiple regulatory matters were raised – to address how the regulatory system works in practice, and to see if these cases demonstrate pattern within themselves over the impact of social media.

Most cases involved six or seven items; that is, an audience member or a public interest body complained about a single case on a single medium for a single reason. In nine cases, however, 10–11 issues were raised by campaigns that crossed genres and activated concerns from public bodies and consumers alike over multiple issues. This provides criteria to report on specific cases; what made them so controversial, and how might these controversies reflect trends introduced by social marketing, if at all?

Closer analysis of these specific cases showed a pattern where youth, social media and sex featured prominently. Seven of the nine cases centred on social media, which was a bigger concern than television in these especially complex cases. Seven of the nine raised the objection that messages were attractive or available to underage audiences. Five complained about connections between alcohol and sex, and four centred on promotions targeted at students.

The emergence of sex as a concern in these data prompted closer scrutiny of complaints about gender representations. There are several scholarly reasons for interrogating this point. A cultural indicators perspective offers that one of the main effects of commercialised storytelling is the production of gender narratives, where women suffer in various ways. In my own previous work on marketing and student identities, two things have been established. First, in pre-social media days, I found women students were concerned about the relationship between sexualised depictions of young women in below the line marketing, and their own experiences of sexual harassment (Ruddock, 2013). Further research on Facebook and student theme nights discovered patterns of female 'performance' in fora where men were largely absent. That is, the way that young women drinkers 'choose' to represent themselves in social media celebrations of drinking, based around organised retailing events, reflects many of the sexualisation concerns frequently directed at advertising proper (Ruddock, 2012). The net conclusion from these studies was that representations of scantily clad women had become normalised in the practice of social media use, but remained an issue of concern for some women students. Thus, there was an organic connection between the experiences of young women drinkers and long-running CIP research on media discourses of gender.

To test this idea further, a word search in the nine case study documents for references to women and men showed the context in which each was represented (as represented by the six-word sequence in which each was based, which can then be traced back to the full complaint to check the reference in context). References were coded to record patterns of representation described in the reports. The sharpest difference revealed about female and male representation was on the issue of bare flesh: 19 references where women exposed parts of the body that are usually clothed, versus only five male examples. Men were more likely to be shown drinking in these promotions than women (eight to three), and women were more likely to be engaged in sexual activity (six to two).

Youth, gender and social media have featured prominently, then, in the most complicated cases that the ASA has addressed since 2010. Yet at the same time, this 'new' situation is consistent with older ideas about media, consumption and identity discussed within the CIP. This enhances the importance of current studies on youth, social media and alcohol as a central case study in research on the influence of media on social well-being.

Drilling down further still, the ASA cases studies also reveal how these trends work in specific instances where complaints are negotiated. In one particular case, we can see how the marketing mix of social media and below the line marketing produced an especially complicated situation demonstrating how social media make it easier to defend potentially offensive or risk-inducing content. Interestingly, much of the controversy surrounded conceptualisation of young people as target markets and knowledgeable consumers.

In 2012, a nightclub in Sheffield, an English town with a large student population, advertised a student-themed night through flyers and its Facebook page. An ASA adjudication report described the content thus:

> Text in a pink circle stated '£1.50 DRINKS ALL NIGHT'. The ad featured a variety of pictures of young people in the club including one of a woman wearing a cropped top and shorts. A speech bubble coming from her shorts had text which stated 'YOU'RE GOING TO GET LAID!'
>
> (Advertising Standards Authority, 2012)

Two complaints resulted. A private individual objected that the people in the ad appeared to be under 16, thus it sexualised minors, and that the ad was generally offensive. The ASA itself charged that the models appeared to be under 25 (where the CAP advises that all significant players in ads must appear to be older), and connected cheap drinks with sex and sexual success.

The appeals panel accepted the ASA's charges, and ordered that the ad should not appear in the same form. Indeed 'Eat My Disco' (EMD), the company who ran the night, agreed that the speech bubble coming from the shorts had been an error, and promised to remove it (Advertising Standards Authority, 2012).

However, on the issue of offensiveness, the ASA panel and EMD agreed that there was no merit to this grievance because of the distribution networks that characterised both flyers and social media, and the savvy-ness of the target group. EMD pointed out that the flyers were distributed in student unions and on a Facebook page that only adults were supposed to access. Further, in their view, the copy would not offend most students. The ASA panel agreed. In other words, there is nothing wrong with advertising for a club night in a licensed venue making direct connections between the event and getting laid, as long as you do not put it on television or radio and do not mention cheap drinks, because that way the target audience are smart enough to see what is going on.

The important point here is to explain how the CIP method outlined in this piece affords a critique that stands on more than anecdotalism and contestable moral objection. The EMD ad, and the adjudication, is at least worthy of debate for sound academic and historical reasons. Empirically, it is one of the most complicated cases the ASA has had to deal with since 2010. Second, it dramatises the complexity that the issue of interpretation introduces to regulatory efforts. Third, it suggests a significant historical trend where alcohol is an especially vivid example of media power that operates by linking media content with the language of pleasure and the opportunity to explore the same. Finally, it shows how youth campus life is an especially rich target for commercial and media interests who seek to combine the language of pleasure and consumption, where the presence of alcohol becomes the natural scenery for the world of youth socialisation – a point that Gerbner made in 1978. In that sense, the EMD case is a concrete example of the blending of commercial and everyday speech (advertisers and students agree there is nothing wrong with using sex to sell retail outlets), and the influence this seems to have on policy (as long as it is not in front of the kids, fine). It is also an example of how social media can operate to continue this particular media tradition.

Conclusion

The advent of new concerns about alcohol marketing brought about by social media illustrates how Gerbner's ideas historically frame the 'change' that seems to have taken place in the second decade of the twenty-first century. Gerbner's basic idea was that corporate storytelling set the tone for the social imagination. The danger was that repetitive stories that linked harm and happiness with particular forms of social organisation affected how audiences understood the world, and what they could do in it. Gerbner was especially concerned that cultural participation, happiness and consumption were continually represented as one and the same, and urged a regulatory system that allowed the public to challenge dominant forms of representation. The topic of media, young people and drinking was foremost in his thoughts. Thus, the issue of how publics speak to media content through mechanisms of regulation that try to hear qualms about new forms of alcohol marketing are highly relevant to Gerbner's predictions about media and democracy, and also serve to show how his work outlines the nature of the regulatory challenges surrounding alcohol promotion.

The question of whether and how various promotional activities affect young people remains challenging, because these activities have changed so dramatically since the advent of social media (Nicholls, 2012). One strategy to address the confusion has been to use quantitative methods to find patterns in social media promotional activities directed at consumers (Carah et al., 2014; Nicholls, 2012). Given this development, it is useful to consider how the current situation articulates with a broader discussion on how media promote consumerism, and how this investigation can be developed by multimethod approaches to different components of the communication system. The idea is to understand how a cultural indicators perspective, already nascent in research on social media and alcohol promotion, can be applied across a broader range of the communication spectrum. Here, the focus is on how the 'effects' suggested in early work on social media can be extended to the analysis of media policy. Previous work explains that drinking is often popularised by promotional activities where brewers and distillers have annexed the language of pleasure (Nicholls, 2006). The suggestion coming from research on social media, youth and alcohol is that alcohol promotion has become a compelling cultural language that people use to make sense of society. In studies from the 1950s to the twenty-first century, George Gerbner identified this as the signature of commercial media.

A cultural indicators perspective shows how alcohol marketing has also affected the language of complaint. By looking at complaints made to the UK's Advertising

Standards Authority over various forms of drinks marketing, this chapter shows how the regulation process limits public debates on this media genre. First, there is very little activity in this regard. Second, what action there is is about exposure not content, where the main regulatory focus seems to be keeping messages away from young people. This is an interesting, and ambiguous finding. On the one hand, empirical studies do suggest that exposure is the problem (Anderson, 2007). On the other, such complaints undermine the logic of the ASA process. If the public think the main problem is exposure, then how can this be addressed through a system that turns on individual complaints about individual messages? Third, there is evidence that social media has added a level of complexity to regulation that exploits the vagaries of interpretation in the adjudication process. Fourth, among the handful of examples that have provoked the most complicated cases in the UK, familiar themes of youth and sexism are apparent. All this shows how an integrated approach to social media marketing, inspired by Gerbner's ideas, promises to show the longevity of the concern that whatever alcohol marketing does, its power rests on the rise of the consumer as the identity that dominates all other modes of social identity.

References

Advertising Standards Authority. (2012). ASA ruling on Eat My Disco. Retrieved 13 December 2015, from www.asa.org.uk/Rulings/Adjudications/2012/1/Eat-My-Disco/SHP_ADJ_171330.aspx#.VmzGEt8rLFw

Advertising Standards Authority. (no date-a). About regulation. Retrieved 13 December 2015, from www.asa.org.uk/About-ASA/About-regulation.aspx

Advertising Standards Authority. (no date-b). Funding. Retrieved 13 December 2015, from www.asa.org.uk/About-ASA/Funding.aspx

Alhabash, S., McAlister, A., Quilliam, E., Richards, J., and Lou, C. (2015). Alcohol's getting a bit more social: When alcohol marketing messages on Facebook increase young adults' intentions to imbibe. *Mass Communication and Society, 18*, 350–375.

Anderson, P. (2007). A safe, sensible and social AHRSE: New Labour and alcohol policy. *Addiction, 102*, 1515–1521.

Carah, N., Brodmerkel, S., and Hernandez, L. (2014). Brands and sociality: Alcohol branding, drinking culture and Facebook. *Convergence: The Journal of Research into New Media Technologies, 20*(3), 259–275.

Gerbner, G. (1958). On content analysis and critical research in mass communication. *Audio-Visual Communication Review, 6*(2), 85–108.

Gerbner, G. (1959a). Mental illness on television: A study of censorship. *Journal of Broadcasting, 4*(3), 293–303.

Gerbner, G. (1959b). Education and the challenge of mass culture. *Audio-Visual Communication Review, 7*(4), 264–278.

Gerbner, G. (1960). The individual in a mass culture. *Saturday Review, 18 June*, 11–13.

Gerbner, G. (1969). Toward 'cultural indicators': The analysis of mass mediated public message. *Audio-Visual Communication Review, 172*, 137–148.

Gerbner, G. (1973). Cultural indicators: The third voice. In G. Gerbner, L. Gross and W. Melody (Eds.), *Communications Technology and Social Policy: Understanding the New Cultural Revolution* (pp. 555–573). New York: John Wiley.

Gerbner, G. (1978). Deviance and power: Symbolic functions of 'drug abuse'. In C. Winick (Ed.), *Deviance and Mass Media* (pp. 13–30). London: Sage.

Gerbner, G. (1980). Social functions of the portrayal of mental illness in the mass media. In J. Rabkin, L. Gelb and J. Lazar (Eds.), *Social Functions of the Portrayal of Mental Illness in the Mass Media* (pp. 45–47). Washington, DC: US Government Printing Office.

Gerbner, G. (1982). The gospel of instant gratification. *Business and Society Review, Spring*, 68.

Gerbner, G. (1984). Political correlates of television viewing. *Public Opinion Quarterly, 1*(48), 283–300.

Gerbner, G. (1990). Stories that hurt: Tobacco, alcohol, and other drugs in the mass media. In H. Resnik (Ed.), *Youth and Drugs: Society's Mixed Messages* (pp. 53–128). Rockville, MD: US Department of Health and Human Services.

Gerbner, G. (1998). Cultivation analysis: An overview. *Mass Communication and Society, 1*(3–4), 175–195.

Gerbner, G. (no date). *TV Rating's Deadly Choice: Violence or Alcohol Annenberg School of Communication*. Philadelphia, PA. http://web.asc.upenn.edu/gerbner/Asset. aspx?assetID=130.

Gerbner, G., Gross, L., Morgan, M., and Signorelli, N. (1980a). The mainstreaming of America: Violence profile #11. *Journal of Communication, 30*, 10–29.

Gerbner, G., Gross, L., Morgan, M., and Signorielli, N. (1980b). Television violence, victimization, and power. *American Behavioral Scientist, 5*, 705–716.

Gerbner, G., Gross, L., Morgan, M., and Signorielli, N. (1980c). Aging with television: Images on television drama and conceptions of social reality. *Journal of Communication, 30*(1), 37–47.

Gerbner, G., Gross, L., Morgan, M., and Signorielli, N. (1982a). Charting the mainstream: Television's contributions to political orientations. *Journal of Communication, 32*, 100–127.

Gerbner, G., Gross, L., Morgan, M., and Signorielli, N. (1982b). What television teaches about physicians and health. *Mobius: A Journal for Continuing Education Professionals in Health Science, April*, 44–49.

Gerbner, G., and Ozyegin, N. (1996). *Alcohol, Tobacco and Illicit Drugs in the Media Mainstream*. Philadelphia, PA: Annenberg School of Communication, University of Pennsylvania.

Griffiths, R., and Casswell, S. (2010). Intoxigenic digital spaces? Youth, social networking sites and alcohol marketing. *Drug and Alcohol Review, 29*, 525–530.

Gunter, B., Hansen, A., and Touri, M. (2010). *Alcohol Advertising and Young People's Drinking*. London: Palgrave Macmillan.

Leiss, W., Kline, S., and Jhally, S. (1997). *Social Communication in Advertising* (2nd edn). London: Routledge.

Lewis, J. (2000). What counts in cultural studies. *Media, Culture and Society, 22*, 629–643.

Lewis, J. (2013). *Beyond Consumer Capitalism: Media and the Limits to Imagination*. London: Polity.

Morgan, M. (2012). *George Gerbner: A Critical Introduction to Media and Communication Theory*. New York: Peter Lang.

Morgan, M., Shanahan, J., and Signorielli, N. (2009). Growing up with television: Cultivation processes. In J. Bryant and M. Oliver (Eds.), *Media Effects: Advances in Theory and Method* (pp. 34–49). London: Routledge.

Morgan, M., Shanahan, J., and Signorielli, N. (Eds.). (2012). *Living with Television Now: Advances in Cultivation Theory and Research.* New York: Peter Lang.

Nicholls, J. (2006). Liberties and licences: Alcohol in liberal thought. *International Journal of Cultural Studies, 9*(2), 131–151.

Nicholls, J. (2012). Everyday, everywhere: Alcohol marketing and social media—current trends. *Alcohol and Alcoholism, 47*(4), 486–493.

Parry, C., Burnhams, N., and London, L. (2012). A total ban on alcohol advertising: Presenting the public health case. *SAMJ: South African Medical Journal, 102*(7), 602–604.

Ruddock, A. (1995). Critical crunching: Cultivation analysis and critical theory. *Commodities, 2,* 22–27.

Ruddock, A. (2001). *Understanding Audiences.* London: Sage.

Ruddock, A. (2012). Cultivated performances: What cultivation analysis says about media and binge drinking. In H. Bilandzic and G. Patriarche (Eds.), *The 'Social' Media User – European Perspectives on Cultural and Social Scientific Audience Research* (pp. 53–68). Chicago: Intellect.

Ruddock, A. (2013). *Youth and Media.* London: Sage.

Seale, C. (2003). Methodology versus scholarship? Overcoming the divide in analysing identity narratives of people with cancer. *Journal of Language and Politics, 2*(2), 289–309.

Shanahan, J., and Morgan, M. (1999). *Television and its Viewers: Cultivation Theory and Research.* Cambridge: Cambridge University Press.

Uzunoğlu, E., and Öksüz, B. (2014). New opportunities in social media for ad-restricted alcohol products: The case of 'Yeni Rakı'. *Journal of Marketing Communications, 20*(4), 270–290.

12 Restricting alcohol marketing on social media in Finland

Marjatta Montonen and Ismo Tuominen

In January 2015, new restrictions on the advertising of alcoholic beverages entered into force in Finland. The restrictions represent a novel approach as they are focused on techniques used in alcohol advertising, rather than the media used or features of the content of advertisements. The Finnish Alcohol Act prohibits the advertising of beverages containing more than 22% alcohol by volume (abv) and restricts the content and placement of advertising for milder beverages. The new restrictions were intended to and do target primarily alcohol advertising in social media. They prohibit advertising, indirect advertising and sales promotion if 'they involve taking part in a game, lottery or contest' or if

> the advertising commercial operator in an information network service administered by itself uses any textual or visual content produced by consumers or places into the service textual or visual content, produced by itself or by consumers, which is intended to be shared by consumers.[1]

The latter, slightly long-winded subsection means that when operating in new media, marketers are not allowed to use any consumer-generated content to advertise alcoholic beverages, or to provide any content for peer-to-peer sharing. This chapter sets the novel approach in the framework of alcohol advertising controls in Finland, reviews justifications for and evidence in support of the new policy, and discusses challenges related to the regulation of alcohol advertising in the digital era.

Brief history of alcohol advertising controls in Finland

The restrictions that came into force in 2015 were the latest in a series of revisions made in the Alcohol Act concerning alcohol advertising. The policy on alcohol advertising in Finland has gone through various stages since the Prohibition era, which in Finland was from 1919 to 1932. In 1932 the Prohibition was followed by an extensive government monopoly system that covered all aspects of the alcohol business, from production to trade and to the control of pricing and sales promotion. There were no legal statutes for alcohol advertising. The monopoly company followed guidance from the State and the advertising of most alcoholic beverages emphasised product information. In 1977, a quasi-total ban on alcohol advertising was introduced. Advertising for low-alcohol beer fell outside the ban as beverages with a maximum alcohol content of up to 2.8% abv are not governed by the Alcohol Act. This provided the breweries a way to promote ordinary-strength beer produced under the same brand name. In the late 1980s, expenditure on low-alcohol beer advertising equalled 20% of the value of low-alcohol beer sales, and low-alcohol beer advertisements were commonly interpreted as promoting stronger beer (Montonen, 1996).

When Finland prepared to join the European Union (EU) in 1995, the all-inclusive alcohol monopoly was dismantled and replaced by a licensing system that was separate for production, wholesale, retail and on-premise sale of alcoholic beverages. The retail monopoly remained in place for beverages above 4.7% abv. The availability of beverages up to 4.7% abv, formerly sold in grocery stores, was expanded by allowing kiosks and gas stations to also sell them, and the range of drinks available was extended from beer only to cider and ready-to-drink mixtures.

Other moves towards liberalisation included lifting the advertising ban for 'mild' beverages, defined as beverages up to a maximum strength of 22% abv. The advertising of 'mild' alcoholic beverages was subjected to content limitations adapted from the EU's *Television without Frontiers* directive (discussed below). These liberalisations contributed to an upward trend in alcohol consumption, accelerated ten years later by three coinciding events (Ministry of Social Affairs and Health, 2006). First, quotas on tax-free imports of alcoholic beverages by travellers arriving from other EU countries were abolished. Second, the neighbouring country Estonia joined the European Union. There was concern the markedly lower price level in Estonia would encourage vast private alcohol imports resulting in loss of alcohol tax revenue in Finland. Third, paradoxically the Finnish government's countermeasure was to cut the alcohol tax by 33% on average, which resulted in an immediate increase in domestic sales and total alcohol consumption. In 2007, when alcohol consumption was at a record high of 12.7 litres pure alcohol per capita (15+ years), the time was ripe for corrective measures.

Starting from 2008, a series of small incremental alcohol tax raises, together with the economic recession, contributed to reversing the trend in total alcohol consumption, recorded sales and travellers' imports (Karlsson et al., 2013). At the same time, the advertising of alcoholic beverages was restricted, in particular but not exclusively, to protect children and young people. In 2008 alcohol advertising on television was limited to the time period from 21:00 to 07:00. Alcohol advertising in cinemas was prohibited, except for movies rated for an adult audience – that is, an age limit of 18 years applied. Mass media advertising for special price offers was prohibited, unless the price was valid for two months without interruption. As a result, special weekend offers and 'happy hours' could only be advertised in store or within serving premises. In 2014 further restrictions were introduced. The television watershed was pushed to 22:00 and the same time restriction was extended to alcohol advertising on radio. Alcohol advertising in outdoor or indoor public places was prohibited. The ban concerned billboards, bus stops, public transport and commercial transportation vehicles, railway stations

Total alcohol consumption, L 100 % alcohol per capita (15+ years), and alcohol policy developments in Finland 1984-2014

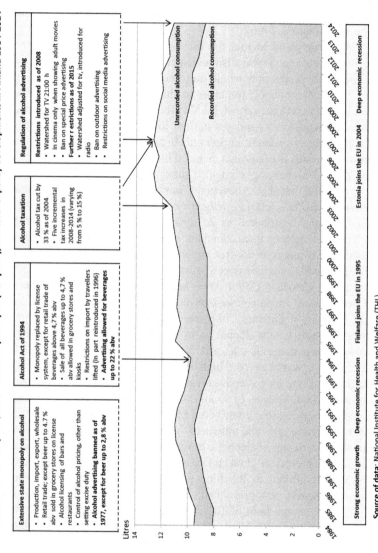

Figure 12.1 Total alcohol consumption L 100% alcohol per capita (15+ years) and alcohol policy developments in finland 1984–2014

and the like, as well as public areas in shopping malls. As a first attempt to curb alcohol advertising on social media, the use of games, lotteries and contests to advertise alcoholic beverages was prohibited as well as the use of any consumer-generated textual or audiovisual materials and the provision of any promotional content for further distribution by consumers when alcohol advertising is carried out via information networks (Figure 12.1).

Different approaches to regulating alcohol advertising

The alcoholic beverages market is highly competitive. With few differences between the products within a category – for example, between lager beers produced by different brewers – the brand image becomes the distinguishing feature and brand advertising becomes central to the commercial success of the product. An argument against the regulation of alcohol advertising is that it does not impact on alcohol consumption but only affects brand shares. Regulation – preferably in the form of self-regulation – would therefore only be needed to weed out content features deemed socially unacceptable, such as portrayal of very young people engaged in drinking or overtly sexual imagery. The downside is, however, that while seeking to increase the market share of their brands, the advertisers collectively disseminate the generic message that alcohol consumption is a pleasurable and rewarding experience without reference to the negative consequences and harms of consumption.

There is varied and robust evidence of the impact of the volume of alcohol marketing – usually measured in terms of exposure – on young people's attitudes and drinking behaviour. The strongest evidence of causal effects comes from longitudinal studies which have found that exposure to alcohol marketing increases the likelihood that adolescents start to drink or, if they have already started, to drink more (Anderson et al., 2009; Gordon et al., 2010a; Gordon et al., 2010b, Jernigan et al., 2016). These studies have taken into account various forms of alcohol advertising – including print, broadcast, outdoor, cinema and branded merchandise – and have examined the cumulative effect of exposure to marketing messages, whether their content is in line with regulatory or self-regulatory guidelines or not. Similarly, studies into the effectiveness of alcohol advertising policies have assessed the impact of reductions in the volume of alcohol advertising rather than modifications of its content (Saffer, 2000; Saffer and Dave, 2006; Sassi, 2015). In contrast, there is no published research available on the effectiveness of content restrictions in influencing young people's attitudes or alcohol consumption.

There is a need for public policy to intervene. The *Global Strategy to Reduce the Harmful Use of Alcohol*, endorsed by WHO member states in 2010, highlights the marketing of alcoholic beverages as a key area of action, in particular to reduce its impact on young people and adolescents (World Health Organisation, 2010). In 2011, the high-level meeting of the United Nations General Assembly called for action by all member states to reduce the burden from non-communicable diseases by addressing their common modifiable risk factors, including the use of alcohol and tobacco (United Nations General Assembly, 2011).

In order to curb the public health harm caused by tobacco, the signatories of the WHO Framework Convention on Tobacco Control have agreed on a clear objective: to eliminate tobacco advertising, promotion and sponsorship effectively at both domestic and international levels (Article 13). This policy aim will become a comprehensive ban that applies to all forms of commercial communication, recommendation or action and all forms of contribution to any event, activity or individual with the aim, effect, or likely effect of promoting a tobacco product or tobacco use either directly or indirectly (World Health Organisation, 2013).

One can ask whether a comprehensive ban on alcohol advertising, promotion and sponsorship would be the most effective for protecting children and young people from alcohol-related harms. While the answer is probably 'yes', when it comes to political feasibility, alcohol and tobacco are not on a par – yet. The most common approaches to regulating the advertising of alcoholic beverages are to prohibit advertising for certain beverage types (typically spirits), to prohibit the placing of advertising messages in certain media (e.g. in youth magazines) or in certain locations (e.g. close to schools), or to restrict the content permitted in the messages (World Health Organisation, 2014). While extensive bans may reduce the exposure to alcohol advertising for the whole population, partial restrictions usually aim at protecting children and young people. Watersheds that limit alcohol advertising on television to time periods where adults are assumed to form the majority audience are a typical example of the latter.

Restrictions on the content of advertising messages have tended to either establish what is prohibited, by giving a 'negative list', or what is permitted, by giving a 'positive list'. The more widely used negative list approach usually aims to protect minors and rule out specific features such as presenting alcohol consumption as a means for social or sexual success. Such restrictions were included in the European Communities' *Television without Frontiers* directive of 1989 (Art. 15)[2] and were integrated in 2010 into the European Union's directive on audiovisual media services (Art. 22),[3] as outlined below:

> In the European Union, television advertising and teleshopping for alcoholic beverages shall comply with the following criteria:
> a) it may not be aimed specifically at minors or, in particular, depict minors consuming these beverages;
> b) it shall not link the consumption of alcohol to enhanced physical performance or to driving;
> c) it shall not create the impression that the consumption of alcohol contributes towards social or sexual success;
> d) it shall not claim that alcohol has therapeutic qualities or that it is a stimulant, a sedative or a means of resolving personal conflicts;
> e) it shall not encourage immoderate consumption of alcohol or present abstinence or moderation in a negative light;
> f) it shall not place emphasis on high alcoholic content as being a positive quality of the beverages.

The content restrictions closely resemble the principles set out in the self-regulatory advertising guidelines issued in the early 1980s by alcohol industry organisations in the United States and in Europe. The approach of enumerating unacceptable types of alcohol advertising content has been found to be ineffective in eliminating youth-appealing content – or has been found to be impossible to objectively assess due to lack of documentation (Jernigan and O'Hara, 2004; STAP, 2007, 2012; Winpenny et al., 2012).

As mentioned above, in Finland the content restrictions of the *Television without Frontiers* directive were incorporated into the Alcohol Act of 1994 and their application extended to all alcohol advertising irrespective of the medium. The 'negative' list approach is a remarkable challenge for any serious attempt at enforcement. The presumption is that what is not forbidden is allowed. In Finland, it is up to the supervisory authority to monitor alcohol advertising in different media and react when needed. If an advertisement appears to be in breach, it is for the authority to point out which content features lead to an 'impression' prohibited by the law – for example, by referring to the screenplay of a television commercial – and to argue intent by the advertiser, rather than unjustified or overzealous 'interpretation' by the authority. If the advertisement in question is found in breach and removed, the same procedure needs to be repeated for the next one. The Finnish supervisory authority has put together guidance for advertisers based on case rulings. The guidance is updated whenever a case lacking precedent emerges and has over the years grown into a 60-page document (Valvira, 2014). Despite the authority's efforts, lifestyle imagery with attractive models, humour, sports and celebrities is common in alcohol advertising in Finland.

French and Swedish legislation governing alcohol advertising takes the 'positive' list approach. In Sweden advertising is only allowed in print media and only for beverages with a maximum strength of 15% alcohol by volume. The size of the print advertisement is limited and 20% of the area has to be reserved for text alerting to health and safety risks. The visual content in the advertisement is limited to the brand logo, a picture of a single consumer package and of raw materials (e.g. grapes as raw material for wine).[4]

In France, advertising of aperitifs and of beverages containing more than 45% alcohol was prohibited in 1941.[5] In 1987, advertising any alcoholic beverages was prohibited on television, in print media for youth, in sports facilities and in the premises of youth associations.[6] In 1991, the so-called Evin law prohibited all direct and indirect mass media advertising for all alcoholic beverages, including alcohol sponsorship, but excluding certain media specified in the law. The permitted media were: print media, except publications directed to youth; radio, in defined time periods; catalogues and brochures issued by alcohol producers and distributors; and billboards, initially only in production areas, and later more widely. Alcohol advertising on television and in cinema is thus prohibited. The content permitted in alcohol advertisements was limited to information about the product: alcoholic strength, origin, composition, taste and aroma, production method, awards received and mode of consumption. All alcohol advertisements are required to carry a text warning about health risks.[7]

The definition of what is allowed is considerably more enforceable than the 'negative' list approach implemented in Finland that requires the assessment of subtle associations created through the interplay of visual, audio and textual elements. The 'positive' list approach can be used in an elegant and economical manner to protect children from alcohol marketing regarding both the media used and the messages transmitted. If a comprehensive ban on alcohol advertising is not feasible, it should be quite possible to limit alcohol advertising to media reaching adults but not children, and to limit the promotional messages to factual and verifiable information on the products to help adult consumers make their choice of drink.

Technological innovation is a challenge for regulation

Alcohol industry has been in the vanguard in taking advantage of the internet and social media to advertise their products (Chester et al., 2010; McCreanor et al., 2013; Nicholls, 2012). Few impact studies so far have examined the effects of these new forms of advertising on young people's alcohol consumption (de Bruijn, 2013; Lin et al., 2012; McClure et al., 2016). Measurement of the volume of alcohol advertising in new media is a challenge because of the multiplicity of websites, social media platforms, mobile applications, virtual communities and varying forms of messaging used. Assessing the scale of youth exposure would require access to website traffic or similar data on content usage and user characteristics (Winpenny et al., 2012).

The move from 'old' to 'new' media presents a challenge for policies to control alcohol advertising. Watersheds set for television advertising lose their meaning when television programming is accessible any time on demand. Rules regarding alcohol advertising in print media may not be applicable when versions of the same content are distributed online. In online shopping, banners have been found to compensate for real-life billboard advertising for alcoholic beverages in jurisdictions where outdoor alcohol advertising is not allowed (Goldfarb and Tucker, 2011). Principles established in the pre-digital era may not automatically be valid for new media or new forms of marketing.

In France, court cases in 2007 and 2008 ruled that the ban on alcohol advertising also applies to alcohol brand websites, non-existent at the time the Evin law was passed.[8] In 2009, however, online communication services were added to the list of permitted media, excluding websites directed to young people or run by sports associations (alcohol sponsorship of sports not being allowed in the first place). The law specifies that online commercials may not be 'interstitial' or 'intrusive'.[9] While interstitials, web pages displaying advertisements during transitions between content pages, are a specific tool of online advertising, 'intrusive' is a characterisation applicable to a broader range of techniques. In 2011, the use of personal Facebook walls to promote a mobile application that enabled the viewing of alcohol advertisements was ruled unlawful; the court considered it an intrusive method used specifically to target a youth audience.[10]

Alcohol is marketed through increasingly sophisticated techniques and increasingly through media that reach across national borders, such as satellite television and the internet (World Health Organisation, 2010). The pace of technological innovations used for commercial promotion of alcoholic beverages is such that regulators have a hard time in catching up. Only a few countries have alcohol advertising regulations specifically for controlling alcohol advertising on the internet or in social media (World Health Organisation, 2014).

Focus on advertising techniques

Focusing on the techniques commonly used to promote alcoholic beverages in digital media is an alternative to regulating media-specific features or the content of advertisements. A number of such techniques have been identified by analysts (Chester et al., 2010; Jernigan, 2010; Mart, 2011; Nicholls, 2012). In social media, interactivity provides the basis for distinct but interlinked and mutually reinforcing techniques, many of which are designed to enhance consumer engagement with the imagery and events created around the brand and with real or imaginary fellow consumers.[11] The techniques are not peculiar to alcohol advertising but are used to market a variety of products, and some of them are common in other areas too – for example, the prominence of contests and games or the merging of 'real' and fictional in television entertainment. Neither are the techniques totally novel in alcohol advertising – for example, testimonials or the bandwagon appeal are familiar from the early days of mass media advertising. Social media platforms and mobile applications have, however, opened up unforeseen dimensions for their use, not least by enabling behavioural targeting, that is personalised messaging based on information gathered on media users' background characteristics and their media content preferences.

'Gamification' is one common technique, apparent in the range of contests, quizzes, surveys and interactive games offered to website visitors and brand followers. Rewards and giveaways used to enhance engagement may have a linkage to real-life events – for example, a chance to win a ticket to a concert – or may require the visitor to disseminate marketing messages to their social network. The reach of branded real-life events – clubs, concerts sports events and the like – is expanded through online sharing of experiences.

Interaction between consumers in the form of conversations and sharing pictures, videos or stories contributes to creating virtual communities. Virtual communities and social networks provide the ground for peer-to-peer recommendations and for conceiving the brand as a means for belonging and identity building. The marketing messages are fed in by advertisers as viral content or created by the consumers themselves. Mobile technologies and applications that provide suggestions for use or enable users to locate people, events and services linked with the brand contribute to integrating alcoholic beverages as a normative part of daily life.

Young people are at the centre of these interactive digital advertising activities because of the penetration and heavy use of new media among them (Jernigan and Rushman, 2014). Young people tend to be the most savvy when it comes to using digital communication media but this does not protect them from the impacts of marketing, in particular when commercial promotion of products and brands is no longer easily recognisable as such. Alcohol marketing in the digital space reaches under-age youth but mostly stays under the radar of parental awareness and control. Online age check mechanisms used by alcohol advertisers usually require visitors to confirm being of legal age but include no attempt at verification, not even in countries where online identity verification services are available (Winpenny et al., 2012).

Interactive digital advertising is inherently engaging, and immersive virtual environments may be even more so. In research to develop marketing tools, methods such as eye movement tracking are being rivalled by innovations such as neuroimaging to gauge brain activation (Ariely and Berns, 2010). It has been suggested that the 'consequences of interacting with products and brands in cyberspace might be even more profound than the known risks of exposure to traditional alcohol marketing' (Chester et al., 2010).

Although much of the nature of digital alcohol marketing and its effects remains unknown, a precautionary approach was deemed justified in Finland. The restrictions adopted focus on two key techniques used in digital alcohol advertising: gamification and social influence advertising where consumers become promoters of the product. The prohibition on the use of games, lotteries or contests to advertise alcoholic beverages is media neutral: it would also apply, for example, to an alcohol-branded trivia quiz on TV or radio. The prohibition concerning the use of consumer-generated content and peer-to-peer sharing (viral advertising) refers specifically to 'information network services'. This allows the restrictions to apply to any digital technology or mode of electronic communication that may be introduced in the future.

Advertising techniques are commonly the focus in consumer protection legislation. In the Finnish Consumer Protection Act, for example, hidden advertising, aggressive marketing, and the use of false claims or misleading information are singled out as inappropriate conduct. Comparative advertising and advertising using raffles, competitions or games are subject to specific provisions. Advertising targeted to under-18s or commonly reaching them is deemed inappropriate if it makes use of the recipient's inexperience or gullibility, or may harm their development or seeks to reduce the opportunity for parents to protect and guide their children.[12] The Finnish Information Society Code highlights that digital direct marketing messages shall be recognisable as marketing, shall indicate the identity of the sender and shall include an address through which the recipient can decline to receive such communications.[13]

The Finnish Consumer Ombudsman has issued guidelines (Kuluttaja-asiamies, 2015) on the use of the 'share this with your friends' technique in marketing. The Ombudsman stresses that when a marketer urges or enables sharing the purpose is always to influence consumer decisions and actions, thereby this is subject to the Consumer Protection Act and to the Information Society Code. As this legislation does not apply to private communication between individuals, a key question for the Ombudsman concerns distinguishing between marketing communication and private sharing. Upholding the Consumer Protection Act's principle that 'marketing must clearly show its commercial purpose and on whose behalf marketing is implemented' may become even more challenging with the move towards 'native' advertising where marketing messages are embedded in digital communication streams – for example, where web articles are formatted to resemble the surrounding editorial content or Twitter is used to disseminate advertiser-generated messages (Lieb et al., 2013).

The issue of impact

There are important points to note about the Finnish restrictions concerning the advertising of alcoholic beverages in information networks. First, the restrictions only apply to commercial communications. To make it clear that private free speech is not being restricted, the Constitutional Committee of the Finnish parliament added to the Bill an explicit mention that it only concerns commercial operators' advertising activities. Marketers can no longer use any material produced by consumers or offer material to be shared by consumers. Consumers' private communications about an alcoholic beverage brand, for example in their own Facebook-page or in a chat service, is by definition not considered advertising. Any private person can share a picture showing them drinking beer or email to friends suggestions on drinks or places to drink. For alcohol marketers, on the other hand, the law allows them to continue using, for example, 'conventional' banner advertisements and run brand websites stripped of games and contests and of anything created by consumers.

Second, the restrictions only apply to domestic advertising and, additionally, to advertising of foreign origin which is targeted to Finnish consumers. With a language such as Finnish, practically not spoken outside Finland, it is quite easy for the supervisory authority to distinguish between alcohol brand websites or social media communications directed to Finns – which are not allowed – and commercial activities targeting markets in other countries – which are not affected by the Finnish ban.

No attempt has been made in Finland to measure how the four new restrictions on alcohol advertising might affect young people's perceptions, attitudes or drinking behaviour and it would, in fact, be extremely difficult to disaggregate each of their roles. The adjustment of the television watershed and the introduction of the same watershed for radio were minor changes. The other two measures do make a difference in the way alcoholic beverages are present in young people's lives: all outdoor advertising for alcoholic beverages has been removed, and the range of techniques available for consumer engagement in social media has been restricted.

More importantly, restrictions on alcohol advertising are just one component of wider public health policies on alcohol and are meant to work in concert with measures to influence alcohol pricing. Advertising is only part of the integrated marketing mix where the bottom line also depends on the consumer appeal of the product, as such, as well as its price and retail accessibility (BMA, 2009). The accumulated evidence on the potential for impact of alcohol control policies strongly suggests that advertising restrictions have synergistic value when used in combination with other measures to reduce alcohol-related harm (Booth et al., 2008; Nelson et al., 2005).

Among 16-year-old students in Finland, the prevalence of drinking and binge drinking and the amounts of alcoholic beverages consumed have decreased throughout this millennium (Raitasalo et al., 2015). Contributing factors may have included tighter enforcement of minimum age limits, more restrictive attitudes among parents, and changes in the way drunkenness is valued among youth. Restrictions on alcohol advertising were meant to and likely have played a role in the shift in attitudes among both adults and young people.

The future for alcohol marketing regulation

The *Global Strategy to Reduce the Harmful Use of Alcohol*, endorsed by WHO member states in 2010, highlights that 'alcohol is being marketed through increasingly sophisticated advertising and promotion techniques, including linking alcohol brands to sports and cultural activities, sponsorships and product placements, and new marketing techniques such as e-mails, SMS and podcasting, social media and other communication techniques.' A precautionary approach would address both the content and the volume of alcohol marketing and would regulate new forms of marketing.

The move from 'old' media to 'new' digital media has profoundly changed both interpersonal and mass communication. While communication technology has become more personal, its uses have become more social in the sense that individuals are able to publish their own content. The distinction between producer and consumer of communication is blurred when the masses have access to means of mass communication. The distinction between editorial content and advertising is fading away with phenomena such as blogging or 'native' advertising. 'Old' mass media are forced to transform themselves, and categories such as print and broadcast media become obsolete when content is being disseminated through multiple technologies and platforms. Even the distinction between online and offline media is melting away.

The parameters of regulation and control have also changed. Established standards are losing their validity in many areas: open sourcing challenges intellectual property rights and crowdsourcing undermines control by the funder. Once released on the internet, content keeps circulating in an uncontrollable fashion. Filtering and blocking content is possible to some extent and has been done on political or moral grounds.

Paradoxically, while keeping track of communication content has become difficult, monitoring users of communication has become easier than ever. Electronic surveillance is being used by governments for social control and by companies to gather data for behavioural targeting of marketing messages. The practices of internet, social media and other digital communication have evolved without public scrutiny or regulatory oversight (van Dijck, 2013).

All these changes require a rethinking of how to regulate the advertising of alcoholic beverages to protect young people and the wider population against commercial pressure to drink. Technological development and the ways people integrate communication technologies into their lives will continue to provide new opportunities for commercial communication, the forms of which are hard to anticipate. One possibility is to identify techniques that are used across communication services – such as gamification – and regulate their use in a media-neutral manner. Supervision and enforcement will remain a challenge, so long as advertisers of alcoholic beverages do not refrain from looking for loopholes and stretching the limits of the rules. If commitment to responsible business in this area is lacking, no enforcement machinery can guarantee that the objective of the law is realised. Probably the only effective way to prevent cross-border advertising from undermining national restrictions is to follow the model of the Framework Convention on Tobacco Control, that is, having signatories agree to apply the same restrictions to domestic and out-flowing advertising and recognise the right of others to take action to limit in-flowing advertising (World Health Organisation, 2013).

The factual and political 'degree of difficulty' for regulating alcohol advertising with an international agreement is apparently higher than for banning tobacco advertising. Apart from constitutional restrictions for some countries to limit free (commercial) speech, it is in the producer's interest to inform consumers about products offered for sale and in the consumer's interest to obtain factual information for purchasing decisions.

If some alcohol advertising is to be allowed in order to allow product information to be communicated to adult customers, based on the Finnish experience the recommended approach should consist of a 'positive list' of content restrictions. The law could, for example, limit the content to a still photograph or sketch of the beverage or the package and to the following factual information, part of which may be mandatory label information:

1 The name, price and distribution channel of the beverage;
2 Basic information on the product as indicated on the package, such as alcohol content and quantity in the package;
3 The name and contact information of the manufacturer or distributor;
4 Information on the geographical origin of the beverage, the method of production and ingredients;
5 Specific instructions for use and health hazards; and
6 Characterisation of the colour, taste and aroma of the beverage, as well as awards the product may have received.

This kind of 'positive list' would by itself eliminate much of the advertising content and techniques that contribute to the appeal of alcoholic beverages to children and young people. If only still pictures of the product are allowed, there is no room for any audiovisual content or in fact for anything interesting enough to be shared with friends. If only truthful product information is allowed, there is no possibility to organise contests or games for the promotion of the beverage.

According to the evidence there is a dose-response relationship between young people's exposure to alcohol marketing through multiple marketing channels and the likelihood that they will start drinking (Anderson et al., 2009; Babor et al., 2010; Jernigan et al. 2016). While the direction of the causal association has been confirmed by longitudinal studies, findings regarding its strength and consistency vary, not least due to variation in ways of operationalising exposure, ranging from measurement of (subjective) advertising recall (Unger et al., 2003) to measurement of (objective) advertising expenditure (Saffer and Dave, 2006).

Optimal regulation would in any case curtail at least the most visible forms of alcohol marketing. In order to balance the need to minimise the harmful effects of alcohol advertising on the one hand, and the commercial needs of alcohol industry and the needs of adult consumers on the other, the legislation should cover both different media and techniques. For example the following restrictions, which for the most part are currently in place in Finland, could serve as a model for legislation on alcohol marketing in other countries:

1   advertising on television (except from 23:00 to 07:00)
2   advertising in cinemas (except when showing films with an 18-year age limit)
3   advertising in public places indoors or outdoors (except in retail and on-premise sites)
4   using sponsorship
5   using games, lotteries or contests
6   using consumer-created content
7   using consumers as distributors of advertising.

Although such steps towards optimal regulation would enable marketers to reach adult consumers through print media and alcoholic beverage outlets, they would not be easy or painless. The alcohol industry will oppose any attempts to restrict one of the core elements of their business. Even the best legislation needs credible surveillance and meaningful sanctions. Until a sufficient number of countries are willing and capable of protecting their young ones from the harmful effects of alcohol advertising, cross-border advertising, which cannot be completely governed by national legislation, will remain a challenge. However difficult it may be, the only way to proceed is for countries one by one to begin to regulate alcohol advertising in a way that makes a difference. This will also be the way to build political pressure towards international treaties to curb alcohol advertising.

Legislation to control alcohol advertising and marketing mainly dates from the period before the advent of the World Wide Web and social networking services. Examples of regulation that specifically take into account the nature of new digital media are scarce. Whereas laws should ideally be precise and straightforward, the rapid pace of innovation and technological development in this area means that there will continue to be room for different interpretations in the application of advertising restrictions in the borderline between commercial and non-commercial communication.

Notes

1 [Alkoholilaki] The Finnish Alcohol Act, No. 1143/1994, as amended by act No. 152/2014.
2 Council Directive 89/552/EEC of 3 October 1989 on the coordination of certain provisions laid down by law, regulation or administrative action in Member States concerning the pursuit of television broadcasting activities.
3 Directive 2010/13/EU of the European Parliament and of the Council of 10 March 2010 on the coordination of certain provisions laid down by law, regulation or administrative action in Member States concerning the provision of audiovisual media services (Audiovisual Media Services Directive).
4 Alkohollag 1622/2010, Kapitel 7.
5 Loi du 24 septembre 1941 modifiant la loi du 23 août 1940 contre l'alcoolisme, Article 9.
6 Loi n°87–588 du 30 juillet 1987 portant diverses mesures d'ordre social, Article 97.
7 Code de la santé publique, Articles L3323–2, L3323–4.
8 Tribunal de grande instance de Paris: Ordonnance de référé 02 avril 2007: Anpaa / Bacardi Martini France, Bacardi Martini Production; Tribunal de grande instance de Paris: Ordonnance de référé 08 janvier 2008: Anpaa / Heineken.
9 Loi n°2009–879 du 21 juillet 2009, Article 97.
10 ANPAA: Publicités illicites. Loi Evin. Décisions rendues en 2013. http://www.anpaa. asso.fr/agir/publicites-illicites-loi-evin.
11 For further discussion and examples, see DigitalAds (digitalads.org), a website operated by the Center for Digital Democracy and Berkeley Media Studies Group.
12 [Kuluttajansuojalaki] The Consumer Protection Act 38/1978/38, as amended by the act 561/2008.
13 [Tietoyhteiskuntakaari] The Information Society Code 917/2014.

References

Anderson, P., de Bruijn, A., Angus, K., Gordon, R., and Hastings, G. (2009). Impact of alcohol advertising and media exposure on adolescent alcohol use: A systematic review of longitudinal studies. *Alcohol and Alcoholism, 44*(3), 229–243.

Ariely, D., and Berns, G. (2010). Neuromarketing: The hope and hype of neuroimaging in business. *National Review of Neuroscience, 11*(4), 284–292.

Babor, T., Caetano, R., Casswell, S., Edwards, G., Giesbrecht, N., Graham, K., Grube, J., Hill, L., Holder, H., Homel, R., Livingston, M., Osterberg, E., Rehm, J., Room, R., and Rossow, I. (2010). *Alcohol: No Ordinary Commodity Research and Public Policy* (2nd edn). Oxford: Oxford University Press.

BMA. (2009). *Under the Influence: The Damaging Effect of Alcohol Marketing on Young People*. London: British Medical Association.

Booth, A., Meier, P., Stockwell, T., Sutton, A., Wilkinson, A., and Wong, R. (2008). *Independent Review of the Effects of Alcohol Pricing and Promotion. Part A: Systematic Reviews*. Sheffield: School of Health and Related Research, University of Sheffield. www.shef.ac.uk/polopoly_fs/1.95617!/file/PartA.pdf

Chester, J., Montgomery, K., and Dorfman, L. (2010). *Alcohol Marketing in the Digital Age*. Center for Digital Democracy and Berkeley Media Studies Group, a project of the Public Health Institute. Retrieved 18 April 2016, from www.digitalads.org/documents/ BMSG-CDD-Digital-Alcohol-Marketing.pdf

de Bruijn, A. (2013). Exposure to online alcohol marketing and adolescents' binge drinking: A cross-sectional study in four European countries. In P. Anderson, F. Braddick, J.

Reynolds et al. (Eds.), *Alcohol Policy in Europe: Evidence from AMPHORA. The AMPHORA Project* (2nd edn). http://amphoraproject.net/w2box/data/e-book/Chapter%208%20-%20AM_E-BOOK_2nd%20edition%20-%20June%202013.pdf

Goldfarb, A., and Tucker, C. (2011). Advertising bans and the substitutability of online and offline advertising. *Journal of Marketing Research, 48*(2), 207–227.

Gordon, R., Hastings, G., and Moodie, C. (2010a). Alcohol marketing and young people's drinking: What the evidence base suggests for policy. *Journal of Public Affairs, 10*(1–2), 88–101.

Gordon, R., MacKintosh, A., and Moodie, C. (2010b). The impact of alcohol marketing on youth drinking behaviour: A two-stage cohort study. *Alcohol and Alcoholism, 45*(5), 470–480.

Jernigan, D. (2010). The extent of global alcohol marketing and its impact on youth. *Contemporary Drug Problems, 37*, 57–89.

Jernigan, D., and O'Hara, J. (2004). Advertising and promotion. In R. Bonnie and M. O'Connell (Eds.), *Reducing Underage Drinking*. Washington, DC: National Academies Press.

Jernigan, D., and Rushman, A. (2014). Measuring youth exposure to alcohol marketing on social networking sites: Challenges and prospects. *Journal of Public Health Policy, 35*(1), 91–104.

Jernigan, D., Noel, J., Landon, J., Thornton, N. and Lobstein, T. (2016) Alcohol marketing and youth alcohol consumption: a systematic review of longitudinal studies published since 2008. *Addiction*, 2016 Aug 26. doi: 10.1111/add.13591. [Epub ahead of print]

Karlsson, T., Kotovirta, E., Tigerstedt, C., and Warpenius, K. (2013). *Alkoholi Suomessa: Kulutus, Haitat ja Politiikkatoimet [Alcohol in Finland: Consumption, Harms and Policy Measures]*. Helsinki: National Institute for Health and Welfare.

Kuluttaja-asiamies. (2015). Kerro kaverille -toiminnossa noudatettavat periaatteet [Guidelines on share-with-your friends functions]. Retrieved 13 April 2016, from www.kkv.fi/ratkaisut-ja-julkaisut/julkaisut/kuluttaja-asiamiehen-linjaukset/aihekohtaiset/kerro-kaverille-toiminnossa-noudatettavat-periaatteet/

Lieb, R., Szymanski, J., and Etlinger, S. (2013). *Defining and Mapping the Native Advertising Landscape*. San Mateo, CA: Altimeter Group.

Lin, E.-Y., Casswell, S., You, R. Q., and Huckle, T. (2012). Engagement with alcohol marketing and early brand allegiance in relation to early years of drinking. *Addiction Research and Theory, 20*(4), 329–338.

Mart, S. (2011). Alcohol marketing in the 21st century: New methods, old problems. *Substance Use and Misuse, 46*(7), 889–892. www.scopus.com/inward/record.url?eid=2-s2.0-79957523498andpartnerID=40andmd5=bd9f019dad2437703f1172f3f6bbe596

McClure, A., Tanski, S., Li, Z., Jackson, K., Morgenstern, M., Li, Z., and Sargent, J. (2016). Internet alcohol marketing and underage alcohol use. *Pediatrics, 137*(2).

McCreanor, T., Lyons, A., Griffin, C., Goodwin, I., Moewaka Barnes, H., and Hutton, F. (2013). Youth drinking cultures, social networking and alcohol marketing: Implications for public health. *Critical Public Health, 23*(1), 110–120.

Ministry of Social Affairs and Health. (2006). *Alcohol Issues in Finland after Accession to the EU: Consumption, Harm and Policy Framework 1990–2005*. Helsinki.

Montonen, M. (1996). *Alcohol and the Media*. Copenhagen: World Health Organisation.

Nelson, T., Naimi, T., Brewer, R., and Wechsler, H. (2005). The state sets the rate: The relationship among state-specific college binge drinking rates, and selected alcohol control policies. *American Journal of Public Health, 95*(2), 441–446.

Nicholls, J. (2012). Everyday, everywhere: Alcohol marketing and social media—current trends. *Alcohol and Alcoholism, 47*(4), 486–493.

Raitasalo, K., Huhtanen, P., and Miekkala, M. (2015). *Nuorten Päihteiden Käyttö Suomessa 1995–2015: ESPAD-tutkimusten Tulokset [Alcohol and Drug Use Among Adolescents in Finland 1995–2015: ESPAD Survey Results]*. Helsinki: National Institute for Health and Welfare.

Saffer, H. (2000). *Alcohol Consumption and Alcohol Advertising Bans*. Cambridge, MA: National Bureau of Economic Research.

Saffer, H., and Dave, D. (2006). Alcohol advertising and alcohol consumption by adolescents. *Health Economics, 15*, 617–637.

Sassi, F. (Ed.). (2015). *Tackling Harmful Alcohol Use: Economics and Public Health Policy.* Paris: OECD.

STAP. (2007). *Report on Adherence to Alcohol Marketing Regulations*. Utrecht: National Foundation for Alcohol Prevention (STAP).

STAP. (2012). *Commercial Promotion of Drinking in Europe*. Utrecht: National Foundation for Alcohol Prevention (STAP).

Unger, J., Schuster, D., Zogg, J., Dent, C., and Stacy, A. (2003). Alcohol advertising exposure and adolescent alcohol use: A comparison of exposure measures. *Addiction Research and Theory, 11*(3), 177–193.

United Nations General Assembly. (2011). *Political Declaration of the High-level Meeting of the General Assembly on the Prevention and Control of Non-communicable Diseases* (A/66/L.1), 16 September. www.who.int/entity/nmh/events/un_ncd_summit2011/political_declaration_en.pdf

Valvira. (2014). Ohje alkoholimainonnasta [Guidance on alcohol advertising]. Retrieved 15 April 2016, from www.valvira.fi/-/ohje-alkoholimainonnasta

van Dijck, J. (2013). *The Culture of Connectivity: A Critical History of Social Media*. New York: Oxford University Press.

Winpenny, E., Patil, S., Elliott, M., Villalba van Dijk, L., Hinrichs, S., Marteau, T., and Nolte, E. (2012). *Assessment of Young People's Exposure to Alcohol Marketing in Audiovisual and Online Media*. Cambridge: Rand Europe. http://ec.europa.eu/health/alcohol/docs/alcohol_rand_youth_exposure_marketing_en.pdf

World Health Organisation. (2010). *Global Strategy to Reduce the Harmful Use of Alcohol*. Sixty-Third World Health Assembly WHA 63.13, 21 May. Retrieved 23 December 2010, from http://apps.who.int/iris/bitstream/10665/44395/1/9789241599931_eng.pdf?ua=1

World Health Organisation. (2013). *Guidelines for Implementation of the WHO Framework Convention on Tobacco Control*. Geneva. www.who.int/iris/bitstream/10665/80510/1/9789241505185_eng.pdf?ua=1.

World Health Organisation. (2014). *Global Status Report on Alcohol and Health 2014*. Retrieved 15 December 2015, from http://apps.who.int/iris/bitstream/10665/112736/1/9789240692763_eng.pdf

13 New marketing, new policy?

Emerging debates over regulating alcohol campaigns in social media

Sarah Mart

In 2009 my colleagues and I at Marin Institute (now Alcohol Justice) published what was to our knowledge the first examination of alcohol promotion on Facebook and the platform's policies regarding such promotion (Mart et al., 2009). We found pervasive messages promoting alcohol brands and dangerous drinking behaviours in paid brand advertising and in free brand and product pages, events, groups and user engagement. We made recommendations to alcohol producers, Facebook and other social networking sites (SNS) in the peer-reviewed journal article, as well as directly to company representatives. Six years later, research studies and reports from around the globe have echoed and expanded upon our initial recommendations and documented the continued proliferation of alcohol promotion on SNS. Yet, as of late 2015, corporate entities and governments have largely ignored public health recommendations to protect youth and reduce the risks from oversaturation and overexposure to digital alcohol marketing.

The problems

Alcohol is a causal contributor to more than 200 diseases, injuries and conditions, and a leading cause of death worldwide (Babor et al., 2010). At least 3.3 million deaths (5.9% of total), and 5.1% of the global burden of disease and injury, are attributable to alcohol (Lim et al., 2012; World Health Organisation, 2014). In the United States excessive alcohol use kills approximately 88,000 people annually (Centers for Disease Control and Prevention, 2013), and collectively cost the nation a conservatively estimated $249 billion in 2010 (Sacks et al., 2015). More than $24 billion (9.7%) of the total US cost came from underage drinking. Alcohol-related problems include but are not limited to physical injuries, risky sexual behaviour, unplanned pregnancy, HIV and other sexually transmitted diseases, tobacco and other drug use, and academic failure (Alcohol Justice, 2014; Centers for Disease Control and Prevention, 2015).

An environment saturated with alcohol products and messages promoting alcohol brands along with general drinking behaviours increases the risk of harm, injury and death to children and youth. Exposure to alcohol marketing is associated with early initiation of drinking for youth who have not started drinking, high consumption levels for those who already drink, and increased number and amount of future alcohol-related problems for young drinkers as they age (Anderson et al., 2009). Such exposure also violates their rights as children to grow up free from the influence and negative effects of alcohol.

The theory

Babor and colleagues (2010) remind us that alcohol is an unordinary commodity – unlike products such as toothpaste or jeans, alcohol requires specific attention, consideration and control due to the product's dangers and risks to the public's health and safety. As peer-reviewed research continues to find, certain alcohol policies are the most effective and cost-effective way to improve alcohol and related harm across populations. Examples include policies regarding alcohol pricing and taxation, state monopoly and control of sales and regulation, alcohol outlet density, and alcohol marketing, advertising and promotion. Thus national and international health organisations recommend reducing youth exposure to alcohol advertising and promotion as a best buy in population health policies to reduce alcohol consumption and related harm (World Health Organisation, 2014). Recently the Conference Declaration of the Global Alcohol Policy Conference, held October 2015 in Edinburgh, Scotland, made clear the urgent need to restrict alcohol marketing in all forms (Global Alcohol Policy Conference (GAPC), 2015).

Many international and national organisations address complex public health problems, such as alcohol-related harm, with a social ecological model to describe and understand the systems of relationships between individuals and groups (social) and the organisations, communities, and society/public policy that surround them (environmental). From this model, we can visualise the effects of alcohol in social media on youth: individuals engaging with known and unknown peers, in their schools, communities and around the world, within a global virtual structure/platform offering many kinds of online interaction with alcohol in general, along with specific brands and companies. Some experts have flipped the original social ecological model and placed the development of health policies and environments in relationship with multiple levels of contexts able to be affected by communities, organisations, groups and individuals (Golden et al., 2015). The upended model offers a way to view levels of potential influence on alcohol policy changes by community, organisation, groups and individuals. Yet certain key players must be acknowledged and included in any models of policy and/or behaviour change: the multinational, billion-dollar corporations producing and pushing the products.

The players: alcohol industry

Major alcohol suppliers and producers have constructed multiple trade groups working to defeat effective, evidence-based alcohol policy and protect alcohol producer revenues in the United States and in nations around the world. In the United States, alcohol producer gross revenues in early 2011 were $60 billion (Federal Trade Commission, 2014). Total US spirits supplier revenue nearly doubled from $11.7 billion in 2000 to $23.1 billion in 2014 (Distilled Spirits Council of the United States (DISCUS), 2015a). One of the largest and most influential producer trade organisations is the newly renamed International Alliance for Responsible Drinking (IARD), affiliated with the Global Alcohol Producers Group and previously known as the International Center on Alcohol Policy (ICAP).

IARD is funded by twelve producers and national producer groups: Anheuser-Busch InBev, Bacardi, Beam Suntory, Brewer's Association of Japan, Diageo, Heineken, Japanese Spirits and Liqueurs Makers Association, Pernod Ricard, SABMiller, Brown-Forman, Carlsberg and Molson Coors (International Alliance for Responsible Drinking (IARD), 2015). IARD's tagline refers to action on alcohol and global health and its foci remain the same as ICAP: diverting attention from and defeating the most effective alcohol policies available to reduce alcohol-related harm; contradicting public health research on such topics as alcohol and non-communicable disease or alcohol marketing; and positing the alcohol producer trade group to policy makers as a neutral non-profit organisation with a public health orientation (Jernigan, 2012).

IARD members are also represented domestically by trade organisations at the national level. In the United States, the Beer Institute represents more than 3300 beer producers, both domestic and US arms of global producers. Its more than 50 members include producers/suppliers such as Anheuser-Busch, Constellation Brewers, Heineken and MillerCoors; alcopops producers such as Mike's Hard Lemonade; and industry media and marketing companies (Beer Institute, 2015). The Beer Institute's policy agenda focuses on defeating efforts to adopt effective alcohol policies such as increased taxes and restrictions on alcohol advertising, as well as promoting the personal responsibility of drinkers as public policy.

The US trade group for spirits, the Distilled Spirits Council of the US (DISCUS), represents both producers/suppliers and marketers, with 15 large corporate members: Agave Loco Brands, Bacardi USA, Beam Suntory, Brown-Forman, Campari America, Constellation Brands, Diageo, Edrington, Luxco, Moet Hennessy USA, MGP Ingredients, Patron Spirits, Pernod Ricard USA, Remy Cointreau USA and Sidney Frank Importing (Distilled Spirits Council of the United States (DISCUS), 2015b). DISCUS launched a Small Distiller Affiliate Membership Program in 2010, with more than 135 members in 35 states to date. DISCUS works at legislative, regulatory and public affairs levels to defeat tax increases (to 'protect' the distilled spirits industry from higher taxes) and other public health policies it deems as trade barriers worldwide.

Along with its policy agenda and programmes for large international spirits producers and smaller producer members, DISCUS also runs a domestic policy arm called the Foundation for Advancing Alcohol Responsibility (FAAR), known as the Century Council prior to its rebranding campaign in 2014. Although FAAR states that it works at the state and federal level to support effective policies for underage drinking and drink driving, it neither lists on its website nor advocates for the best buys in alcohol policy supported by global health organisations: increased alcohol prices and taxes, decreased availability and outlet density, and restrictions on alcohol advertising and promotion (Foundation for Advancing Alcohol Responsibility (FAAR), 2015). FAAR's parent organisation, DISCUS, works specifically to protect the industry from higher taxes.

The players: social media

Alcohol producers and their trade associations are not the only corporate entities responsible for exposing young people to an abundance of alcohol promotion. The multibillionaire owners of social networking platforms are there too. Facebook, the eldest of these platforms, was founded less than two decades ago in 2004. It is the world's biggest social network with more than 1.01 billion daily active users, and 894 million mobile daily active users, as of December 2015 (Facebook, 2015b). Facebook bought Instagram, a leading photo-sharing SNS, in 2012. YouTube, the video-sharing site, was launched in 2005 and purchased by Google in 2006. YouTube boasts more than one billion users per day, and 80% of its views are by users outside the United States (You Tube, 2015).

SNS such as Facebook, YouTube, Twitter and their offspring provide low-cost, largely unmeasured, mostly unregulated promotional space where products of all kinds, including alcohol, can grow and strengthen brand relationships with target populations, especially youth. Ninety-two percent of teens in the United States report going online daily, aided by ubiquitous access to smartphones (Lenhart, 2015). Ninety percent of young adults (age 18–29) in the United States use social media, compared to 12% in 2005 (Perrin, 2015). Half of all teens visit SNS daily, and a third of them visit several times a day. Multiple studies have found that the SNS Facebook, Instagram and YouTube are most frequently used by youth (Bennett, 2014; Lenhart, 2015; Winpenny et al., 2014).

Alcohol companies have been active on these and other SNS since the platforms launched, and have significantly increased their presence and spending on alcohol promotion on social media in recent years (Federal Trade Commission, 2014). In addition to paid advertising, alcohol companies rely on free and unmeasured advertising from users of social media sharing branded content (such as posts, photos, videos, links, sponsorship, contests, sweepstakes and giveaways), as well as sharing user-generated content (such as posts, photos, and videos) (Chester et al., 2010; Griffiths and Casswell, 2010; Mart, 2011; Mart, et al., 2009).

The regulatory facade

Alcohol producers and their trade groups refuse to acknowledge the role their product advertising, marketing and promotion plays in youth drinking and associated harm, particularly with regard to digital media used to engage young people and encourage them to share content about their alcohol brands. The Beer Institute and DISCUS, as well as the most prominent US wine trade organization, the Wine Institute, have promulgated their own voluntary self-regulatory advertising and marketing guidelines for decades, and issue periodic statements cheering their effectiveness. The voluntary guidelines originally centred on traditional advertising channels such as television, radio and magazines; audience demographics and exposure; and vague, subjective content advisement. In recent years DISCUS has added a section to its guidelines regarding digital marketing and social networking.

The following gaps have been documented and recommended for regulators to address: the responsibility of alcohol brands for their own messaging, interaction with and management of others who create online content regarding their brands, and audience participation and mediation the brands invite/encourage; acknowledgement that brand messages are often created via interactions between consumers and brands in everyday life; and ways that alcohol brands collect information about consumers, what kind of info they collect, and how brands use the information to target consumers (Brodmerkel and Carah, 2013). Particular challenges with industry self-regulation seen in the United States include: lack of an independent, third-party review body; lack of enforcement power and reasonable, appropriate penalties other than requests to pull ads; lack of enforceable federal law or binding industry agreement; and lack of one standard system of objective standards and consistent monitoring and enforcement for all types of alcohol (Marin Institute, 2008).

Researchers have found many examples of alcohol companies violating the industry's own self-regulatory guidelines, especially within SNS (Barry et al., 2015a; Barry et al., 2015b; Nicholls, 2012; Smith et al., 2013). IARD's own guidelines for alcohol advertising in digital and social media specifically name user-generated content on third-party platforms as out of the control of alcohol producers, and therefore not covered under the IARD guidelines. Yet the guidelines also state that alcohol companies should monitor and clearly communicate about how they are monitoring user engagement (International Alliance for Responsible Drinking (IARD), 2014).

The ineffectiveness of industry self-regulation continues to be documented, and multiple studies rate voluntary/industry self-restrictions at the same level as no restrictions (Jernigan and Esser, 2014). Yet many countries depend on industry self-regulation. Sixteen out of 166 countries in a 2012 study (Australia, Cyprus, Denmark, Germany, Ghana, India, Ireland, Myanmar, Netherlands, New Zealand, Niger, Nigeria, Rwanda, South Africa, the United Kingdom and the United States) reported industry voluntary/self-restrictions on alcohol advertising in social media (Global Information System on Alcohol and Health (GISAH), 2015).

No federal agency, independent external third party, or industry group in the United States comprehensively monitors and evaluates alcohol advertising and promotion with the authority to hold alcohol producers accountable and apply appropriate penalties for violations. The US Alcohol and Tobacco Tax and Trade Bureau (TTB) considers an advertisement any written or verbal statement, illustration or depiction which is in, or calculated to induce sales in, interstate or foreign commerce, or is disseminated by mail. The definition includes websites and other internet-based advertising such as social media (Federal Trade Commission, 2014). Alcohol advertisements are not required to be approved by TTB or any other government or non-governmental organisation before being disseminated.

The US Federal Trade Commission (FTC) Bureau of Consumer Protection is mandated to protect consumers against unfair, deceptive, or fraudulent practices by businesses (US Alcohol and Tobacco Tax and Trade Bureau, 2015). The FTC has released four reports on alcohol advertising practices based on industry-supplied data in the last two decades (1999, 2003, 2008 and 2014). The 2014 report also included information regarding digital and social media trade practices from the 14 companies responding. These companies spent 7.9% of total advertising spending on digital and online advertising in 2011, four times as much as was spent in 2005 (Federal Trade Commission, 2014).

The FTC made several recommendations to alcohol producers and marketers about social media in its 2014 report. It encouraged companies and their respective trade organisations to: use more advanced versions of age-gates on their own websites; use age-gating technology offered by SNS and develop such technologies for newly emerging media; provide better transparency with improved privacy policies and disclosures about the collection and use of consumer data; use blocking technology and frequent live monitoring to identify and remove user-generated content that violates industry guidelines; promote compliance with the industry guidelines, including training and compliance manuals for staff; and participate in cross-company efforts to facilitate compliance. The Beer Institute was specifically urged to allow competitor complaints.

The FTC also urged state alcohol regulators and public health advocates to use industry guidelines and report advertising complaints to the Beer Institute, Wine Institute or DISCUS as appropriate. It promoted the industry-supported 'We Don't Serve Teens' alcohol education materials offered in conjunction with the FTC to anyone concerned about under-age drinking. Finally, the report made clear that the federal agency supports self-regulation of alcohol marketing to reduce underage targeting and stated that the agency actively monitors self-regulation within the alcohol industry, both formally and informally.

However, with no entity responsible for monitoring and enforcement, no penalties for non-compliance, and no evidence to support self-regulation as an effective strategy to protect children and youth from alcohol marketing, the FTC recommendations are essentially meaningless. They are minor tweaks to already-toothless and ineffective industry self-regulation, not tools that will reduce youth exposure to alcohol promotion on social media at a level that matches increased spending and expansion of exposure by alcohol corporations. In the United States and so many other countries, alcohol advertising in measured and unmeasured channels is virtually unregulated, and children and youth are not adequately protected from overexposure to branded alcohol promotion (Hastings and Sheron, 2011).

Solutions: policy, monitoring, enforcement, authority and accountability

Alcohol advertising experts have for years called for more and better measurement of youth exposure to alcohol marketing in digital media (Jernigan and Rushman, 2014). The WHO Global Strategy to Reduce the Harmful Use of Alcohol recommends that countries regulate the content and volume of marketing, sponsorships and promotional activities targeting young people, including new marketing forms such as social media, and set up regulatory or co-regulatory frameworks with a legislative basis to do so (World Health Organisation, 2010). These frameworks would monitor and regulate content of and exposure to branded alcohol advertising. For SNS, they would include ages of users able to access alcohol-related social media, as well as user-generated content and levels of user engagement.

Globally, some countries have attempted to ban alcohol advertising on social media. In 2012, 21 out of 166 total countries reported bans on alcohol ads in social media for beer, wine and spirits (Global Information System on Alcohol and Health (GISAH), 2015). Two countries had bans on alcohol ads in social media for at least one type of alcohol. Russia reported a ban on all online alcohol advertising originating outside the country. Sweden reported partial restrictions on beer and wine advertising content, and a total ban on spirits advertising. France reported partial restrictions on time and place of advertising for beer, wine and spirits.

Finland added social media-specific definitions and regulations to its Alcohol Act that went into effect as of January 2015 (Viita, 2013). The language of the new Act defines and regulates certain alcohol advertising practices on social media, and in particular bans the following: games, lotteries and contests; user-generated content including posts, photos, video clips or ads; and marketing content intended to be shared by users (European Centre for Monitoring Alcohol Monitoring (EUCAM), 2014). The bans do not apply to marketing originating from other countries, but do prohibit the targeting of Finnish internet users from other countries.

In September 2013 the South African Cabinet approved a draft bill to control the marketing of alcoholic beverages, to then be available for public comment (Parry et al., 2014). After calling for a second regulatory impact assessment to follow an initial assessment conducted by the Department of Health, the bill stalled with no further movement, concerning public health advocates and researchers. What originated as hope for effectively addressing alcohol's substantial burden on public health in South Africa, including alcohol costs of harm at an estimated 12% of the country's gross national product (Ramsoomar, 2015), could instead now be undermined by the alcohol industry's formidable influence.

With our 2009 study, Marin Institute called for alcohol companies to be held accountable for the use of their brands and related communications on Facebook and other SNS. We recommended that alcohol companies require Facebook to remove all content about their brands until it revised its advertising policy, instated monitoring and compliance practices, and required demographic restrictions in all Facebook features used to promote alcohol.

Our recommendations to Facebook included that the platform should stop accepting paid advertisements for alcohol products and refuse other types of alcohol-related content across the platform. We also recommended that Facebook immediately restrict messages about both generic dangerous drinking behaviours, as well as paid ads for specific alcohol brands, and place the same demographic restrictions on all parts of the platform as those placed on paid alcohol ads. We called for Facebook to hire external monitors to enforce all these regulations.

While we received immediate contact from a Facebook public relations representative on the day the article was released, the phone meeting did not result in any substantive action. We offered assistance and resources to Facebook staff for professional development on the issue of alcohol marketing and promotion, but that offer was not accepted. In the months following the study's release, Facebook policy changed to state that paid alcohol advertising would be able to be seen by users who, according to their birthdate in their Facebook profile, were as old or older than the minimum legal drinking age in the country where they report residing (Facebook, 2015a). We also noticed in subsequent months that some Facebook pages for alcohol companies included official statements identifying them as official pages and listing home office addresses and websites. Some official alcohol brand pages also added so-called responsible drinking messages to their About Us section.

Facebook and other social media policies regarding alcohol advertising and promotion remain severely lacking. Such policy depends on under-age users to set up their profiles with accurate birthdates so that they will be age-gated and unable to view content from alcohol companies. These policies also depend on alcohol companies to age-gate official alcohol brand pages and purchased ads to protect youth from exposure. Finally, SNS require that individual users report single posts by users or brands. Even then, anonymous monitors or reviewers employed by the SNS may decide that the reported post does not violate the site's community standards, and it will remain.

Solutions: state legislation

One state has taken legislative action to try to protect children from advertising on digital and SNS. The state of Delaware passed the Delaware Online and Personal Privacy Protection Act in 2015 that includes language banning alcohol advertising to youth under the minimum legal drinking age of 21 (State of Delaware, 2015). While it is too soon to see practical outcomes realised from this law, early review indicates that it reinforces restrictions that likely already exist, as knowingly and intentionally advertising alcohol directly to under-age youth is already illegal. The law clearly bans alcohol advertising on internet services directed to children, but only to those specific kinds of services. On SNS such as Facebook, Instagram and YouTube, advertisers cannot direct alcohol advertising to users who have entered their birthdate as younger than their country's minimum legal drinking age. But since users can enter any birthdate for their account without having to verify it, it is easy for underage youth to lie about their age. Finally, the law cannot have a meaningful impact without including the most popular and widely used social media by youth such as Facebook, YouTube and Instagram, and without a comprehensive system to monitor and enforce violations.

Solutions: other policy models from other public health problems

In recent years, Facebook has greatly increased its participation in creating solutions to suicide ideation and self-harm, another public health problem for youth and young adults that will take strategic policy initiatives to change, on its platform. Based on consultation with experts in the field, Facebook created new ways for the platform to help address and hopefully prevent the problem by connecting and referring users who post concerning status updates with people and resources for support (Flynn, 2015).

A behavioural identification and referral model with users posting and sharing about concerning drinking behaviours on Facebook would make individual users responsible for breaking silent bystander norms that support those dangerous behaviours. It would be more than what Facebook and other social networking sites currently do to address alcohol and related harm. However, offering increased options for individual users to try to support or get help for other individuals in their social networks may very well be meaningless in the face of million-dollar deals with alcohol advertisers on the sites that they frequent.

To reduce exposure to alcohol promotion and elevated risk of harm from that exposure, SNS founders and boards of directors could focus on making changes within their own platforms. Doing so would take a policy decision for Facebook/Instagram, YouTube/Google and other SNS to refuse alcohol advertising and promotion across their sites. As Facebook founder Mark Zuckerberg and his wife Dr Patricia Chan have recently shared with the world, health, education, equality and community are major pillars of their future philanthropy plans (Goel and Wingfield, 2015). They have dedicated billions in the coming decades to support and reinvigorate public hospitals and public health programmes, and research to address and eliminate health problems that injure and kill millions of people each year. Other technology moguls (Google, WhatsApp) have recently given substantial amounts for medical and health causes not related to alcohol as well (McBride, 2015). With alcohol the fifth leading cause of death worldwide and the leading cause of death and disability for young people 15–24 in most parts of the world (Global Alcohol Policy Conference (GAPC), 2015), tech philanthropists should see that they can make one of the biggest positive changes within their own realm of control.

With the global nature of the alcohol industry and the universal reach of SNS, partial and voluntary regulation and control in one state or country will not adequately address the problem. The onus is on beer, wine and spirits producers and marketers; founders/owners and boards of directors of social networking sites who provide platforms for alcohol promotion; and elected officials and government leaders – to stop deflecting independent research findings and to start making decisions based on the best public health research available.

References

Alcohol Justice. (2014). Alcohol-related harm in the United States. Retrieved 13 April 2016, from https://alcoholjustice.org/images/factsheets/AlcoholRelatedHarm2014.pdf

Anderson, P., de Bruijn, A., Angus, K., Gordon, R., and Hastings, G. (2009). Impact of alcohol advertising and media exposure on adolescent alcohol use: A systematic review of longitudinal studies. *Alcohol and Alcoholism, 44*(3), 229–243.

Babor, T., Caetano, R., Casswell, S., Edwards, G., Giesbrecht, N., Graham, K., Grube, J., Hill, L., Holder, H., Homel, R., Livingston, M., Osterberg, E., Rehm, J., Room, R., and Rossow, I. (2010). *Alcohol: No Ordinary Commodity Research and Public Policy* (2nd edn). Oxford: Oxford University Press.

Barry, A., Bates, A., Olusanya, O., Vinal, C., Martin, E., Peoples, J., Jackson, Z., Billinger, S., Yusuf, A., Cauley, D., and Montano, J. (2015a). Alcohol marketing on Twitter and Instagram: Evidence of directly advertising to youth/adolescents. *Alcohol and Alcoholism*, first published online: 22 November 2015, doi: http://dx.doi.org/10.1093/alcalc/agv1128.

Barry, A., Johnson, E., Rabre, A., Darville, G., Donovan, K., and Orisatalabi, E. (2015b). Underage access to online alcohol marketing content: A YouTube case study. *Alcohol and Alcoholism, 50*(1), 89–94.

Beer Institute. (2015). About the Beer Institute. Retrieved 10 September 2016, from www.beerinstitute.org/about

Bennett, S. (2014, 24 February). Teens, Millennials prefer YouTube to Facebook, Instagram to Twitter [Study]. *AdWeek*. Retrieved 15 March 2016, from www.adweek.com/socialtimes/teens-millennials-twitter-facebook-youtube/496770

Brodmerkel, S., and Carah, N. (2013). Alcohol brands on Facebook: The challenges of regulating brands on social media. *Journal of Public Affairs, 13*(3), 272–281.

Centers for Disease Control and Prevention. (2013). Alcohol and Public Health: Alcohol-Related Disease Impact (ARDI). Alcohol-attributable deaths due to excessive alcohol use, average for United States 2006–2010 [Alcohol Related Disease Impact (ARDI) Application, 2013]. Retrieved 13 April 2015, from www.cdc.gov/ARDI

Centers for Disease Control and Prevention. (2015). Alcohol and public health. Fact sheets – alcohol use and your health. Retrieved 13 April 2015, from www.cdc.gov/alcohol/fact-sheets/alcohol-use.htm

Chester, J., Montgomery, K., and Dorfman, L. (2010). *Alcohol Marketing in the Digital Age*. Center for Digital Democracy and Berkeley Media Studies Group, a project of the Public Health Institute. http://digitalads.org/how-youre-targeted/publications/alcohol-marketing-digital-age-1

Distilled Spirits Council of the United States (DISCUS). (2015a). *Distilled Spirits Council 2014 Industry Review*. www.discus.org/assets/1/7/Distilled_Spirits_Industry_Briefing_Feb_3_2015_Final.pdf.

Distilled Spirits Council of the United States (DISCUS). (2015b). Home page. Retrieved 10 September 2016, from www.discus.org

European Centre for Monitoring Alcohol Monitoring (EUCAM). (2014). Finland bans alcohol-related social media communication in 2015. Retrieved 15 March 2016, from http://eucam.info/2014/02/27/finland-bans-alcohol-branded-social-media-communication-in-2015/

Facebook. (2015a). Advertising policies. Retrieved 15 March 2016, from www.facebook.com/policies/ads/

Facebook. (2015b). Stats. Retrieved 25 November 2015, from http://newsroom.fb.com/company-info/

Federal Trade Commission. (2014). *Self-Regulation in the Alcohol Industry: Report of the Federal Trade Commission*. Washington, DC: Federal Trade Commission. www.ftc.

gov/system/files/documents/reports/self-regulation-alcohol-industry-report-federal-trade-commission/140320alcoholreport.pdf.

Flynn, K. (2015, 2 December). How Facebook acts to prevent suicide with human connections amid a world of algorithms. [International Business Times]. Retrieved, from http://www.ibtimes.com/how-facebook-acts-prevent-suicide-human-connections-amid-world-algorithms-2206722

Foundation for Advancing Alcohol Responsibility (FAAR). (2015). Home page. Retrieved 13 April 2016, from http://responsibility.org/

Global Alcohol Policy Conference (GAPC). (2015). *Conference Declaration. Edinburgh, Scotland, 9 October.* www.gapc2015.com/uploads/gapc2015/edinburgh_declaration_final2.pdf.

Global Information System on Alcohol and Health (GISAH). (2015). Alcohol control policies. Advertising restrictions. Advertising restrictions on social media. Data by country. Retrieved 15 March 2016, from http://apps.who.int/gho/data/node.main.A1545?lang=enandshowonly=GISAH

Goel, V., and Wingfield, N. (2015, 1 December). Mark Zuckerberg vows to donate 99% of his Facebook shares to charity. *New York Times.* Retrieved 15 March 2016, from www.nytimes.com/2015/12/02/technology/mark-zuckerberg-facebook-charity.html

Golden, S., McLeroy, K., Green, L., Earp, J., and Lieberman, L. (2015). Upending the social ecological model to guide health promotion efforts toward policy and environmental change. *Health Education and Behavior, 42*(Supplement 1), 8S–14S.

Griffiths, R., and Casswell, S. (2010). Intoxigenic digital spaces? Youth, social networking sites and alcohol marketing. *Drug and Alcohol Review, 29,* 525–530.

Hastings, G., and Sheron, N. (2011). Alcohol marketing to children: A new UK private member's bill provides a simple, clear, and effective way forward. *BMJ, 342,* 720–721.

International Alliance for Responsible Drinking (IARD). (2014). *Digital Guiding Principles: Self-regulation of Marketing Communications for Beverage Alcohol. Beer, Wine and Spirits Producers' Commitments to Reduce Harmful Drinking.* Washington, DC: International Council on Alcohol Policy.

International Alliance for Responsible Drinking (IARD). (2015). Members and affiliations. Retrieved 10 September 2016, from www.iard.org/about/members/

Jernigan, D. (2012). Global alcohol producers, science and policy: The case of the International Center for Alcohol Policies. *American Journal of Public Health, 102*(1), 80–89.

Jernigan, D., and Esser, M. (2014). Assessing restrictiveness of national alcohol marketing policies. *Alcohol and Alcoholism, 49*(5), 557–562.

Jernigan, D., and Rushman, A. (2014). Measuring youth exposure to alcohol marketing on social networking sites: Challenges and prospects. *Journal of Public Health Policy, 35*(1), 91–104.

Lenhart, A. (2015). *Teen, Social Media and Technology Overview 2015.* Washington, DC: Pew Research Center. www.pewinternet.org/files/2015/04/PI_TeensandTech_Update2015_0409151.pdf

Lim, S., Vos, T., Flaxman, A., Danaei, G., Shibuya, K., and Adair-Rohani, H., et al. (2012). A comparative risk assessment of burden of disease and injury attributable to 67 risk factors and risk factor clusters in 21 regions, 1990–2010: A systematic analysis for the Global Burden of Disease Study 2010 [Corrected version]. *Lancet, 380,* 2224–2260. http://ac.els-cdn.com/S0140673612617668/1-s2.0-S0140673612617668-main.pdf?_

tid=c95c4b2e-03b4–11e3–81a2–00000aab0f27andacdnat=1376356255_162c0fcb344 2b57b9b3da8563377405a

Marin Institute. (2008). *Why Big Alcohol Can't Police Itself: A Review of Advertising Self-Regulation in the Distilled Spirits Industry.* San Rafael, CA: Marin Institute.

Mart, S. (2011). Alcohol marketing in the 21st century: New methods, old problems. *Substance Use and Misuse, 46*(7), 889–892.

Mart, S., Mergendoller, J., and Simon, M. (2009). Alcohol promotion on facebook. *Journal of Global Drug Policy and Practice, 3*(3). http://globaldrugpolicy.org/3/3/1.php

McBride, S. (2015, 1 December). Zuckerberg's donation latest in string of gifts by technology mavens. *Reuters.* Retrieved 15 March 2016, from www.reuters.com/article/us-markzuckerberg-baby-donors-idUSKBN0TL03720151202

Nicholls, J. (2012). Everyday, everywhere: Alcohol marketing and social media—current trends. *Alcohol and Alcoholism, 47*(4), 486–493.

Parry, C., London, L., and Myers, B. (2014). Delays in South Africa's plans to ban alcohol advertising. *Lancet, 383*(9933), 1972.

Perrin, A. (2015, 8 October). Social networking usage: 2005–2015. *Pew Research Center.* Retrieved 15 March 2016, from www.pewinternet.org/2015/10/08/2015/Social-Networking-Usage-2005–2015/

Ramsoomar, L. (2015, 26 February). The ban on alcohol advertising on South Africa. *Public Health Association of South Africa.* Retrieved 15 March 2016, from www.phasa.org.za/ban-alcohol-advertising-south-africa/

Sacks, J., Gonzales, K., Bouchery, E., Tomedi, L., and Brewer, R. (2015). 2010 national and state costs of excessive alcohol consumption. *American Journal of Preventive Medicine, 49*(5), e73–79.

Smith, K., Cukier, S., and Jernigan, D. (2013). Regulating alcohol advertising: Content analysis of the adequacy of federal and self-regulation of magazine advertisements, 2008–2010. *American Journal of Public Health, 104*(10), 1901–1911.

State of Delaware. (2015, 7 August). Internet privacy and safety agenda becomes law with governor's signature. Retrieved 15 March 2016, from http://news.delaware.gov/2015/08/07/internet-privacy-and-safety-agenda-becomes-law-with-governors-signature/

US Alcohol and Tobacco Tax and Trade Bureau. (2015). About the FTC. Bureaus and Offices. *US Department of the Treasury.* Retrieved 15 March 2016, from www.ftc.gov/about-ftc/bureaus-offices

Viita, K. (2013, 12 April). Finland plans alcohol-ad ban in public places to shield children. *Bloomberg Business.* Retrieved 15 March 2016, from www.bloomberg.com/news/articles/2013–04–12/finland-plans-alcohol-ad-ban-in-public-places-to-shield-children

Winpenny, E., Marteau, T., and Nolte, E. (2014). Exposure of children and adolescents to alcohol marketing on social media websites. *Alcohol and Alcoholism, 49*(2), 154–159. doi: http://dx.doi.org/10.1093/alcalc/agt174

World Health Organisation. (2010). Global strategy to reduce the harmful use of alcohol. Sixty-Third World Health Assembly WHA 63.13, 21 May. Archived by WebCite® at www.webcitation.org/5vB5AX2e8. Retrieved 23 December 2010, from http://apps.who.int/gb/ebwha/pdf_files/WHA63/A63_R13-en.pdf

World Health Organisation. (2014). Global status report on alcohol and health 2014. Retrieved 15 December 2015, from http://apps.who.int/iris/bitstream/10665/112736/1/9789240692763_eng.pdf

You Tube. (2015). Statistics. Retrieved 15 March 2016, from www.youtube.com/yt/press/statistics.html

14 Digital alcohol marketing and the public good

Industry, research and ethics

Tim McCreanor, Helen Moewaka Barnes,
Antonia C. Lyons and Ian Goodwin

Introduction

The writings in this volume present some of the diverse interests that public good researchers and policy makers have in the confluence of alcohol marketing and social media. The commitment to the health and well-being of populations and a determination to value these community assets above business goals and profits underpins this work. This means that public health needs to understand the potentials and threats entailed in the emerging social phenomena, particularly in the face of apprehension and even hostility by some commercial interests. Public good science in this domain asks questions about the links between social media marketing of alcohol and its influence on consumption, as well as the associated harms and costs at population level. This primary focus sits within a wider context of concerns about how the development of digital life is changing social environments and their relationships to drinking cultures.

Social researchers have commenced investigation of the dynamic, complex, emergent, technologically mediated and commercially driven social practices at work within society, building on decades of scholarship especially in media studies, social psychology and sociology. Within the field of alcohol marketing, itself a long-standing concern to public health as a driver of population-level alcohol consumption, the research is mostly less than five years old. At this point we know very little and while what we have gleaned is striking and not a little alarming, it is still more interpretative than empirical. To progress the broad aims articulated throughout this book, more energy, resources and innovation are required.

The research tools we have at our disposal are emergent. One of our key roles as researchers is to adapt existing methods and create new approaches that can help to address critical research questions. The chapters throughout this volume canvass multiple theories, methods and approaches, and the last section in particular reflects on the ethical and social goals of public good science in this domain. This final chapter aims to foreground the contributions of the diverse contributions, point to gaps where new efforts seem likely to be rewarding and discuss some of the challenges inherent to the field. We encourage the emerging efforts to collaborate, using collective skills and experience, along with those of wider social science communities, to create a new body of knowledge to inform policy and political practices that can mitigate the effects of alcohol marketing within social media. We begin by exploring some of the contours of this uneven and contested field before turning our attention to the methods, approaches and challenges that public good science can work with, around and innovatively on from.

As often happens where public good interests clash with the interests of commercial parties, the domain of digital marketing and alcohol consumption is characterised by a frustrating imbalance in power and resources. Alcohol and media corporations control vast and critical datasets that could be used to answer some of the important questions about the effectiveness of their digital marketing campaigns and the mechanisms by which alcohol promotions in a digital environment influence consumption. However, this proprietary information is protected by the powerful vested interests that both platform owners and alcohol corporations have in retaining private ownership of data, making it largely inaccessible to interrogation by health and other public good researchers. Coupled with this information blockade is the megalith of resources and business drivers that corporations have available to invest in, to improve their systems, in a continuous programme of software development and research, mounted upon the digital commons. Pro-industry activity, with minimal public oversight or governmental restraint (as befits advanced neoliberalism), outruns and outguns the marginalised, fragmented, ethically bound efforts that public good research has thus far mustered to anticipate problems and develop societal responses.

We begin this chapter by focusing on what we can discern (from a distance) of developments and activities within corporate sectors that bear on alcohol marketing in the digital domain. Then we turn to a brief overview of the primary methods used within the field by public good research. We aim to promote discussion around the development of new, theory-driven empirical approaches to understanding the issues from a public good perspective.

Industry ethics and research

What has come to be known as 'the Facebook experiment' is a highly relevant example of the kind of imbalance apparent across public and private sectors, and it also illustrates the lack of oversight in the commercial sector around research ethics. In 2012, without notification and relying only on Facebook's Data Use Policy for consent, researchers for the corporation accessed and systematically altered the newsfeed functions of nearly 690,000 users (Booth, 2014). They used algorithms to classify some three million posts as negative or positive according to a published content analytic program. They then manipulated the emotional content of items arriving in the newsfeeds of the subjects differently across two groups. For the first group, they reduced the positive emotional content of incoming posts by withholding a proportion of such items from the newsfeed, while in the second group they reduced negative content in the same way. Subsequent measures of negativity and positivity in the posts of subjects found significantly lower measures of positivity in group one and significantly lower levels of negativity in group two compared to control groups who experienced only random withholding of inward posts (Kramer et al., 2014). The findings were taken as evidence of 'emotional contagion' in the absence of non-verbal cuing and published in the US Proceedings of the National Academy of Sciences. Predictably there was an outcry of criticism from social scientists and public watchdogs and a muted apology from Facebook (Rushe, 2014). Facebook has undoubtedly benefited from this knowledge that seems likely to feed into their expertise in relation to platform design, their ongoing push towards the perfection of profit-orientated, real-time algorithmic agency, and possibly marketing advice to clients. Together these actions clearly signal the lack of user protection against manipulation and commercial exploitation in social media.

The outcomes of this unethical experiment may be but the tip of the iceberg given the proprietary ownership of all user data by such corporations. The point here is to illustrate platform owners' ability to control, manipulate and innovate on a massive scale with the marketing needs of their corporate clients, which include alcohol corporations, foremost in mind. If public health scientists had the same access to the digital datasets of social media and alcohol corporations, they would be able to generate a plethora of insights and understandings that would vastly improve our ability to protect users from the effects of digital alcohol marketing and better control alcohol consumption at population level.

The history of efforts to regulate the use of alcohol (Babor et al., 2010; Edwards et al., 1994) is one of long-standing conflict between alcohol research and policy sectors, and the diverse commercial enterprises engaged in the production and sale of alcohol. Where the former have created and implemented effective regulatory controls on consumption, the latter have argued and lobbied with great success for deregulated environments in which consumers exercise a right of 'choice' over consumption. Particularly under the auspices of neoliberal political reforms (see Goodwin and Griffin, this volume), this has led to the undermining of control and often to rising consumption, risky drinking practices and population-wide harm (Babor, et al., 2010).

The alcohol industry, along with other sectors associated with significant harms to society, attempts to reduce perceived constraints such as ethics and regulation on what they see as legitimate business activities. 'Corporate Social Responsibility' (Wikipedia, 2016) manoeuvres may make it seem that big alcohol has grown some conscience but while key players are keen to appear and be recognised as philanthropic and socially oriented, their major goal remains growth in consumption to drive increased profits to shareholders. Fundamental to neoliberal business logic is a notion that policy and regulation, the main source of effective intervention by public authority in reducing consumption (Anderson et al., 2009), is to be avoided, eroded and revoked. In this sense even the considerable costs of investment in lobbying political structures, supporting potentially industry-influenced research, and attempting to undermine robust research findings, are regarded as acceptable practices. For decades corporate responsibility organisations, such as the Portman Group in the UK, the International Centre for Alcohol Policies in the United States, Drinkwise in Australia and many similar groups attached to particular corporations, have carried these roles (Casswell and

Thamarangsi, 2009; Miller et al., 2011). They are funded by big alcohol to actively prosecute the maintenance of business-friendly policy climates in many jurisdictions. The main ethical characteristics of the corporate alcohol sector focus on privilege, profits and power without concerns for the negative impacts on society.

Within this environment, alcohol marketing has been particularly contested via longitudinal studies that are able to strongly link exposure to marketing in conventional media with subsequent measures of consumption (Anderson et al., 2009; Smith and Foxcroft, 2009). As outlined earlier, the alcohol industry response has been to promote an industry-friendly focus on consumer responsibility, along with ineffective approaches for the control of alcohol marketing, particularly via 'self-regulation' (Casswell, 2004; Jones and Gordon, 2013) built around precarious notions of corporate responsibility. Here the emphasis has been on 'independent' monitoring bodies (usually firmly controlled by corporate media interests), inconclusive complaint practices that are too delayed to prevent exposure and relentless pressure on politicians and public figures for more business-friendly policy settings (Babor, et al., 2010; Casswell and Thamarangsi, 2009). The elements relating to alcohol marketing in the 'Dublin Principles' devised by the International Centre for Alcohol Policies (a major industry-funded body) in the late 1990s (Caetano, 2008) are an early expression of how the corporate alcohol sector sees these issues.

As the potential of social media became apparent to marketers through the mid-2000s, and big alcohol began to invest in the new channels (Jernigan and Rushman, 2014; Mosher, 2012; Nicholls, 2012), it was only a matter of time before similar formulations would be generated to cover new developments and pre-empt government policy interventions. To realise their proposed extension of light touch regulation in the digital domain, a coalition of 13 giant alcohol corporations put together a new document to define their preferred approach to marketing in social media as a set of 'Digital Guiding Principles' (Beer Wine and Spirits Producers, 2014) to self-regulation of alcohol marketing in September 2014.

Apart from being entirely voluntary for signatories and other users, the principles turn primarily on the inherently ineffectual notion of the 'age-affirmation mechanism'. This easily avoided gateway would have under-age viewers of alcohol marketing disqualify themselves on the basis of being under legal age of purchase. Aside from the demonstrable evasion of such mechanisms on alcohol sellers' websites through simple misrepresentation of date of birth, this represents a highly selective scenario for how alcohol marketing in a digital world operates. In particular it ignores the architecture and affordances of social media; for example, Facebook users (as the Facebook Experiment illustrates) do not control what messages appear in their newsfeeds or those that appear from 'friends' on their posting wall, so, depending on their network settings, exposure to marketing materials from diverse sources can be omnipresent.

A second notion highlighted in the framework is that alcohol marketing materials should only be placed in media where there is a reasonable expectation that 70% or more of the audience will be of legal purchase age, an almost futile proviso given the level of uptake by children and the networked connectivity of social media. Other suggestions are the inclusion of messages in digital promotions requesting content not be forwarded to persons under the legal purchase age and the embedding of 'responsible drinking' slogans. Equally ineffective are calls for transparency that prevent the masking of sources of marketing and that privacy of social media users be upheld by requiring that marketers obtain consent before sending marketing materials. Given the precedents forged by established social media corporations and the entrenched practices of alcohol corporations, it is hard to see their 'digital guiding principles' framework as offering any protections to society.

As we have argued elsewhere (McCreanor et al., 2013), in some senses, social media are an ideal vehicle for marketers keen to operate unfettered by public health and other social concerns. They are commercial platforms by design, where the business model turns critically upon selling detailed user information about interests, preferences, identity and so on to third parties interested in targeting consumers (Fuchs, 2010; van Dijck, 2013). The one-to-one relationships that social media enable between marketers and platform users are widely understood as being an invaluable advance on the one-to-many relationships of conventional broadcast and print media. The links between platform owners and marketers are business relationships that are easily obscured from regulators on the grounds of 'commercial sensitivity'. This means it is almost impossible to get reliable data to understand measures of exposure to alcohol marketing. Combined with the power of social media corporations to control issues such as 'privacy', access, marketing standards and so on, this creates a 'perfect storm' of deregulated conditions that gives marketers ungoverned and potentially ungovernable advantages and channels.

Research has tracked the active engagement of corporate alcohol in social media and the internet at large (e.g. Carah, 2014; Mart et al., 2009; Nicholls, 2012) and the linkages are increasingly obvious in public documents. The case of Diageo, one of the largest alcohol corporates, is instructive. Attributing the resuscitation of their dying Smirnoff brand to marketing via Facebook from about 2008 (Mosher, 2012), the company quickly moved nearly one-fifth of its marketing budget to social media. While the significance is difficult to judge, the Annual Report (Diageo, 2015) shows that by September 2014 Facebook Vice-President Nicola Mendelson was a non-executive director on the board.

It may be that, even working with the expansive access that social media corporations can deliver in terms of communication with mass markets, alcohol corporations are dissatisfied with aspects of such partnerships, which may perhaps be seen as diluting their profits. Diageo's annual report appears to hint that the corporation may develop its own independent digital media capabilities:

> In support of our marketing agenda, a market-leading cloud-based digital infrastructure has been established, providing a cost effective, scalable and secure platform for our digital assets. Using external benchmarking, a comprehensive plan has been developed with our marketing function to accelerate digital capability building on this core platform.

Whatever the actual intention of this move, this statement demonstrates that Diageo is embracing a paradigm shift, with the digital revolution underpinning their marketing portfolio. As CEO Ivan Menzes commented in 2015, 'It is not about doing "digital marketing", it is about marketing effectively in a digital world' (Joseph, 2015). Clearly anticipating ongoing success at building alcohol brand strength (and thereby consumption) worldwide, this observation sends a clear signal to those concerned with public health approaches to alcohol of the magnitude of the unprecedented challenges ahead.

Public health ethics and research

As public good research interest in the role of digital technologies in marketing alcohol has grown, scholars have adapted or created multiple techniques for exploring the constitution and dynamics of the phenomena. Beginning with informal observation of alcohol-related behaviours in digital media and the enthusiasm of alcohol corporations for engagement and investment in the space, researchers worked with multiple approaches, sometimes in combination (e.g. Lyons et al., 2015). Over a relatively short trajectory, methods have ranged sparsely over a territory that includes critical commentary, content analysis, discursive inquiry, online ethnography, digital technologies, survey approaches, experiments and longitudinal studies. For the most part these applications are conventional forms adapted to digital research contexts. Key challenges lie ahead in the development of native methodologies, methods and ethics for a digital world.

Although this is a new area of research, it is worth noting that approaches are not yet unified by any specific theory, working instead from broad understandings of public health alcohol science (Babor et al., 2010) and emerging frameworks created by social media scholars (boyd, 2007; Fuchs, 2010; van Dijck, 2013). There is considerable promise in Ruddock's (this volume) observation of the power and relevance of Gerbner's Cultural Indicators approach, which is a broader media theory with a specific interest in marketing, alcohol and youth. Carah (this volume) develops valuable conceptual work on access and privacy from wider theorising about the roles and rights of social media corporations in society. There remains an urgent need to advance our theorising of the mechanisms that fuel associations between digital exposure to alcohol marketing and alcohol consumption and to fit such insights within more general understandings of social media and society.

Another characteristic of public good (as distinct from commercial) research life is that for several decades now universities, hospitals and other research institutions in many Western jurisdictions have become active in advising, guiding and enforcing articulated ethical practices especially for publicly funded research. While it is fair to say that the central concern is for the rights, confidentiality and well-being of research participants, the protection of researchers and the standing of institutions is also at issue. If the procedures and requirements of ethics committees are often seen as a bureaucratic restraint on public good researchers, overall the debates, 'case-law' and application of ethical principles have been beneficial to the development of protective best practice within diverse social research communities. We are working in a domain where the ground rules about privacy, consent and research integrity are set and manipulated by commercial interests. In contrast to the commercialised approaches set into their systems by social media corporations, public good ethics frameworks and practices take on additional value as a marker of respect between researchers and participants. Such attributes matter in practical terms, since the kinds of change required to make a difference to the complex issues at stake around alcohol and social media may require the mobilisation of populations to adopt resistant practices, demand political change and re-assert community rather than commercial values.

Every field of research brings its own particular challenges. The chapters in this volume touch on some of these as they report their own studies or those of others. In part this reflects the overall ethics of the private sector where notions such as privacy and confidentiality are publicly rejected within the operating principles of corporations such as Facebook, Google and Twitter (van Dijck, 2013). Many users may be instrumentally ignorant of the point that becoming a member of most social media systems (and indeed other commercial platforms) entails agreeing that their personal data becomes available to the corporation for its commercial use. This potentially creates a very different set of understandings and expectations around data ownership (and who has the right to decide what happens to such data). In contrast, the institutional ethics and processes that shape public good research function to be explicit about issues of participant privacy, confidentiality and anonymity.

The emerging literature around alcohol marketing and social media demonstrates that multiple styles of research are employed by public health and other independent researchers, in an attempt to gauge the influence of these practices on consumption. Currently most research effort has been concentrated on user profiles and interview-based studies, with some work in online ethnography and mining industry data but to date there have been very few longitudinal studies of the kind that have been invaluable in relation to understanding the impacts of alcohol marketing in conventional media. As far as we know, while social media platforms and their corporate clients routinely use 'big data', no independent research has used such information to examine this domain. We briefly consider what is entailed in the research approaches listed above and discuss some of the ethical challenges and the implications for public good alcohol research.

Methods

New technologies – we agree with Monk and Heim (this volume) and other commentators that there is potentially much of value for researchers in the technologies that social media have developed. The ability to gather data using cheaply available affordances such as time-stamping, geocoding and app-driven automation is a welcome extension of what has previously been carried out through valuable but labour-intensive and costly ethnographic work. A doctoral study in which we are involved is using such methods to try to quantify and qualify the marketing materials that arrive in volunteer participants' smartphones in the course of a night of socialising in New Zealand towns and cities. In practice many current approaches hybridise multiple methods in innovative combinations; what follows is an indicative sketch of some of the possibilities.

User profiles – Griffiths and Casswell (2010) were pioneering in providing a qualitative study of links between alcohol display and various expressions of intention to drink. Ethical issues around the use of the materials were addressed by use of pseudonyms and not displaying pictorial materials that could in any way lead to identification of volunteer participants. Moreno and her colleagues (Moreno et al., 2012a; Moreno et al., 2012b) carried out multiple studies that were invaluable in building up a consistent picture of how often and in what ways users reference and mark alcohol-related content and alcohol use in their pages. The treatment of data was primarily quantitative so the summary nature of reporting meant that individual identities were not exposed.

Critical analysis – several scholars have used critical analysis to provide formative leadership and direction to the field. Two in particular stand out: Thomas Mosher's (2012) deconstruction of the use of social media by Diageo to rescue the failing brand Smirnoff and James Nicholls' (2012) piece that highlights the invasive omnipresence of alcohol marketing on- and offline. Without recourse to scientific method, specific disciplinary approach or particular datasets, these papers take questioning, challenging approaches to the evidence and actions of marketers to describe and critique their impacts. In doing so they highlight the power of social media in particular to access, influence and encourage users to purchase and consume alcohol. Both provide evidence and support for the need for public health to engage with and take seriously the emerging threat of alcohol marketing in cyberspace.

Web search – a pioneering paper from Mart et al. (2009) attempted to explore the quantitative dimensions of alcohol marketing online by searching the web for pages promoting alcohol. The key insight here was that the sheer volume of material in circulation in multiple genres was such that several searches were cut off at 5000+ items because the material simply could not be dealt with given the available resources. Marketing materials were obvious in the websites of alcohol producers and sellers but also appeared in multiple user-controlled channels such as YouTube clips, brand fan clubs and user-generated content. Carah (2014) made excellent use of a range of data on marketing drawn from commercial research houses, such as Socialbakers, to show the levels of incursion of alcohol brands into social media.

Interviews/focus groups – these are ideal for gathering both shared and individually nuanced experiential data from participants. While often limited to relatively small numbers of participants, interviews are excellent for understanding the personal meanings that attach to alcohol marketing in terms of identity, values and excitement. Focus groups provide more insight into shared social meanings and experiences. Analysis is generally thematic, seeking to highlight commonalities, participants' meaning-making and the range of experiences reported in data. Such qualitative data also lend themselves to discursive analyses of various kinds that can dissect the subtle, codified meanings that participants employ in their talk. Here complexity, nuance and contradictions become resources to identify conflicted or unstable understandings and interpretations of the influences at work in intoxigenic environments.

Online ethnography – ethnographic approaches include what has become known as netnography; exploring the online environment as participants experience it. A feature is an increasing use of digital tracking and capture data so that participant accounts, as well as their navigation of sites in synchronised streams, can be analysed providing rich and detailed accounts of online life and engagements/use of alcohol marketing materials (Lyons et al., 2015). This approach directly links the participant, individual profile materials and online images and is central to understanding the associations between alcohol marketing and personal consumption. Existing studies shed useful light on participants' responses, providing insights into the complexities of alcohol identification, brand relationships and practices, allowing real-time exploration of impacts of alcohol marketing, participant meanings and the informed unpacking of interactions between online and offline alcohol practices. This approach could usefully be sharply expanded to cover different jurisdictions, niche diversity within social settings and variability across key social divisions such as ethnicity, gender and class before we can begin to interpret the wider significance of the findings.

Policy studies – to date most jurisdictions have invested very little energy in attempting to come to grips with the policy implications of online alcohol marketing. For example, in New Zealand a 2014 ministerial review of alcohol marketing ruled that web-based activity was outside its brief and would not be considered in updates to existing controls. An independent panel of academics and public health practitioners (Independent Expert Committee on Alcohol Advertising and Sponsorship (IECAAS), 2015) carried out a complementary review that cited strong scientific evidence about the high efficacy of online alcohol marketing and argued:

> The online social media environment is absolutely crucial to consider in any review of alcohol advertising and sponsorship, especially as it relates to younger people.
>
> (p. 7)

In Finland efforts are being made to address the problems. In this volume, Montonen and Tuominen report on the process of banning alcohol marketing in social media, although it is too early to begin to measure the impact. It is hoped that other jurisdictions within Europe and elsewhere will observe the changes and outcomes as they develop and consider how they might work in their own policy frameworks.

Surveys – in the United States, Moreno and colleagues used a combination of stratified cross-sectional surveys, particularly of young people, that provided strong evidence of associations between alcohol-related social media activity such as mentions of brands and drinking on profiles and independent measures of alcohol problems collected via AUDIT scales of participants. This quantitative work has been invaluable in establishing the extent and prevalence of associative influences of the marketing on behaviour.

Longitudinal studies – while expensive and demanding to carry out, longitudinal studies are able to provide evidence about causal relationships. They have been used to identify the link between alcohol marketing in conventional media and subsequent consumption (Anderson et al., 2009; Smith and Foxcroft, 2009). To date the only longitudinal investigation of the effects of online alcohol marketing comes from McClure et al. (2016). They recruited 2000 US 15–20 year olds of whom 59% reported seeing alcohol marketing online while 5% or less had visited an alcohol site or become a fan. Their analysis and showed a 'prospective association' between receptiveness to online alcohol marketing and subsequent alcohol-related problems at one-year follow-up.

Big data – probably the most challenging arena for public research is the possibility of using the very detailed mass digital data recorded by social media platforms themselves to better understand the levels of activity of alcohol marketing and consumption. Such 'big data' approaches, hitherto mainly used by the social media corporations themselves (Kennedy and Moss, 2015), where algorithms are used to search digital user data for pattern and variation, have much potential. Focused on marketing exposures and independent measures of alcohol consumption in longitudinal designs, these methods could provide the ability to drill down into associations and, possibly, causal chains activated through social media.

The ethical issues are highly significant given the level of information social media provide about individuals and, while these issues are practically and legally of little importance in commercial settings, different values, particularly around privacy, are important to social research. Potentially there are also risks or sensitivities in relation to specific marketers who may be aggrieved at having their practices unexpectedly exposed to scrutiny, and possible reactions from platform owners who may be distressed at irritations to their commercial client base.

Conclusion

The case for the need to gather empirical evidence about the impact of alcohol marketing in online spaces and social media in particular is strong and growing. Effective policy and other actions are dependent on the quality and breadth of research findings in the area. As with many other clashes between corporate interests and the public good, there is a radical imbalance in resources and data access. Nevertheless, the thoughtful application and adaptation of existing techniques and the development of new approaches are already gathering momentum on the public good front. With determination, commitment, publication and presentation, international peak bodies responsible for controlling and reducing population-level consumption and harms from alcohol will become informed about the need for greater efforts in this domain. At the country level, researchers are already raising their voices to express concerns over developments and some jurisdictions are producing policy interventions.

As the chapters of this volume, along with the growing international literatures on the topic demonstrate, the issues are complex, power-saturated and a matter of considerable concern to public good alcohol science. As researchers, policy makers and practitioners, we have some tools and the potential to develop new approaches centred in the theories, practices and architectures of cyberspace. We also have an ethics of public respect and engagement that differs sharply from the approach of the corporate sector. Our research and ethics, maintained and extended, will prove an important resource for the engagement and mobilisation of communities and populations to join in the protection of, and defence against, the impacts of online commercial alcohol marketing.

References

Anderson, P., de Bruijn, A., Angus, K., Gordon, R., & Hastings, G. (2009). Impact of alcohol advertising and media exposure on adolescent alcohol use: A systematic review of longitudinal studies. *Alcohol and Alcoholism*, 44, 229–243.

Babor, T., Caetano, R., Casswell, S., Edwards, G., Giesbrecht, N., Graham, K., Grube, J., Hill, L., Holder, H., Homel, R., Livingston, M., Osterberg, E., Rehm, J., Room, R., and Rossow, I. (2010). *Alcohol: No Ordinary Commodity Research and Public Policy* (2nd edn). Oxford: Oxford University Press.

Beer Wine and Spirits Producers. (2014). Digital guiding principles self-regulation of marketing communications for beverage alcohol. Retrieved May 2016, from www.k-message.com/wp-content/uploads/2014/10/Digital-Guiding-Principles-DGPs.pdf

Booth, A. (2014, 30 June). Facebook reveals news feed experiment to control emotions. *The Guardian*. Retrieved 1 June 2016, from www.theguardian.com/technology/2014/jun/29/facebook-users-emotions-news-feeds

boyd, d. (2007). Why youth (heart) social network sites: The role of networked publics in teenage social life. In D. Buckingham (Ed.), *Youth, Identity and Digital Media Volume* (pp. 119–142, McArthur Foundation Series on Digital Learning). Cambridge, MA: MIT Press.

Caetano, R. (2008). About smoke and mirrors: The alcohol industry and the promotion of science. *Addiction*, *103*, 175–178.

Carah, N. (2014). *Like, Comment, Share: Alcohol Brand Activity on Facebook*. Brisbane: Foundation for Alcohol Research and Evaluation, University of Queensland.

Casswell, S. (2004). Alcohol brands in young peoples everyday lives: New developments in marketing. *Alcohol and Alcoholism*, *39*(6), 471–476.

Casswell, S., and Thamarangsi, T. (2009). Reducing the harm from alcohol: Call to action. *Lancet (Series)*, *373*, 2247–2257.

Diageo. (2015). Annual report. Retrieved June 2016, from www.diageo.com/en-row/newsmedia/pages/resource.aspx?resourceid=2814

Edwards, G., Anderson, P., Babor, T., Casswell, S., Ferrence, R., Giesbrecht, N., Godfrey, C., Holder, H., Lemmens, P., Makela, K., Midanik, L., Norstrom, T., Osterberg, E., Romelsjo, A., Room, R., Simpura, J., and Skog, O.-J. (1994). *Alcohol Policy and the Public Good*. Oxford: Oxford University Press.

Fuchs, C. (2010). Labor in informational capitalism and on the internet. *The Information Society*, *26*(3), 179–196.

Griffiths, R., and Casswell, S. (2010). Intoxigenic digital spaces? Youth, social networking sites and alcohol marketing. *Drug and Alcohol Review*, *29*, 525–530.

Independent Expert Committee on Alcohol Advertising and Sponsorship (IECAAS). (2015). Response to the report of the Ministerial Forum on Alcohol Advertising and Sponsorship (MFAAS). Retrieved June 2016, from http://img.scoop.co.nz/media/pdfs/1507/IECAAS_report_21_July_2015.pdf

Jernigan, D., and Rushman, A. (2014). Measuring youth exposure to alcohol marketing on social networking sites: Challenges and prospects. *Journal of Public Health Policy*, *35*(1), 91–104.

Jones, S., and Gordon, R. (2013). Regulation of alcohol advertising: Policy options for Australia. *Evidence Base*, *2*, 1–37.

Joseph, S. (2015, 30 July). Diageo: 'We're marketing for a digital world, not doing digital marketing'. *The Drum*. Retrieved June 2016, from www.thedrum.com/news/2015/07/30/diageo-were-marketing-digital-world-not-doing-digital-marketing

Kennedy, H., and Moss, G. (2015). Known or knowing publics? Social media data mining and the question of public agency. *Big Data and Society*, *October*, doi: 10.1177/2053951715611145.

Kramer, A., Guillory, J., and Hancock, J. (2014). Experimental evidence of massive-scale emotional contagion through social networks. *PNAS*, *111*(24), 8788–8790.

Lyons, A., Goodwin, I., McCreanor, T., and Griffin, C. (2015). Social networking and young adults' drinking practices: Innovative qualitative methods for health behavior research. *Health Psychology*, *34*(4), 293–302.

Mart, S., Mergendoller, J., and Simon, M. (2009). Alcohol promotion on facebook. *Journal of Global Drug Policy and Practice*, *3*(3). http://globaldrugpolicy.org/3/3/1.php

McClure, A., Tanski, S., Li, Z., Jackson, K., Morgenstern, M., Li, Z., and Sargent, J. (2016). Internet alcohol marketing and underage alcohol use. *Pediatrics*, *137*(2).

McCreanor, T., Lyons, A., Griffin, C., Goodwin, I., Moewaka Barnes, H., and Hutton, F. (2013). Youth drinking cultures, social networking and alcohol marketing: Implications for public health. *Critical Public Health*, *23*(1), 110–120.

Miller, P., de Groot, F., McKenzie, S., and Droste, N. (2011). Vested interests in addiction research and policy. Alcohol industry use of social aspect public relations organizations against preventative health measures. *Addiction*, *106*(9), 1560–1567.

Moreno, M., Christakis, D., Egan, K., Brockman, L., and Becker, T. (2012a). Associations between displayed alcohol references on Facebook and problem drinking among college students. *Archives of Paediatric and Adolescent Medicine*, *166*(2), 157–163.

Moreno, M., Grant, A., Kacvinsky, L., Egan, K., and Fleming, M. (2012b). College students' alcohol displays on Facebook: Intervention considerations. *Journal of American College Health*, *60*(5), 388–394.

Mosher, J. (2012). Joe Camel in a bottle: Diageo, the Smirnoff Brand, and the transformation of the youth alcohol market. *American Journal of Public Health*, *102*(1), 56–63.

Nicholls, J. (2012). Everyday, everywhere: Alcohol marketing and social media—current trends. *Alcohol and Alcoholism*, *47*(4), 486–493.

Rushe, D. (2014, 2 October). Facebook sorry – almost – for secret psychological experiment on users. *The Guardian*. Retrieved 17 June 2016, from www.theguardian.com/technology/2014/oct/02/facebook-sorry-secret-psychological-experiment-users

Smith, L., and Foxcroft, D. (2009). The effect of alcohol advertising, marketing and portrayal on drinking behaviour in young people: Systematic review of prospective cohort studies. *BMC Public Health*, *9*(51), 1–11. www.biomedcentral.com/1471–2458/1479/1451

van Dijck, J. (2013). *The Culture of Connectivity: A Critical History of Social Media*. New York: Oxford University Press.

Wikipedia. (2016, 4 June). Corporate social responsibility. Retrieved 17 June 2016, from https://en.wikipedia.org/wiki/Corporate_social_responsibility

Index